THE
MILF
diet

Also by Jessica Porter
The Hip Chick's Guide to Macrobiotics

THE
MILF
diet

· · · · · · · · · · · · · · · · · ·

Let the Power of Whole Foods Transform
Your Body, Mind, and Spirit . . .
Deliciously

Jessica Porter

EMILY BESTLER BOOKS
—
ATRIA

NEW YORK   LONDON   TORONTO   SYDNEY   NEW DELHI

ATRIA BOOKS

A Division of Simon & Schuster, Inc.
1230 Avenue of the Americas
New York, NY 10020

Copyright © 2012 by Jessica Porter

All rights reserved, including the right to reproduce this book or portions thereof in any form whatsoever. For information, address Atria Books Subsidiary Rights Department, 1230 Avenue of the Americas, New York, NY 10020.

First Emily Bestler Books/Atria Books hardcover edition January 2013

EMILY BESTLER BOOKS / ATRIA BOOKS and colophons are trademarks of Simon & Schuster, Inc.

For information about special discounts for bulk purchases, please contact Simon & Schuster Special Sales at 1-866-506-1949 or business@simonandschuster.com.

The Simon & Schuster Speakers Bureau can bring authors to your live event. For more information or to book an event, contact the Simon & Schuster Speakers Bureau at 1-866-248-3049 or visit our website at www.simonspeakers.com.

Designed by Elizabeth Van Itallie

Photographs: Joshua Shaub

Manufactured in China

10 9 8 7 6 5 4 3 2 1

Library of Congress Cataloging-in-Publication Data

Porter, Jessica.
The MILF diet : Let the power of whole foods transform your body, mind, and spirit . . . deliciously / Jessica Porter.
    p.   cm.
1. Vegetarian cooking.   2. Organic foods.   3. Women—Health and hygiene.   4. Cookbooks.   I. Title.
TX837.P67   2012
641.5'636—dc23   2011044437

ISBN 978-1-4516-5568-1
ISBN 978-1-4516-5571-1 (ebook)

This book is dedicated to the late Michael Simpson,
who had a beautiful body, a shimmering soul, and uncanny MILFdar.

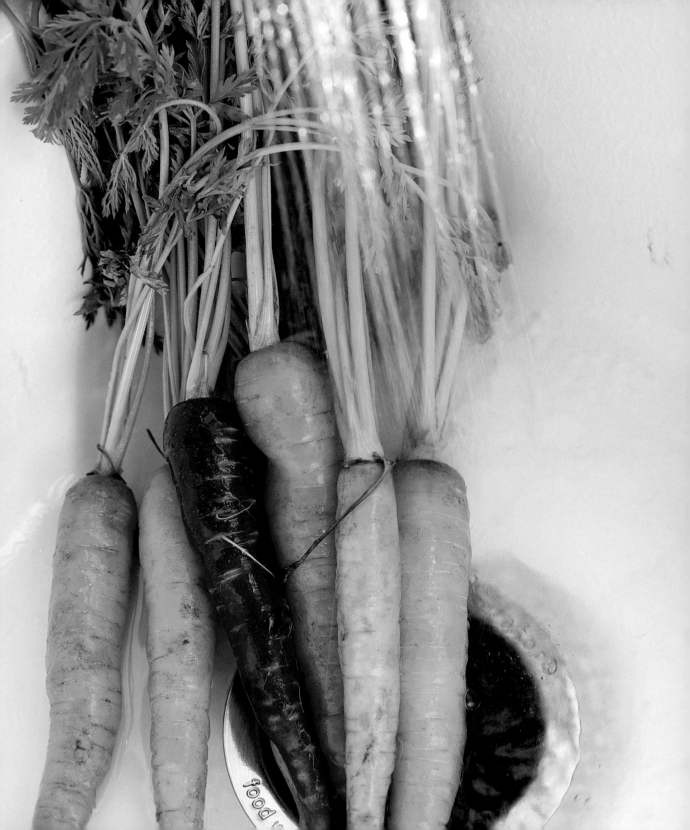

Contents

1

....

What Is a MILF?

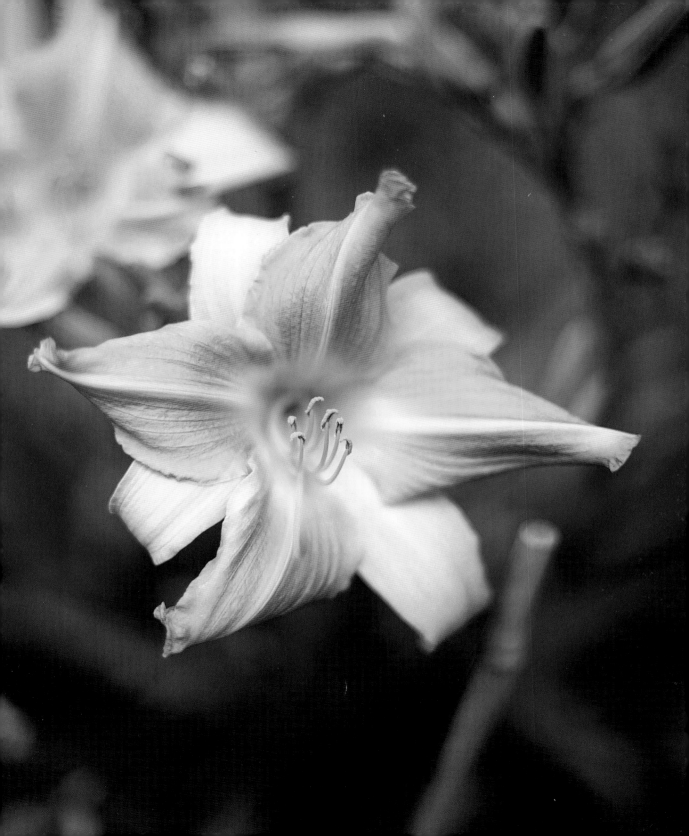

The term "MILF" means, in slightly more titillating verbiage, "*mother with whom I'd like to fornicate*." According to Wikipedia,

> "M.I.L.F." denotes a sexually attractive older female, generally between 30 and 50 in age and not necessarily an actual mother. The term was popularized by the film *American Pie* (1999), though the origin of the term predates this {as it was} already used for years on the Internet.

These days, "MILF" has become a compliment. While other names for sexy women have remained stuck to the brothel floor, "MILF" has picked itself up, crawled out the door, and marched with pride into the local health food store. That's because there's something more to "MILF." Something almost magical about it. I've seen it in the eyes of every woman whom I've told about *The MILF Diet*. First the teensiest bit of shock and then a wonderful expression of joy. "I love it!" they said, time and time again. Nine out of ten women surveyed had good feelings about the term "MILF."

And then it revealed itself in a flash of neurological lightning: "MILF" is evolutionary. "MILF" acknowledges that women can—and do—stay sexy and vital, and that mothers can turn heads as well. Clean, pure, and the Madonnas of a certain Madonna/whore complex: *MOTHERS*.

Finally. We MILFs have been waiting for the last two thousand years to get our sexuality back. Ever since Mary played the Immaculate card in Bethlehem, our culture has been struggling with a fundamental split: women are unconsciously perceived as either good girls or good-*time* girls, either naughty or nice.

What a drag for us MILFs! We knew that our C cups were for fun *and* function. We knew that we could change a diaper *and* look smoking hot—just not always at the same time, thank you very much. There was no actual split in us. And, frankly, it's been painful to constantly—and often unconsciously—have to choose one side of ourselves over the other.

But "MILF" saves the day! Suddenly we can be mothers (or the age of mothers) *and* be considered frisky in the bedroom. With "MILF" comes the acknowledgment of the complexity and beauty of womanhood.

And what's best about "MILF" is that the term was generated by men, for men. It's not some politically correct label we're trying to shove down their throats. Perhaps the term "MILF" is evidence that a healing is going on in our newly minted males. Maybe it's because they were brought up by sexy, cool, independent women . . . MILFs themselves. Maybe it's because there are just some very sexy mothers out there, pushing their carts at Whole Foods. No matter its origins, I'm suggesting we co-opt this term and wear it with pride. Because it reunites sexuality and the great maternal gifts of womanhood, it's a four-letter word we can get behind.

Okay, okay. "MILF" may not save marriages. Or heal nations. But it does, like the Madonna/whore complex, do its work quietly and subconsciously within the culture. With "MILF" comes a positive, deep, and pleasurable recognition that we women are fantastic in our fecundity, are wired to love deeply, and can be thoroughly naughty in bed. Stuff we knew all along. Finally, the men are figuring it out.

And these days, with yoga classes on every corner and Eckhart Tolle on every bedside table, your average MILF is working on her higher self, too. She is exploring another dimension that takes her personal power to the next level. In this book, we address that plane of consciousness and unite it again, appropriately, with motherhood, sexuality, and the other lovely attributes of MILFiness.

The age of the MILF is upon us, and it's about freaking time.

How Does a MILF Stay MILFy?

One of the quickest routes to natural MILFiness is through food; by eating whole, natural foods and letting go of processed, crappy "food," the female body finds its peaceful home again. Extra pounds simply fall away. Inner hardness softens. The plumbing works much better. You step off that horrible emotional roller coaster and a wonderful clarity descends.

Happily, these foods will also significantly reduce your risk of decidedly un-MILFy conditions like osteoporosis, diabetes, heart disease, and breast cancer. Whole grains will leave you feeling energized, yet relaxed and clearheaded. Sea vegetables will make your skin all dewy and your hair stronger and shinier. Bye-bye, tracksuits! Hello, cute tennis outfits! Your DILF won't know what hit 'im.

But that's not all; by sticking close to Mother Nature in our food choices, that "witchipoo" intuition we each carry inside becomes sharp, dependable, and loud. You will become more sensitive to vibrations and less a victim of the material world and its follies. You will start working more from the creative right hemisphere of your brain and less from the noisy, logical left. You will find your own inner balance and a whole new dimension to your feminine power. This is cruising at high MILFitude.

And the sex? Well, sex changes, too. The MILF diet will bring you back home to your body. Every single buzzing cell of it. So instead of focusing on the finish, you will relish the journey again. Rubbing up against your DILF will blow your mind, because by merely being in his presence, open and MILFy, your opposite energy fields collide and start their fireworks. Remember, you radiate a powerful, womanly, nourishing force. Your very essence makes a man feel strong and alive.

To stay MILFy is to keep a certain feminine je ne sais quoi alive and kicking. And yet, that mysterious element may not be so mysterious. In Chinese philosophy, the feminine principle is called yin, a soft and receptive force. In the West, the closest we come to describing the feminine might be Mother Nature, as we acknowledge her uniquely female qualities.

Natural femininity exists—perfectly intact—inside of you. You don't need to chant about it, or wear the right fertility amulet, or even understand it in an intellectual way. This energy *is* you. You are it. By being born with a set of ovaries, a uterus, and a functional set of boobs, you are a card-carrying member of the Yin Club, and head pom-pom waver on Mother Nature's cheerleading squad.

In Taoist thought, opposite (yet complementary) forces come together to make all things. Although we in the West recognize sets of opposites like sperm and egg, man and woman, oil and vinegar, we tend to reduce them to their material, mechanical components. We love to whip out the microscope and analyze them, reducing them further to ittier and bittier parts. But in the East, each member of any duality is thought to be backed by a fundamental force of nature: yin or yang. To the Eastern mind, everything can be seen through this lens of yin and yang. And if that language is too weird, let's swap it for "expansion and contraction." For instance, plants expand in the summer and contract in the winter. The tide rolls in and the tide rolls out. At this very moment, your heart is expanding and contracting. Ditto your lungs. All these rhythms are created by the natural attraction between these two opposite forces, which are at play on every level of existence.

No matter where we look, we continually find layer after layer of this duality—more expanded elements connecting with more contracted elements—whether it's electrons balancing protons, hydrogen meeting oxygen, or Fred Astaire spinning Ginger Rogers. This simple, elegant dance is taking place in, around, and throughout our bodies every moment of the day.

So, if men and women make up one of the great, dynamic, and mysterious dualities of nature, we—as MILFs—are governed by one side of the energy spectrum. We represent, if you will, the more expanded side of things: Our bodies are naturally softer. We get fat more easily. Our breasts and butts and hips are lovely and expanded. We open and expand to receive a lover. We expand to grow babies and we expand even more to give birth to them. And once the little darlings are born, we expand, emotionally and psychically—again and again and again—to make room for them and give them what they need.

In terms of communication, we express ourselves more easily and, whereas men can at times seem linear, analytical, or locked up inside themselves (contracted), women are generally bursting forth (expanded) with feelings, or words, or heartfelt advice for a friend.

Even science is showing that men's and women's brains are significantly different; men tend to stay a little more stuck in their left hemisphere, while the female connects back and forth between hemispheres more quickly and easily. With larger deep limbic systems, we tend to be more connected to our feelings, to other people, and to our internal worlds. We are sensitive creatures, easily bruised, and all our estrogen makes us eager to diffuse tension. Whereas men are coded to defend and protect (contract), we women bond and connect (expand)—that's our thing. Of course, we all have access to both sides of the spectrum (men express love; women can defend), but, just as it's naturally easier to write with one of your hands than the other, each gender has its dominant mode.[1]

And these natural feminine gifts are powerful; one could argue that the world needs more of them these days. It is connection that makes a strong family, a healthy neighborhood, or a united world. It is this feminine principle that forges communication, empathy, and love. A woman in touch with her natural femininity creates a space for others to be welcomed and received. She helps people to grow into themselves. She nourishes and supports.

But modern eating has messed with us. With the dubious "luxury" of convenience foods, we are ingesting decidedly unnatural chemicals, preservatives, dyes, and stabilizers. By eating animal products at every meal, day in and day out, we're developing a dull insulation of saturated fat and stressing out our internal organs. Thanks to the factory farming of livestock, our bodies have been bombarded with excess hormones that interrupt the delicate balance of our own endocrine systems. With white sugar creeping into everything, our immune systems are weakening, our bones are becoming brittle, and we can be reduced to emotional wrecks by the loss of a good parking spot. Caffeine—the most popular drug on the planet—is messing with our hearts and our precious fertility and making us wrinkly and anxiety-ridden. Some of us are becoming too hard: rigid, tight, and aggressive—sort of like men. Other women are getting weak—physically and emotionally—and becoming needy and dependent. But many of us indulge in all extremes, so we're a mixed bag of weird vibes; angry and weepy, arrogant and scared.

Because the MILF diet is made up of whole foods, cooked according to simple, natural principles, it will bring your body, mind, and spirit back into balance. You will begin to connect with the fundamental rhythms of your body, the seasons, and the natural world.

If you have a hard time connecting with your sensitivity and inner softness, this diet will help you stop and smell the roses. If you give endlessly and feel as if you're disappearing, MILFy

---

1. If you find these gender generalizations simplistic, or even offensive, I understand; I did, too, for quite a while. And, yes, what I've written—although it represents a big picture—does not make room for the complexities of each individual. Like any other woman, I resist being pigeonholed. Fear not. It's okay to let all this energy gobbledygook go. Feel free to explore the MILF diet because it will make you healthier, happier, and sexier. Aren't those reasons enough?

foods will help you rediscover that line between yourself and others, and you will begin to dance it happily. Nature is continually seeking balance; you should be, too. As you cook MILF-ier foods for your family, you will begin to wield an ancient womanly power. You will begin to create a stronger, saner, and happier world.

But don't worry. The MILF diet won't render you Birkenstocked (unless that's your thing), nor will you grow your hair too long with a bad case of the frizzies. By realigning with this energy, you will become more beautiful, powerful, and ridiculously alive than you've ever been. And finally, by eating this way, you will start to turn back the clock; your skin will glow, you will drop pounds effortlessly, and you will have the energy of a teenager. Instead of Father Time having his way with you, you will turn on your stiletto and deliver him a saucy little slap in the face.

Long live the MILF.

What Is the MILF Diet?

The MILF diet is designed to help you stay balanced, happy, and healthy by helping you harmonize with nature. It includes the following:

Whole grains: It begins with organic whole grains. Brown rice, millet, quinoa, whole oats, barley, spelt, and other cereal grains, in their whole, unpolished form, make up the center of the diet. Packed with slow-burning complex carbohydrates, fiber, vitamins, and minerals, these lovely graceful seeds keep the body feeling both energized and relaxed. Whole-grain products, like bread and pasta, are totally legal, but take a backseat to the whole grains themselves.

Vegetables: Grains are balanced by lots and lots of vegetables. And in order to support her feeling truly balanced, the MILF selects a variety of vegetables that grow in various ways: upward-growing leafy greens like kale, collard greens, and bok choy (rich in chlorophyll, calcium, vitamin K, and other nutrients); round vegetables such as onions, squash, and cabbage (sweeter, full of complex carbohydrates and antioxidants); and downward-growing root vegetables such as carrots, parsnips, and burdock (satisfying, grounding, and also rich in minerals and vitamins). Ideally, vegetables are organic, locally grown, and eaten in season.

Proteins: For protein, the MILF diet reaches in the plant-based direction, but not exclusively. Beans such as kidney, pinto, adzuki, garbanzo, lentil, and Great Northern, along with soybeans and their products (tofu, tempeh), make up the greatest source of protein in the MILF diet. Nuts and seeds play an important role by adding protein, as well as a satisfying richness, and can be made into butters or sauces or just sprinkled on dishes.

The MILF diet can be practiced vegan-style but doesn't have to be. In terms of meat, the diet leans toward white-fleshed fish, because it is easily digested and lower in fat (and therefore lower in toxins). No food is a strict no-no on the MILF diet, because every MILF is a free agent, encouraged to explore her body's relationship to all foods; but for the purposes of her optimum health, the suggested serving of fish is one or two servings per week, if any.

Sea vegetables: The MILF diet also harvests plants from the sea: sea vegetables such as nori, wakame, and arame play a consistent and important role in the MILF diet. Rich in easily absorbed minerals, sea vegetables build stronger bones and hair and beautify the skin. They even perform quite magical acts like discharging heavy metals and radioactive isotopes from the body.

Natural sweets: Because girls are made of sugar and spice and everything nice, the MILF diet does not wag its finger at sweets. Using sweeteners that are high in complex carbohydrates, like rice syrup and barley malt, MILFs stay satisfied without experiencing all the nasty problems associated with white, refined sugar. From natural sweeteners come cookies, pies, cakes, and creamy desserts. Fruit and fruit juices keep the average MILF sweet and happy as well.

Fermented foods: Finally, the MILF diet includes fermented foods, in the forms of unpasteurized pickles, soy sauce, and miso. Natural fermentation helps build immune-boosting intestinal flora and adds digestive enzymes to the mix. Like sea vegetables, miso is a total superfood with rich nutritional benefits and tumor-inhibiting properties. Using the basic ingredients of the MILF diet, many supplemental dishes can be concocted; whether it's a bean dip, a creamy vegetable spread, or a luscious pesto sauce, whole foods can form the base for all the foods that make life delicious, fun, and celebratory.

The MILF diet is easily made kosher and gluten-free and fits within the Weight Watchers PointsPlus program.

How to Use This Book

Now, I know some of you out there are what we like to call type A's, and it is your nature to start a new regime at once and to do it perfectly. God bless you. I have spent many years of my life and trillions of neurons trying to be like you. But no matter how many lists I make, they end up crumpled and carrot juice–stained in the giant purse I call my car. My journey has been slower, and messier, than those of most type A's. I like to feel things out a bit, be convinced that the water is safe, and then step in, toe by toe.

Luckily for us, both approaches work. But just so you know, this book is laid out in a very particular way: The first third of *The MILF Diet* contains information that is designed to appeal to your intuition. In it, we will consider the big picture and how nature, your body, and food work together. The right hemisphere of your brain—the more holistic one—will love it. This section will introduce lots of new ideas and will engage your intuition. The front of the book should, fingers crossed, get you all inspired to eat good food.

Meanwhile, the hard facts—about the deleterious effects of extreme foods and the nutritional benefits of your new MILFy foods—are all at the back, in the last third of the book. There you will find the scientific stuff, translated by Yours Truly, and it should satisfy both the left hemisphere of your brain and your sexy inner librarian. The back of the book should make you feel very good about what you're doing because the jury is in: this way of eating works, on every level.

I've kept the right- and left-brain stuff separated because each side of your brain has a very different way of processing information, and both sides deserve their own time and space. The middle of the book contains all the recipes and the practical tips on how to do this and that.

For you type A's, if you want to get some brown rice on the stove ASAP, then go straight to page 107. Cleanse your kitchen of the bad stuff, stock it to the brim with the good, and get cracking. You will also find the specifics of the MILF diet, a shopping list, and other practical tips beginning on page 52. All the recipes are sorted by category, so you're good there, and I have no doubt you will be feeling some results within a few days. And when that happens, be sure to read page 94 on detox and changes you might encounter. You'll need that if you dive in fast. And I hope, as you experience profound physical shifts, you will come back to the

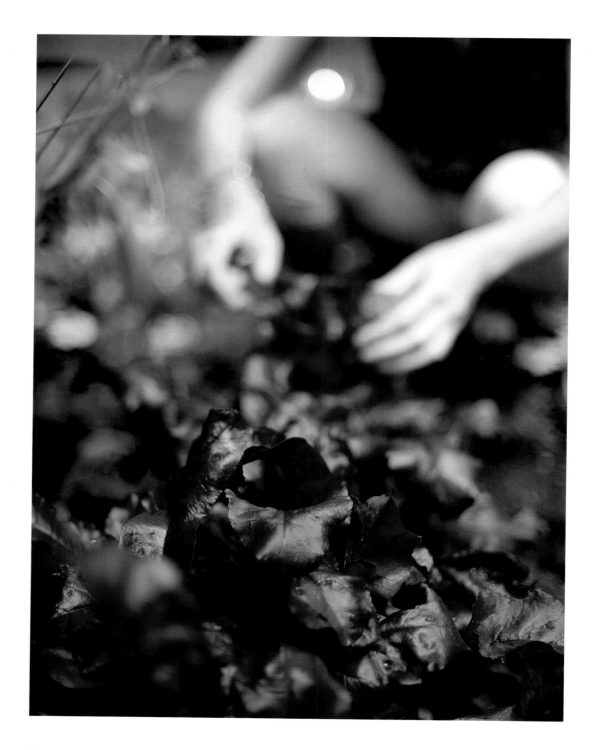

beginning of the book and start to see the bigger picture of your exciting adventure. Having this perspective will help you to sustain your practice.

For the meanderers like me, I encourage you to sit back and enjoy the ride. I have designed a gentle path for you that is doable and allows for reflection and integration. Remember, this is not a normal "diet"; it is a way of eating that will transform your life from the cells on up, and meandering is a perfectly respectable way to approach it. You will find that whole grains and vegetables, charged with the vital oomph of life, will push you along your journey.

And in terms of the practical, let me make it clear to the meanderers and the A's from the beginning: If you do nothing more than introduce whole grains and more vegetables into your and your family's diet on a regular basis, you will have turned your lives around. You will feel better, look better, and begin moving in nature's direction. That's it. You can toss this book, or use it as a doorstop, or shove it under the butt of a toddler at the dinner table, and I will still be overjoyed knowing that you've let the magic of whole grains and vegetables into your life. They are *that* powerful.

Take your time and do some thinking, feeling, and experimenting as you read this book. Pick it up, put it down, and be sure to pick it up again. Let your heart crawl into it and your intuition judge it. *The MILF Diet* is designed to open you up and reveal the ocean of power inside of you; but remember that every ocean comes in waves, is governed by the moon, and is a beautiful, sparkling collection of single drops.

Non Credo

Non credo means, in Latin, "I do not believe." And I recommend that. Please, please, *please,* don't believe a word I say just because I say it. I am not a doctor, nor a nutritionist. Heck, I'm not even a mother.

But *waaaaay* more important than those things . . . I am not *you.*

Only *you* live within your body and can feel its strengths and limits. Only *you* can experience the lovely peaceful ride of whole grains and other natural foods. Only *you* can find out if yin and yang make any sense. When it comes to exploring the physical world, all our lovely lady talk can get us only so far. At some point, it's between you and your fork.

And, hey, while you're at it, why not apply a little *non credo* to doctors, nutritionists, and other mothers, as well? I'm not suggesting that you disrespect them or reject their suggestions, only that you recognize the inherent limits of "expertise" coming from the outside. No matter how many degrees they have, the so-called authorities will never live inside your body and hear your precious intuition. They cannot chew your food for you. Nor feel the lovely tug of your heart. It is both a privilege and a responsibility to live in a body—constantly being created and uncreated by nature—and only you can decide what feels right, what needs to be released, and what remains to be discovered.

And if it seems daring to question external authority, remember this: the MILF diet is only asking you to get closer to nature. That's it. No funky pills. No crazy regimens. The MILF diet is based on the fact that Mother Nature has always provided for you and that—if you lean on her—you will strengthen yourself physically, emotionally, and spiritually. It's not rocket science . . .

Just *magic*.

My Story

I grew up on TV dinners and Tang crystals. At six, I was caught stealing chocolate cupcakes from the family refrigerator, and I pathetically pleaded my case by saying, "I *needed* one." For my eleventh birthday, my mother's gift to me was two tubs of Baskin-Robbins ice cream (Rocky Road and Pink Bubblegum)—the huge ones they scoop from at the store. I am not the groovy child of peaceniks who grew up thinking raisins were a treat.

Around the age of thirteen, I started to worry about my weight. Not because I felt fat, but because I stood on the scale one day, and the number I saw was *not,* funnily enough, the one they kept mentioning in *Vogue.* I panicked and started my first diet. I think I lost seven pounds . . . and gained twelve.

So I tried harder. More diets ensued, and more pounds snuck on. Noisy aerobics classes—a form of torture unique to the 1980s—were endured. Over time, I started to gain some real weight. I became deeply miserable, doing kicks and jumps in the exact opposite direction of my truth. But that's what I had to do, right? I didn't care if I was happy as long as I was SKINNY!

Fast-forward to college graduation. With a head full of expensive ideas, I still couldn't handle food like a normal person. I felt like I had earned a BA in bingeing. Having moved to Manhattan, surrounded by all-night corner markets and twenty-four-hour delis, I was a mess. I looked in the mirror one day, peered into my dead eyes, and thought, "This isn't the way it's supposed to be."

I signed up for a healthy cooking class, almost as a lark. It seemed ridiculous that I would even cook, let alone cook actual *food,* but something got me there. I arrived in the room, sweaty and tired, and with more contempt than a normal twentysomething should have, I crossed my arms and waited to see what the ridiculous hippies were up to.

The first thing I noticed was that the class didn't concentrate on weight loss. Or calories. Or even nutritional science. This class explored the basics of the energetics of food: Is it cooling or warming? Does it grow in the spring or the fall? Is it whole or is it processed? I heard a commonsense approach that a child could have understood and my grandmothers would have applauded. The teacher talked about eating to harmonize with the seasons—longer cooking in winter, lighter dishes in summer. She extolled the virtues of eating what grows nearby. Not murdering a dish with seasoning. She even questioned the wisdom of drinking milk. Huh?

And she was so serene! As she moved from task to task, there was a fluidity to it all that was strangely hypnotic. I couldn't keep my eyes off her knife going through the squash . . . the seeds getting spooned out . . . the flame being carefully raised.

Weirdly, she handled food as if it had a spirit. As if it was more than the sum of its parts calculated on some nutrition fact sheet. As if each carrot, or bean, or freakin' grain of barley contained some magical code from Mother Nature that we were supposed to crack—first with our mouths and then with our souls.

And it wasn't lost on me that she was thin. Not crazy thin, like eating-disorder skinny, just I'm-exactly-the-way-I-should-be-in-the-economy-of-the-universe thin. Her whole body fit into the flow, in this weird, natural way.

I had no previous template for this type of creature. She defied every diet book I had ever read. She was not bouncing up and down in a Lycra bodysuit. She didn't have a scrunched-up, sweaty face and she wasn't yelling at me to "Feel the burn!!!" She was just there, doing her thing, all thin and beautiful and serene. I guess, looking back on her now, she was a kind of MILF.

I hated her.

But I couldn't hate the food. I didn't expect it, but the stuff she cooked tasted amazing—yes, even better than Baskin-Robbins. The meal consisted of brown rice cooked with chestnuts, a sweet-and-sour bean stew, a couple of simple yet elegant vegetable dishes, and a lovely, fruity pudding. It left me feeling light, clean, and yet totally satisfied. Miraculously, after all those years of junk, my body could still recognize real food. I went home with my sarcasm bruised.

I took my sweet time getting into it. I was a little too cool to be roasting seeds and buying barley malt. But my body—and, I suppose, my spirit—couldn't forget how peaceful and calm she was. How warm and relaxed the room had been. How well I'd felt after eating the food. Slowly but surely, I started my experiments: buying a pressure cooker and burning some rice. Trying strange new vegetables. Daring to make miso soup from scratch.

It became obvious, very quickly, that these natural foods had power. Suddenly, I knew where my colon was and felt its happy wave. Certain foods made me break out in a sweat, while others gave me tons of energy. Still others helped me lose weight more easily than ever before. And when I journeyed back to my regular fare—the ice cream and the sugary baked goods—I just felt crummy. Worse than ever, in fact. As if something inside of me was curling up to die.

Over the next few months, I bought cookbooks and started really digging into this way of eating. My life began to revolve around food again, but now it was in a positive, empowering way. Although my diet sometimes swayed between old and new habits, with every vicissitude, I was learning things about my body and its relationship to what I put inside it. And I wasn't just learning with my head; as my appetite for healthy food increased, I developed a sixth sense about what I needed. If I just relaxed and let go in the kitchen, I could feel a palpable pull from within my body toward certain foods and seasonings and cooking styles. One day, I was attracted to red foods, the next day to green: "This should be steamed . . . no, sautéed!" My inner compass was bringing me to balance, again and again, and I had never felt anything like it in my life. My bigwig university hadn't taught *that*.

And over time, I started to lose weight. Although it took me a while to develop some real consistency with my new way of eating—I didn't get off the roller coaster overnight—this time, when I came back to my "diet," instead of some crazy deprivation-based calorie-counting nightmare, it was a return to satisfying, nutritious foods that made me feel strangely balanced. Returning to them felt like coming home to my body. And I discovered the happy paradox that the foods that made me feel full and satisfied were also the ones that were making me smaller.

Although I was delighted with the weight loss, I came to see that it was the least dramatic of the changes taking place inside of me: whereas I had felt scared and lost inside, I was now feeling peaceful and strangely whole. I realize now that the whole grains, rich in complex carbohydrates, were stabilizing my blood sugar and their B vitamins were calming my nervous system. Previously harsh and quick to judge, I was now quick to forgive and even laugh things off. Turns out that, with fewer toxins in my body, I was happier and more relaxed. I knew I was in some serious New Age trouble when a beloved ceramic bowl fell from the top of my refrigerator, shattering on the kitchen floor, and what passed through my mind was simply: "Bowl dropping." No anger. No anxiety. Whoa.

I was in deep.

I would walk down the streets of New York feeling a sort of stupid happiness, not brought about by anything in particular, just an essential buoyancy that came from eating foods that supported my vitality. The wellness I was experiencing went beyond my ego or events in my life. I was simply availing myself of good fuel . . . principally whole grains, which boost serotonin levels in the brain. I wanted to hold up a sign: "Grain for the Brain!" They have that much power.

Of course, I had to wrestle with all of this in therapy. I wasn't exactly ready to learn that my deepest happiness came from the next meal. Didn't I have to have a fancy car? The perfect boyfriend? At least more money? But meal after meal, it became clear that not only were whole foods determining my mental and emotional states, they were actually pushing my life forward. Causing me to make healthy choices. Forcing me to grow.

I started embracing my spirituality, which was downright weird, having come from a family that looked down on faith as a crutch for the weak-minded. But I was feeling a real pull toward a higher plane of perception—one that transcended the duality of the material world. I began to perceive—in trippy little moments—that everything was connected. I didn't realize it then, but the foods—whole and created not in factories, but by nature—were helping me to feel a part of the Bigger Picture.

The Birth of the MILF Diet

After a few years of eating this way, I moved to Massachusetts to study whole foods cooking more deeply. At the school I attended, I met students and teachers equally as immersed in this lovely new reality. They confirmed for me what I had experienced, and the scientific truth behind it, and assured me it was only the beginning of the positive changes to come. I saw in all of them the elegance of my first cooking teacher and I felt the same peace emanating from their bodies. They laughed easily. I could sense that they weren't weighed down by tons of gunk, physically or emotionally; and that seemed pretty cool.

I paid special attention to the women and noted a few interesting things: First, they were naturally thin. Every single one of them. And none of them was babbling mindlessly about calories, or self-control, or cardio workouts. Second, they were beautiful. Okay, maybe they weren't all genetic goddesses (I'm certainly not), but they all had glowing skin, beautiful hair, sparkly eyes, and a lovely poise that women in this modern world seem to be losing.

They were strong, but never pushy. Instead of relying on their personalities, their power issued forth, gently and invisibly, from deep inside . . . more a vibrational strength that I sensed with my body. And perhaps most important, although these ladies were cooking a lot, they were the furthest thing from "Stepford wives," or cowed domestic slaves. It became clear to me that by cooking, simply *cooking,* they were actually running the joint. On every level. These ladies were wise and deep and strong in a way that was totally new to me.

Not to mention sexy. This wasn't a chaste home economics class. Because sex was considered a healthy part of a healthy life, the topic was discussed with a certain nonchalance. It made sense; everyone was fully in their bodies. There was no sludginess around their midsections. No hiding out from the energy. If good sex is about one's central nervous system responding with a certain electricity to its opposite pole in a loved one, these people were simply givers and receivers of clear signals. Good-quality minerals—from whole grains, vegetables, and especially sea vegetables—plus a lack of insulating saturated fat kept their bodies sensitive and highly charged; their antennae were working.

But it wasn't sleazy. Like the female power deep inside each woman, the energy was just there. Part of life. Just as a plant contains seeds, we contain sexuality. Yes, pleasurable and powerful and potentially life-giving, but, really, no big deal in the grand scheme of things.

Nothing to be ashamed of or get all freaked out about. Sex was just part of the yin and yang of being alive.

And, boy, were these ladies alive, reproductively speaking. Some of them had five children. Others eight. I have a friend in Alaska who's been eating whole, natural foods since she was six, and now—at my age—she has thirteen children. Of course, I'm not advocating that kind of reproduction; it's hard to argue for it in today's world. But the fact that these women had the energy and vitality to conceive, gestate, birth, nurse, cook for, and wrangle multiple children was a testament to the power of the food. And, honest to God, they were happy, enjoying that stupid happiness I had stumbled upon in Manhattan. Finally, these supermoms even looked good—all a-sparkle with the life force.

Because I entered this world in my mid-twenties, I wasn't paying much attention to the signs of aging; that just wasn't on my radar. I was much more interested in how I felt, looking good, and forging a career path. But ten years later, things changed. You know you've crossed the Rubicon into middle age when you start to notice other women's skin; you detect that discoloration, that roughness, or that wrinkle. Sure enough, in my late thirties, I began to pay attention to the little gifties of time showing up not just on my face, but on the faces of all of my friends. My gaze went from their eyes to the crow's-feet emerging next to them.

But the results of my surveys were not uniform across the board; my friends eating a standard American diet were looking a little tired. Their skin seemed duller, and they issued universal complaints about the difficulty they had losing weight. Some of them were on medications for depression, or anxiety, while others had a hard time sleeping. As we all aged, talk turned to fertility, breast cancer, and bone health. Many of my friends seemed to be checking out of their bodies, as if their midsections were stiff and simply structurally functional—something to keep their legs and arms attached to. Yes, there were those MILFier ones, usually those who worked out a lot, but often they carried a taut tension in their bodies that exhausted everyone around them.

Although I didn't know it at the time, it turns out my observations had some backup; processed foods, laden with chemicals and preservatives, as well as meat, sugar, and caffeine, were taking their toll on my friends' health and vitality. They were losing their natural balance.

On the other hand, my lady friends eating whole, natural, predominantly plant-based foods were simply looking better. They had ridiculous amounts of energy while remaining soft and flexible. Sure, they might have gained a wrinkle or two, but their inner lights had just gotten brighter with age. And the electricity of life—their sexuality or womanhood—still pulsed through them. You could just feel it. They were, in a word, MILFy.

I leaned on my MILF friends to write this book. They all gave me tips, recipes, and their very real wisdom about living a MILFy life, feeding their kids, and even insights into their sex lives. Some of them have been eating this way for over forty years, while others are relative newbies. The vast majority of them are mothers, but a couple of them are not. They range in age from thirty to eighty-three, so I've thrown a GILF or two in there. I even had the opportunity to photograph a handful of them, and I consider them models for living sane, peaceful, and happy lives in this world that tells us that to age is to decay, that women shrivel and disappear. Well, these ladies aren't disappearing, on any level. Whole foods keep them vibrant and sexy. You'll see that in their photographs.

I also noticed a pronounced difference in how each group of women *thought* about their health; those eating conventional foods seemed caught up in the powerlessness of Western medicine: if you're unlucky, you get "struck" by something. It was just a matter of good fortune and ardent crossing of fingers to avoid some nasty disease. But women who had studied whole foods cooking felt more confident; they knew the medicinal properties of many foods and applied them as needed. Because their intuitions were sharp, and their bodies' signals strong, they knew better when they felt out of balance, and generally treated themselves by tweaking their diets. Not only did they have a much greater feeling of control over their health, they were not, in fact, falling prey to as many colds, allergies, and aches and pains as my other girlfriends. I saw no pills when I snooped in their medicine cabinets. It seemed that, by sticking close to nature, they were staying in the flow of life.

But before I go on, let me clarify: I'm not trying to suggest that the world divides itself between two groups of women—good and bad, right and wrong. I have been blessed with a ridiculous number of female friends and I cherish each and every one of them deeply, no matter what they eat. Because of my own struggles with food, I've felt the sting of judgment and the futility of someone giving me advice about what I put in my mouth. Therefore, I follow a policy of *never* wagging my finger at a friend's cheeseburger—unless I want to wreck a perfectly good relationship. No, as far as I'm concerned, the eighteen inches between a woman's hand and her mouth is a sacred space as personal as certain erogenous zones. I deal in information, not judgment. We all have to explore to find out what works for us.

But that doesn't mean I haven't observed the overall trends I'm describing. They are consistent and obvious. Just as someone who lives in a green, wooded area is going to get more oxygen than a downtown city-dweller, these are simple physical realities. When people eat fresh, clean, unprocessed food, they tend to feel better—and often look better—than someone who regularly eats out of a box. Period.

And just as moving from the city to the country will bring you fresher air at any age, altering the course of your food journey pays off no matter how old you are; women I've known who started eating MILFy foods in their forties, their fifties, and even their sixties looked and felt better very quickly. After just a couple of weeks of eating whole grains, they increased their energy dramatically. With a few servings of sea vegetables, their skin started to glow. A nice, soft peace began to emanate from their beings. After reducing their consumption of meat and dairy, years of tension and heaviness and sludge fell away. It's never too late to MILFify.

Since I got turned on to this stuff, I've been a private chef, written books, and traveled far and wide teaching about this way of eating. I'm not going to pretend that this is a panacea, nor that the MILF diet is going to appeal to everyone. If anything, nature shows us that different creatures need different things and that rigid adherence to any dogma can lead to big problems. Using whole food, your intelligence, and your intuition, you need to find out what's right for you. But I will say that, with only incredibly rare exceptions, when someone tells me she's gone in the MILFy direction, it's followed by an enthusiastic report about the ways in which she started to feel, and look, better. Quickly. And that the benefits keep right on coming.

And those women I've been observing for the last twenty years? The ones with kids hanging off them while they stir their soups? One thing I know for sure: those chicks don't age. They just don't.

I wrote this book for all the women out there who want to crack the code.

Here's to our great adventure.

2

· · · · · · · · · ·

Your MILFification, Phase One

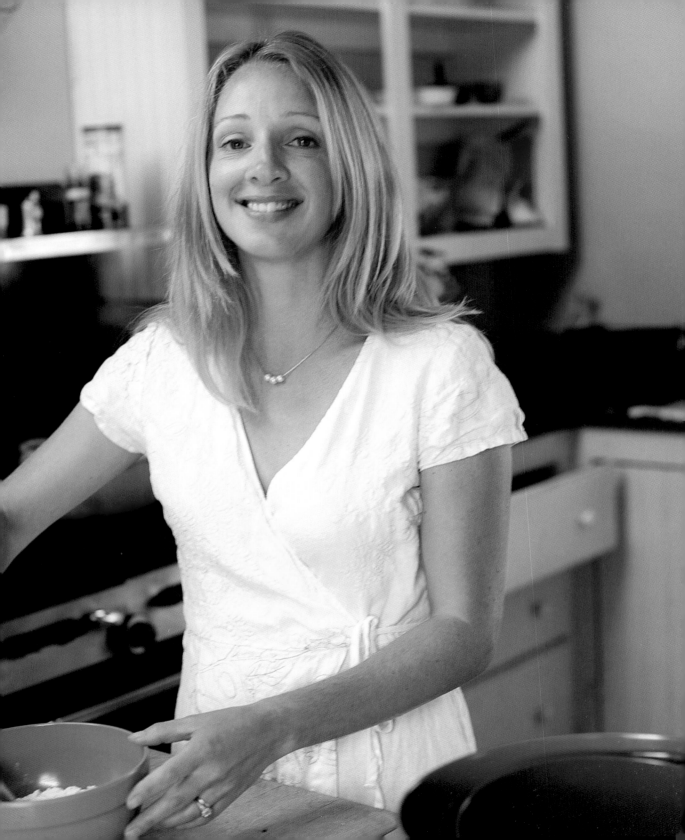

Remember when Alice fell down the rabbit hole? When Neo chose the red pill over the blue one in *The Matrix*? Well, this is that moment for you, Ms. MILF. It's time for you to start your great adventure.

You need to eat whole grains. Whole grains will help you find your inner compass and bring you to balance. And from there your journey will simply unfold quite intuitively. But if you just keep reading this book without putting some whole grains into your brain, you may never take this ride.

You're going to begin with brown rice. I don't care how you get it; maybe a Chinese or Japanese restaurant near you serves it. Maybe you can find some at the deli at Whole Foods or a local health food store. It's best if you buy some dry and cook it yourself, but it really doesn't matter as long as you start eating brown rice.[1] Right now.

If you're cooking, go to the recipe on page 107 and make it. You need organic brown rice, some sea salt, and water. That's it. If you don't have a heavy pot with a heavy lid, don't worry about it right now. You can skip soaking the rice this time, and I don't care if you burn the bottom or if it's a little mushy; just make your brown rice and start eating it. The rest of this book will make much more sense to you when your brain is bathed in the lovely nourishing glow of brown rice.

Oh, wait. One more thing: you need to chew it really well.

This is how you fall down the rabbit hole, Alice. By chewing brown rice really, really well . . . until it's a sweet liquid in your mouth . . . you will start to have your trippy, MILFy experience. You see, whole grains contain lots of complex carbohydrates and they are the *perfect* fuel for the human body. But unlike the simple carbs found in candies and chocolate, complex carbohydrates need to be broken down—in your mouth—before they can be absorbed into your body to do their work. You won't feel the amazing peace, steadiness, and stupid happiness of whole grains until you chew them really well.

---

1. You should be able to find brown rice produced by a company called Lundberg on the shelves of nearly every grocery store in the country. If you can't, ask your store to order it.

Chewing Instructions

1. First, make sure you are not too hungry. Being hungry will make you wolf down the rice and that's exactly the opposite of what we're trying to achieve here.

2. Do this experiment alone. It's difficult to relax enough to chew properly when there are other people around, trying to get your attention or engage you in conversation.

3. If you have any unsweetened pickle (a dill pickle, sauerkraut, olive, ginger pickle, or other) in the house, dole out about a tablespoon and slice it up into little pieces. If you don't have it, don't worry. It's not a deal breaker.

4. Place a reasonably sized mouthful of not-so-hot rice in your mouth. Add a very small piece of the pickle or sauerkraut to the mouthful. This will help you produce lots of saliva. With the first few bites, make sure to get a little piece of the pickle or condiment on your fork with the rice.

5. Before you start to chomp down, close the back of your throat the way you do when you savor a sip of wine. This throat-closing is important, and will feel counterintuitive for a while. Don't worry. You'll get better at it. With your throat closed, start chewing the rice.

6. *Try not to swallow.* Not even the saliva you're generating. You will add more and more saliva to the mix; that's good. Keep going. You are going to chew this mouthful of rice until every grain has been dissolved into a sweet liquid. I know it feels weird, but you can do it. . . . Imagine a lovely serene cow. She chews this much.

Oops! You swallowed! I know. It's hard. If you got to twenty chews, or even thirty, that is excellent. Try again with the next mouthful. This takes practice.

As you continue, aim to eventually chew the rice fifty times per mouthful. And when you get good at that, go for 100. By doing this, your body will begin to relax, your breath will drop lower into your belly, and you will heave a great sigh as you sink into your parasympathetic nervous system. By chewing the rice, you are adding a special digestive enzyme called ptyalin—found only in your saliva—that will help to convert the rice into glucose in your mouth. Then the glucose will be absorbed slowly and smoothly into your bloodstream, eventually making its way up into your brain, which will get all dopey and satisfied. So chewing is not just about taking more time to eat; it's about stimulating the proper digestive enzymes. If ptyalin is not produced in your mouth—through proper chewing—none of your other digestive enzymes work as well. You walk away from a meal feeling cranky and dissatisfied.

7. Stop when you're satisfied. This should happen automatically. You don't need to have some insane conversation in your head, or with your stomach, or a calorie chart. If you're really chewing your rice, you will simply push the plate away when you've had enough.

Before I learned how to chew, I was never really satisfied after I ate. I could wolf down a big meal and feel stuffed but still find myself cruising for the knockout punch of a candy bar or some other strong sweet. Learning to chew complex carbs is the single most powerful tool I've ever discovered for beating my eating disorder. If I feel like I'm getting wacky with food, I just sit down and chew some grains and/or vegetables really well and I fall back into my body and into the moment. The crazies just disappear. Poof!

Chew on This

I got up to twelve chews before everything went down the hatch.

But I kept trying. And the next day it happened. By the end of my bowl of rice and roasted winter vegetables, I had made it to thirty-six.

And something else happened, or should I say, didn't happen.

I didn't crave a dessert after my meal.

I didn't dread going to bed for fear I would lie there trying to decide whether or not to make a big pot of pasta, or go get the Ben & Jerry's . . . or the peanut butter.

You see, I've been a binge eater all my life.

I've bitten my finger shoving food into my mouth.

I've gone out in lousy weather, in bad neighborhoods, at ungodly hours to get something to eat.

I used to beg for sugar.

Beg.

So since dedicating myself to chewing my food thoroughly till everything becomes a slightly sweet liquid, those late night tremors, that sheer hell of climbing the walls trying to feed that animal inside . . .

Well, it just doesn't happen.

And it hasn't happened for the last several weeks.

I just chew.

And I'm up to sixty.

I. Feel. Amazing.

Chew your food.

Anna Romer, Los Angeles MILF

Please understand that no MILF chews every bite of every meal; life just doesn't allow for that. But by chewing at least some of your food very well, you will:

- Start to get a sense of inner balance
- Feel more coordinated in your body
- Experience smooth, calm energy that lasts for hours
- Experience greater mental clarity
- Be totally in the moment
- Feel truly satisfied after a meal
- Experience fewer cravings for sweets
- Have great poops
- Begin a completely new relationship with food, yourself, and nature

Ta-da! One food. Eaten the way nature intended. *That's* how powerful food can be.

Welcome home.

Now keep reading. . . .

Balance

MILFiness is all about balance. By staying balanced, MILFs are healthier, are sexier, and have more fun.

Your body is constantly finding balance for you. By pumping your heart, exhaling toxic gases, and keeping your blood at a proper pH, it maintains a delicate balance called homeostasis. This system can handle a remarkable number of twists and turns on the road of your existence, adapting to stress, challenges, and the trillions of mind-blowing shifts that happen every second on a cellular level. This internal balancing act is one of the great miracles of life.

And balance isn't happening just inside of you: you are a product of a vast network of organic systems all striking their natural balances; they include the soil, the oceans, the atmosphere, and space itself. So naturally your inner world seeks to balance with the outer world; you relax into sunlight and shiver when it's cold. You experience teenage joy in the spring and mature melancholy in the fall. You give love to your family and receive it back from them in kind. That's healthy. You are meant to harmonize with the bigger systems of nature. You are meant to feel connected to all of life.

Yin and Yang

Here's a little secret: nature strikes this continual balance through systems of opposing forces. Your lungs inhale and exhale. Your blood moves away from your heart, only to come back to it again. Your nervous system goes on high alert and then it relaxes. Every organic system works on its own rhythm, repeating its cycle—in concert with all sorts of other cycles—the way nature intends it to.

So from now on, we're going to describe the opposing forces of each cycle using two simple words we're borrowing from the Taoists: "yin" and "yang." Yin represents the more expansive, upward, or diffuse side of the spectrum, while yang represents contracting, downward, or gathering force.

Because our bodies are made up of many different systems, all cycling at their individual rates, it makes sense that we need good-quality natural yang force and good-quality natural yin force to keep everything moving along nicely. A heart that *only* contracts is a problem. Lungs that *only* expand are a no-no. Every cycle needs both forces in order to fulfill its purpose.

Yang is the contracting, gathering, downward, and inward force. It is centripetal. It comes down from the cosmos and governs the composition of physical matter. It creates heat, speed, intensity, dryness, and hardness and causes things to be compact. It is considered more male.

Yin is the expanding, diffusing, upward, and outward force. It is centrifugal and it governs decomposition and spiritualization. It comes up, out of the earth, as the planet spins on its axis. Yin force supports coolness, slowness, relaxation, wetness, softness, and things being expanded. It is considered more female.

To see yin and yang in all their glory, go to page 346 and look at the chart of all sorts of different attributes sorted by their yinness and yangness. If you really fall in love with yin and yang, check out my first book, *The Hip Chick's Guide to Macrobiotics,* where I go into this dynamic duo in more detail.

Do the Twist

Yin and yang are powerfully attracted to each other, and when they come together, they form a spiral of energy. In fact, as you read these very words, you are spinning on a planet, orbiting the sun, which is part of a huge twisted corkscrew of a galaxy. Look around you: pinecones, spiderwebs, seashells . . . even the water flushing down your toilet, all spirals. Think about how plants comes out of the earth—unfurling or twisting. Bite into a carrot and you'll see a spiral.

We humans have been intrigued by spirals from the get-go, and a gut-level attraction to spirals makes a lot of sense when you consider your own beginning: your father's lucky sperm rotated like a microscopic drill toward your mother's gently spinning egg. From their union, you arrived, a tiny fetal spiral. Your umbilical cord contained veins and arteries twisting gently toward the placenta. For months, you were tucked in a little spiral, big head forward and tiny knees up, and sometimes in the dark of night, you assume this position again . . . it just feels *right.*

Your fingerprints are tight spirals, while your bones and muscles twist as well, but with greater length and extension. And let us not forget the hair spiral on the top of your head. Or your ears. Even your DNA, the very code from which you continually re-create yourself, is written on a spiraling double helix. How elegant.

Imagine an invisible spring of energy—like a Slinky toy—that runs along the midline of your body. Imagine that it can contract tightly or extend out beyond your aura. The contracting part of the spiral (yang) helps to make you a physical being; it concentrates energy, brings you into the world, and keeps you engaged in the material aspects of your life. It is reaching toward the earth. This yang force governs your body.

The expansive (yin) part of the spiral pushes against all that contraction; it is energy that wants to move beyond your body, to release, and to connect with the invisible, more vibrational aspects of the world. It helps you to express thought, emotions, and the more subtle aspects of your being. It is reaching out to other people and up into the heavens. This yin force governs your spirit.

As these contracting and expanding forces unite along your midline, they make secondary spirals of energy, aka "chakras," that charge the crown of your head, your third eye, throat, heart, solar plexus, uterus, and perineum with the precious life force. These chakras also move energy out into the world and exchange it with the energy of others. This invisible energy is known in India as "prana" and in China as "chi," and good health depends upon both its strength and its ability to flow in natural ways.[2]

Because the MILF diet is composed of whole, natural foods, it will strengthen your chi while moving it where nature needs it to go. Whole foods also help all the yins and yangs in your body maintain balance: your heart will beat with gusto while its arteries stay relaxed and open. Your nervous system will tense for a deadline and relax into a candelit dinner. Your chakras will shut down in the presence of an enemy and open happily to receive a lover. You get my drift.

And while we're speaking of love, perhaps the spiral we're most familiar with is the powerful vortex of energy that's created when a man and woman fall into it.[3] We even refer to these romantic relationships as "whirlwinds," intuiting in some way their helical nature. On a physical level, the woman brings more yin force to the table, while the man brings more yang, causing a strong magnetic pull between them. And when they embrace, they feel the lovely warm energy of the spiral they create together. Energy is also exchanged on mental and emotional levels as the relationship becomes more bonded, and on a soul plane, yin and yang are working out their special, secret projects as well.

Sex occurs when the spiral the lovers create becomes so charged with force that it needs to release its pent-up electricity. And sex is much more than the meeting of body parts; it is yin force and yang force reaching out to each other, connecting and coursing powerfully through the body of each partner. Chakras open fully . . . heartbeats thunder . . . climaxes are reached . . . and deep, dammed-up rivers of energy are freed to flow. Sex is healing and balancing. But more on that later . . .

---

2. From now on, I will refer to this invisible life force as "chi." It's just a great word.
3. Of course, all types of love—heterosexual and homosexual, parental and platonic—create spirals of energy, but the male/female one is uniquely charged so that it can create a new life. Although I will be concentrating on the male/female spiral, there are yin and yang forces in every relationship. Look for them.

Everything is relative, so yinness and yangness can be assessed only through comparison. For instance, your diamond ring may be more expanded than your sister's, but it's a contracted little joke compared with Elizabeth Taylor's. And even *hers* may seem small and contracted compared with the Queen of England's. Yinness and yangness are never absolute, so don't worry about identifying them perfectly.*

Exercises: Identify three things that fold up, unfold, or are shaped in spirals. Notice the yin and yang forces within each spiral and how they are both happening at once. Compare one spiral with another in terms of yinness and yangness.

Examine three different objects around you. In which ways are they yang (hard, straight, dry, small, heavy) and in which ways are they yin (soft, curved, moist, expanded, and light)? Although things may appear to be governed by one force or the other, all things contain both forces, in varying degrees. Find them.

* By the way, this interpretation of yin and yang, borrowed from the macrobiotic diet, is not exactly the same as the one your acupuncturist might use, but that shouldn't stop you from applying it to your eating and your life.

The Yin and Yang of Food

Of course, the things we put into our mouths are made of yin and yang forces too, and they impart their distinct energies to us. Some natural foods create more contraction, heat, and pressure (more yang), while others have a relaxing, expanding, and cooling (more yin) effect on the body. Still others hang out in the middle. Natural foods help us maintain our balance.

But when we eat too many foods that contain *extreme* yin or *extreme* yang force, they make us lose our balance.

Let's take a look. Here are foods and substances that carry strong, or extreme, yang force:

EXTREME YANG FOODS
- Meat (beef, pork, lamb, venison, etc.)
- Poultry
- Eggs
- Salty cheeses
- Too much or bad-quality salt (and sodium in processed foods)
- Hard, dry baked flour products

- Caffeine (has strong yin, too)
- Some food additives and preservatives

Yang foods tend to contain more sodium and less potassium. They are saltier and denser, and have a contracting or drying effect on the body. Of course, you can eat some of these foods some of the time, but daily use and/or overuse of these substances causes the systems of your body to tip into excess tightness and contraction. Eating too much of them can make your overall energy too tight, intense, or overheated and may even make things clot, harden, or close. Consumed in excess, over long periods of time, these foods can help fuel conditions like high blood pressure, muscle stiffness, constipation, kidney stones or gallstones, atherosclerosis (or anything ending in *sclerosis,* which means "hardening"), heart disease, and cancers that are hard and found in the lower parts of, or deep within, the body, such as ovarian, prostate, pancreatic, and bone.

Clearly, we don't want that.

But extreme yang force doesn't work just on physical systems; it has some emotional and behavioral side effects, too:

- Chronic aggression
- Rigidity in thinking and behavior
- Being controlling and overly competitive
- Sexual obsession or compulsivity
- Materialism
- Inability to relax
- Self-absorption
- Closed-mindedness
- Lack of sensitivity to one's inner world, one's emotions, or other people
- The desire to dominate nature and others

Do you know anyone who fits this checklist? And how does he or she eat? Think about it.

On the other end of the spectrum are the foods and substances that carry strong, or extreme, yin force:

EXTREME YIN FOODS

- White sugar and other refined carbohydrates
- Milk, cream, butter, ice cream, and soft cheeses
- Tropical fruits and fruit juices (unless you live in the tropics)
- Tropical spices (unless you live in the tropics)
- Nightshade vegetables (potatoes, tomatoes, eggplants, and bell peppers)
- Chocolate
- Alcohol
- Marijuana and other recreational drugs
- Caffeine (has strong yang impact, too)
- Artificial sweeteners
- Most prescription drugs
- Birth control pills
- Some food additives and preservatives

Yin foods often contain more potassium than sodium. Tropical foods are considered more yin because they have a more expansive and cooling effect on the body. Many extreme yin foods are highly processed and have been stripped of their minerals, and as you may have noticed, lots of yin things we ingest on a regular basis aren't actually foods at all. For the most part, yin substances tend to release energy and send it to the periphery.

As with the yang extremes, it's okay to have some of these foods some of the time, but daily consumption and/or overconsumption of extremely yin substances can cause your body to become weak, loose, and overly expanded. Ingested over time, extremely yin food can fuel conditions like fatigue, depression, diarrhea, anemia, inflammation, arthritis (or anything ending in *itis*, which is a suffix that denotes inflammation), diabetes, and even cancers found in the upper or peripheral regions of the body, such as cancers of the breast, skin, brain, lungs, or lymphatic system. When tumors burst and spread to other regions of the body, that's yin force, too. Recent research is leaning toward the idea that heart disease is caused by yin factors as well.

These extreme yin substances cause emotional and behavioral issues as well:

- Depression
- Chronic fear
- Physical and emotional weakness
- Ineffectiveness
- Laziness
- Being spacey or scatterbrained
- Having no boundaries
- Being too sensitive to vibrations
- Getting lost in spirituality
- Lack of interest in sex
- Being self-absorbed in a low-self-esteem-y way

Know anyone who exhibits many of these characteristics? How does he or she eat?

Chances are you've pegged someone who exhibits characteristics from both lists, and that's okay. Because yin and yang attract each other, most of us are choosing from both ends of the spectrum and we may exhibit extreme qualities in both directions.

In fact, Western cuisine balances extreme yin and yang elements all the time. Here's a list of dishes or snacks that contain extreme yins and yangs:

Yang	Yin
Pretzels	Beer
Cheese	Wine
Hamburger	French fries
Ham	Cooked with pineapple
Steak	Potatoes
Turkey	Cranberry sauce
Scrambled eggs	Hash browns
Meat tacos	Salsa
Lamb	Mint jelly
Hot dogs	Ketchup, mustard, or sweet relish

We find these combinations satisfying not just because they taste good together, but because they strike a feeling of balance in our bodies.[4] However, because these foods are extreme, the balance we are striking is a wide and precarious one.

Extreme foods and substances test the limits of our natural balancing mechanisms, forcing the body to go to equally extreme measures to maintain homeostasis. Meat builds up acids that tax internal organs and cause bone loss; sugar causes weakness and decay; dairy foods stress the immune system; caffeine keeps our world in chronic freak-out mode. When we ingest these things on a regular basis, it doesn't take long for the body to become stressed and tired and to begin to age prematurely. Systems start to sputter, weaken, or even break down. The lovely body—doing its utmost to stay balanced—gets overworked and its inner seesaw collapses.

It's the same story with emotional and even mental conditions; over time, extreme foods overwork the system until things get out of whack on every level. If that sounds weird, consider this: we accept that drugs and alcohol can push the body and mind to extremes, so why not foods eaten day after day, week after week, year after year?

FYI: If the yin and yang of extreme foods don't make intuitive sense (yet), read about these foods beginning on page 256. I discuss meat, sugar, dairy, caffeine, and processed foods and their impact from a more historical, nutritional, and scientific point of view. You'll also find practical tips on kicking them out of your life.

4. Of course, some people hang out on one end of the spectrum exclusively. Vegans who eat lots of white flour, sugar, chocolate, and fruit become extremely yin, and carnivores who rarely touch a vegetable or piece of fruit—and also abstain from sweets and alcohol—become super yang. These individuals may experience imbalance more quickly and obviously than those choosing from both sides.

The Good News

Luckily for us, Mother Nature has concocted foods to help our bodies run all their systems optimally, and you have just eaten one of them: brown rice. The MILF diet is all about eating foods that are uniquely suited to the human body—foods that contain good-quality yin and good-quality yang—helping the body to buzz along smoothly and MILFily without becoming too stressed out or breaking down.

MILFy foods are natural. Because they are whole, unprocessed (or minimally processed), and organic whenever possible, they will bring you back to your lovely balanced center. They are:

- Whole grains and whole-grain products
- Vegetables (both land and sea), cooked, fermented, and sometimes raw
- Beans and other plant-based proteins
- Natural sweeteners
- Fruit (local and in season)
- Unrefined vegetable oils
- Unrefined sea salt and minimally processed seasonings

For more on the MILFy foods and the science behind their effectiveness, go to page 311.

When we eat these naturally balanced foods, not only do our bodies work better, we feel better on every level and we begin to exhibit nice, sane, and balanced yin and yang characteristics. Healthy yang characteristics:

- Physical strength
- Stability
- Positivity
- Orderliness
- Persistence
- Effective rational and analytical thinking
- The desire to defend and protect
- The ability to work with nature without abusing it

But balanced foods also nurture healthy yin characteristics:

- Softness
- Flexibility
- Intuition
- Receptivity
- The ability to multitask
- The ability to self-reflect
- Spiritual connection
- Patience
- The ability and desire to nurture
- Sensitivity to vibrations and invisible information

Because MILFs eat good-quality, balanced foods, they exhibit characteristics from both ends of the spectrum. MILFs are strong and flexible, patient and persistent, emotional and rational. Because MILFs are women, they lean toward the yin side of things more often than men do, but it is their inner balancing mechanism that makes them truly healthy. Life presents a situation, and a balanced MILF adapts accordingly. Life changes again, and the MILF finds balance once more. That's health. And these days, we need this MILFy balance because . . .

Our Culture Is Very Yang

If you've found it a little difficult to find spirals while sitting in your cubicle at work, I'm not surprised. The spiral is nature's shape, not man's. We have constructed a world full of straight lines, hard surfaces, and orderly schedules.

But nature doesn't work that way. Go outside . . . there are very few perfectly straight lines in the natural world. For the last few thousand years, however, we have been hell-bent on dominating Mother Nature. Figuring her out. Conquering her. Drilling down into her core and exploiting her resources. Instead of respecting and cooperating with the system we are a part of, we just keep hammering away at it. That's pretty yang.

We live in little squares in hard concrete buildings. On straight streets. In crowded cities. And from our rooms, we either watch little boxes of flickering light or peer into rectangular screens that offer the illusion of release from our yang little boxes.

We work. Hard. Hour after hour, we apply ourselves to tasks that squeeze us of our energy. The yin expansion comes at the end of the day, with that glass of wine; or on the weekend; or once a year on that blessed vacation.

Even our bodies have become yang. We go to gyms and work out on machines, pushing ourselves as if we're running from hungry tigers. Curves are bad. Jiggles are weak. That little belly you have? Disgusting. We drive ourselves to be thinner, prettier, stronger, and better in every way, when all we really want to do is relax, yin out, and enjoy some chocolate cake.

And our minds have become yang, too. We are encouraged to analyze with our left hemispheres instead of intuiting with our right ones. We are told to depend exclusively on "the facts" and never on our guts. Emotions are considered weak—the stuff of wimps. Detached, we look at nature as a set of mechanical puzzles to be solved in order to serve humans, instead of experiencing it as a throbbing, magical field of energy in which we are participants and cocreators.

Even the lovely relaxation we get from a good gab with a MILFy girlfriend is drying up. We text instead of calling, or we tweet the minutiae of our lives, sending 140 characters into a cybercloud in which everyone else is spinning and chattering and spewing their bons mots and witty wisecracks as well. We've become so yang and self-absorbed that we don't care who's listening . . . our "friends" and "followers" are merely numbers. We seem together, but we are really all alone.

Instead of being whole human beings treating one other with care and respect, we're turning into hostile, defensive, depressed people. Just watch the news for five minutes and see the screaming heads battling it out to shout one another down. If you prefer drama, you can watch one of the many prime-time shows starring murder and rape. If you don't have a TV, you can just cruise the Internet for porn for the next ten thousand years. Our appetites have become dark, bloody, and hypersexualized. All this aggression and objectifying lust is bad-quality yang.

Maybe it is because our modern diet is pushing our bodies and minds faster than ever before; in the last sixty years, our per capita consumption of meat has increased by more than 50 percent, breaking the 200 pounds per year mark. But we're not just big carnivores; the average American eats more processed food than any other citizen on the planet, with store-bought goodies making up a historically unprecedented 57 percent of the average American diet. And what do we chase all our burgers and cookies down with? Soda after soda after soda, replete with chemicals and high fructose corn syrup. It should come as no surprise that we are experiencing an internal pressure—and chaos—caused by toxins, excess hormones, refined foods, and record amounts of animal protein.

I ask you: Does your life feel faster or slower than it did twenty years ago? Do you feel more pressure or less? Do you have three channels on your television or five hundred? Is the planet warmer or cooler? Is your nervous system poked more times per day—from more angles—than it was fifteen years ago? Are you speeding up or slowing down?

Time to take a deep breath.

It's important to remember that there's nothing wrong with yang force; we've just taken it to an extreme. Our cultural spiral is *too* yang and contracting. But we need good-quality yang energy to protect ourselves, to build shelter, to start projects, to move forward. In fact, we can't do anything at all without yang force. But the yang force we're exerting these days is too intense; instead of being productive and positive, it has tipped into aggression and control. It's meant to contain and protect; instead it dominates and suffocates.

And because extreme yang attracts extreme yin, all this contraction is making for unusually expanded yin as well. Instead of relaxing, we take pills and black out. Instead of being soft, we're flabby and flaccid. Instead of relating to one another, we disappear behind a computer screen.

So it's time to make balance. And, ladies, because men are naturally more yang, we can't trust them to get us out of this mess. More yang force will not balance this spiral.

But yin will. The MILF diet will bring natural balance back into your body, your life, your family, and your world. And because you are a woman—naturally more yin—you will bring back the soft, receptive, intuitive force we've all been waiting for. It's about time we created some juicy, gorgeous, and powerful MILFs.

Only yin can win.

3

......

Your MILFification, Phase Two: Grains and Greens

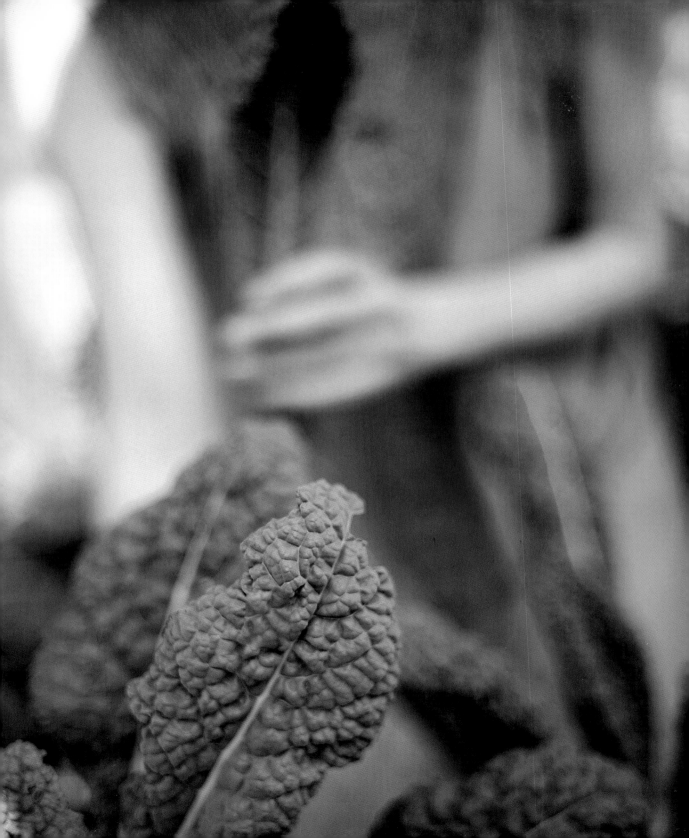

So you've chewed your rice really well and felt some peace, balance, and clarity from that. Well, we're just going to build from there. I'd like you to begin eating some kind of whole grain every day—even twice a day. And we're going to add some leafy greens to those grains. Leafy green vegetables like kale, collard greens, napa cabbage, and bok choy—blanched, sautéed, or steamed—will give you a light, upward, and relaxing energy while the grains continue to make you feel grounded and centered. Grains and greens are your first foundation. Eat anything else you normally would,[1] but place grains and greens at the center of your life, letting them into your body at least once a day and chewing them well. Twice is even better.

You will find grain recipes starting on page 102 and a vegetable blanching recipe on page 126.

That's it. Rinse and repeat. You will be amazed. If you never do anything else, you will have changed a lot.

If you'd like to barrel ahead with the rest of the MILF diet, that's okay. However, it's really important to check in with yourself and any tendency you might have to move quickly on to new projects and burn out just as fast. The MILF diet is meant to be practiced—with a spirit of exploration and play—over a lifetime, so there's no real hurry here. I would rather you take small steps, letting yourself really *feel* the benefits of daily whole grains and greens, so that your body—and not your chattering mind—starts making the next set of decisions. It is your body that will learn, improve, change, and adapt, because it has an intelligence all its own. It is your body that will say, "I like that . . . Do it again." Your mind has been running the show for long enough. Give it a rest.

---

1. I mean that. Grains and greens are not enough. Make sure you get your protein, fats, and other foods. I want you to simply feel that these grains and vegetables create balance *within* your current regime.

And because you're eating natural foods—with actual power—they will propel you. You will know when it's time to start playing with sea vegetables. You will know when you're suddenly turned on by a turnip. You will know when it's time to drive on past the Starbucks. Your body will demand that you up the ante because wellness begets wellness. Extreme foods will start to feel uncomfortable and your body will begin to shake them off. If you normally feel as though you have no time, the peace and calm of whole grains and vegetables will miraculously *make* time, as your energy increases and your priorities naturally rearrange themselves. Grains and greens are that powerful. So just eat them . . . every day . . . for the next week. This transition should be easy and doable. Any kid could cook rice. A monkey could steam greens! Introducing these foods should feel like the easiest, least dramatic exercise on the outside and a shift of life-changing proportions on the inside.

FYI: Some MILFs are in phase two for up to a year without ever diving deeper into cooking or the diet, and they see amazing results: more energy, clearer skin, increased flexibility, and stable moods. They experience an inner balance that becomes downright addictive. My friend Victoria made just the Chocolate Chip Rice Treats on page 223 for her family (on top of all their regular foods) *for a year* before she got in deeper. Now she's studying to become a healer. It's okay to take your time.

Phase Two Dos and Don'ts

DO: Plan. Even though phase two is simple, it always helps to plan your food for the day ahead. Write it down and it will happen.

DO: Keep reading this book. Especially the stuff at the back. Learn about the foods you're eating and the power they have on page 311. Start learning about the extreme foods and what they're doing as well on page 257.

DO: Practice your chewing. You will get more from this experience, on every level, if you absorb all the nutrients from the foods by chewing them thoroughly. Chewing grains is a little easier than greens, so concentrate on your grain dishes. If you don't have time to chew every mouthful, just make sure to chew one-third of the grain on your plate, preferably at the end of the meal. That will help everything else be digested better, retroactively.

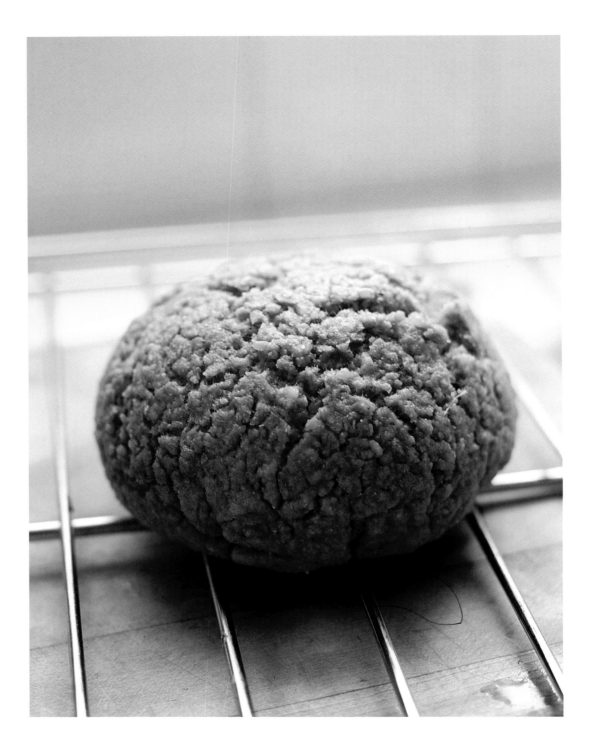

DO: Cook ahead. Grain dishes last two to three days, so make enough for a while. Keep leftovers interesting by frying them up with vegetables, rolling them into burritos, or chucking them into soup.

Greens should be cooked fresh daily, which isn't hard.

DO: Explore local health food restaurants, the deli counters at health food stores, and any other MILFy resource you might have in your area. Maybe there's a farmers' market you've never shopped at. Check out Happycow.net to find vegan or vegetarian restaurants that might serve whole grains and Yelp.com for reviews of other places in your stomping ground.

DON'T cook a big pot of grain and eat from it for the entire week. After a couple of days, it loses its mojo, so you need to cook a new grain dish every couple of days.

DON'T push this on the family unless they're actively interested. Just let yourself have your personal experience for a while. It will give you more confidence and authority when you start introducing these foods into the family fare.

So, as you spend this next week chewing on grains and greens, here's some food for your soul.

Yin Is In

MILFs enjoy what I like to call "natural femininity." They understand yin force and embrace its special powers.

Of course, we are all on a continuum of gender, and nothing is ever completely fixed; some women have unusually strong yang force and some men are pretty yin. That makes life interesting. But it's obvious that nature made two distinct sexes to come together to create new energy and new life. That's a fact. And as long as we are in one side's body or the other, it behooves us to understand—and even nourish—our role in the play of life.

MILFs are more yin. Actually, women—as a whole—are more yin than men, but MILFs embrace this reality. Let's examine our yinness on the physical level.

Women	Men
More fat and less muscle	Less fat and more muscle
Softer skin	Harder skin
Less body hair	More body hair
Bigger pelvis, smaller shoulders	Bigger shoulders, smaller pelvis
Physical center of gravity closer to earth	Physical center of gravity closer to heaven
Fewer red blood cells per pint of blood	More red blood cells per pint of blood
Lighter bones	Heavier bones
Perspire less	Perspire more
More sensitive to pain	Less sensitive to pain
Genitals are upward, inward, and hollow	Genitals are downward, outward, and dense
More estrogen and oxytocin	More testosterone
More hormonal cycling	Less hormonal cycling
Higher voices	Lower voices
Motivated by relationships (upper chakras)	Motivated by sex (lower chakras)

If you look closely at the female characteristics, they all represent an underlying yinness: fatness, softness, lightness, sensitivity, variability, and a desire to forge relationships are all yin characteristics. A woman's underlying spiral of energy is looser, more expanded, and more outward than a man's.

Men, with more muscle and denser blood and bones, squeezed to perspire more, being less sensitive, less variable, and driven like heat-seeking missiles to inseminate, are simply more governed by yang force than we are. Their underlying spirals of energy are tighter, more contracted, and downward.

But the differences don't stop there. In the last decade or so, we've been studying the brains of men and women. Instead of finding superficial disparities, the differences the neuroscientists have discovered are profound. Yin and yang forces show up in the most basic wiring of our brains. Opposite is a very short list of our significant differences.

Women	Men
Bigger communication and emotion centers in the brain	Bigger sex and aggression centers in the brain
Multitask	Focus on one thing at a time
Problem-solve through empathy	Problem-solve through analysis
Experience stress through parasympathetic nervous system	Experience stress through sympathetic nervous system
More intuitive	More analytical
More generous	More self-contained
Motivated to share	Motivated to compete
Get high on relating	Get high on winning
Natural peacemakers	Wired to defend and protect

These characteristics as well—generosity, communication, the tendency to emote, and the inclination to make peace—seem to point to an expansive, outward force moving through us. The men are just the opposite: their focused, competitive, and analytical minds steer more aggressive, sexually charged, and hunter-type bodies. They are governed by contraction.[2]

Together, you and your DILF make a spiral of energy; he brings a little more contraction to the table while you bring a little more expansion.

The key to long-lasting MILFiness is celebrating this soft, expanding force within us. Not only is it powerful in its own ways, it works in perfect harmony with good-quality yang force. Both sides are needed to keep the electricity of humanity crackling.

Using Your Yin

You are probably already using your yin force intuitively. You naturally diffuse your DILF's tension just by being in his presence. Your sex life allows him to relax and open up. Your children feel a space inside you where they are loved and truly known. By stroking heads, rubbing

---

2. Of course both genders contain both forces, but just as one of your hands is naturally dominant, you, as a female, are governed by yin force.

backs, and kissing boo-boos, you are lightening loads and infusing your home with a soft, gently expanding force.

While your DILF may be the steward of the more physical aspects of family—he protects, locks the door, fixes the roof[3]—you may naturally handle the more invisible aspects of family; you blow on the tiny embers of confidence and nourish from the inside out. While contracting force protects bodies, expanding force lifts souls.

If you don't feel as though you're good at channeling yin yet, don't try. Yin can't be found through trying. It is through relaxation, letting go, and *allowing* that yin force works its magic. But rest assured, your double X chromosomes are programmed to channel it, and when you eat whole, natural foods—reducing yang foods like meat and processed foods—your contracting force will take a backseat, allowing your inner expansion to breathe and bloom. You will eventually relax and feel a peaceful energy flowing from inside of you out into the world.

Of course, modern life and motherhood require a lot of yang force, too; wrangling children takes a ton of contracting energy; jobs are more than sitting around eating bonbons. But that contraction needn't come from heavy animal food, excess salt, or processed foods. Whole grains will keep your energy nicely contracted and forward-moving, while vegetables will keep you relaxed, fluid, and open.

And lest you should think that yin force is weak, or plays second fiddle to yang, think again. It was by channeling the feminine that Gandhi, Martin Luther King Jr., and Nelson Mandela did their good work in the world. Good-quality yin holds the space for nonviolence, moral integrity, and unconditional love.

Because yin force lifts and liberates, it is the stuff of great religions and all stirrings of the spirit. Even Jesus Christ and the Buddha, who taught us the power of compassion, charity, and peace, were basically showing us their girlie sides.

Because when it comes to love, empathy, and compassion? Let's face it, ladies: we do this stuff in our *sleep.*

As the world spirals down into its extreme yangness—faster, hotter, more self-absorbed, and hypersexualized—we can't afford to get on the bandwagon. We need to use our natural

---

3. I realize that there are lots of single moms out there who do both the yin and the yang jobs in the family. Ditto single dads. Bless you.

yin—balancing our personal energy, connecting with one another, and lifting the vibe of the world. And although what I'm suggesting is radical, these changes won't come from making speeches or attending rallies; this revolution must begin in your kitchen and transform you on a cellular level. By cooking like MILFs, we pull in our husbands and our children and make them more balanced human beings as well. We save the world from the inside out.

Ladies, it's time to honor this exquisite power we possess and to step into it. No more competing with men, or even comparing ourselves with them. Our mission is entirely different from theirs.

It may be a man's world . . . but it's a MILF's universe.

4

Your MILFification, Phase Three: Power

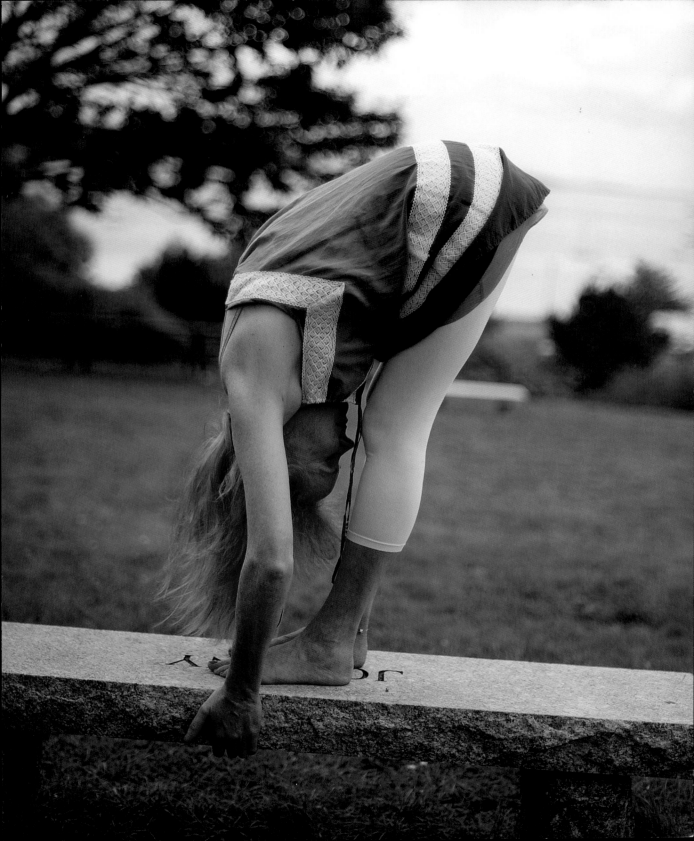

I named this phase "Power" because that's what you'll get by cooking healthy MILFy balanced foods. You will have more energy, more personal influence, more clarity and creativity. Your intuition will become razor sharp and you will begin to really feel the potency of food. This phase is powerful because, by stepping fully into the MILF diet, you are inviting in the energy of the universe. By cooking balanced foods, you are becoming a healthier woman who can bring good-quality yin force to your family and the world. Thank goodness.

And remember, although others may have power in your life—like your boss, or your congressman, or the president—their powers are actually quite limited; they don't control the vital, dynamic, and sparkly vibe that gets unleashed in your body and your kitchen. And they never will. That's yours.

In order to begin phase three, let's discuss what a MILFy balanced meal looks like. A balanced meal contains:

- 30 percent: Whole grain (or grain product, on occasion)
- 50 percent: A variety of vegetables (upward, round, and downward growing), cooked in a variety of ways
- 20 percent: Beans or bean product

These percentages are not hard-and-fast rules; some days you'll crave more vegetables, some days more grain. Ditto beans. You may skip a food group entirely at a certain meal but come back to it at the next. Look to these percentages as simple, gentle guidelines.

Those are the basics. And you can mess with those basic ingredients in thousands of different and interesting ways, starting today.

When you get good at handling the basics, you'll be ready for more: balanced meals become real powerhouses of health and well-being when they are rounded out by

- Soup (three to seven times a week)
- Small servings of sea vegetables (cooked into soups or into bean dishes, plus an arame or hijiki side dish two times per week)
- A sauce or dressing (whenever you feel like it)
- Naturally sweetened dessert (three to four times a week)
- A small serving of pickle (1 tablespoon total per day)

If you're not ready to dive in this deep, that's fine. It takes many a MILF a little while to get up to speed. If you'd prefer to hang out in phase two and slowly kick meat, sugar, dairy, and caffeine—one at a time—go to the back of the book (starting on page 271) for tips on making those transitions.

Kitchen Setup

You don't need much to get started. The bones of the MILFy kitchen are:

A good vegetable knife
A wooden cutting board
A couple of heavy pots with heavy lids (enameled cast iron is ideal)
A couple of stainless steel pots
A cast-iron or stainless steel frying pan
Wooden and stainless steel spoons
Mixing bowls

That's really it. You can make a ton of great stuff with just that. If you have only a plastic cutting board, or aluminum pots, don't let that stop you.[1]

---

1. Do get rid of aluminum cookware, however, as you budget permits. Not only might it carry risk to your health, it's simply too light; most stainless steel and all cast-iron pots and pans have thicker bottoms that hold heat better for cooking.

To dive deep into the MILF diet, it's best to have the following:

A stainless steel or enameled cast-iron pressure cooker
A suribachi (ceramic serrated mortar and pestle)
Flame deflectors (aka simmer rings)
A blender
Steamer baskets
Glass jars for storing grains and beans
Sushi mats
Rice paddles
A fine grater, for ginger and daikon
Cake pans
Cookie sheets

And I'm assuming you have stuff like strainers, can openers, and whisks. The itty-bitty things.

I'm also crossing my fingers that you have a gas stove. Gas flames are much easier to control than electric elements, and the food generally tastes much better when cooked over a flame. If gas is an option, I encourage you to sock away some cash for your future gas stove (used ones can be very reasonable), but if natural gas isn't piped through your neighborhood, that's okay. Don't let that stop your MILFiness.

To order a starter kit that includes a good vegetable knife, a wooden cutting board, flame deflector, rice, good sea salt, and some other goodies, go to my website at milfdietbook.com.

Planning

Planning is important. As they say, "Fail to plan . . . plan to fail!" And I find that's very true. When I have a plan for the next day's (or week's) menus, however rough, the chances of my eating well increase exponentially. Whether you sit down on a Sunday and think through the week or just do it every night, make your plan and do your best to stick with it. You'll find that, plan in hand, you can relax as you make it happen.

You may also want to plan to reach out and get support. Beginning phase three can be a big shift in habits, so it's helpful to get a team assembled. Find a MILFy friend who wants to step into the kitchen as well. Make a plan to call each other once a day to share tips and download about how it's going. If you live near each other, share the cooking and deliver!

Don't be afraid to hire a teenager (your own or someone else's), as you would a babysitter, to do some of the kitchen chores. Whether it's cleaning up after you, chopping vegetables, shopping, or stirring things, an hour of a teenager's time is cheap and can lighten your load considerably. As an added bonus, he or she will gain more respect for food and cooking.

Chat on my website. This is a great resource for MILFs all over the world to share recipes, tips, and even cooking woes. You'll find lots of recipes and even a meal planner that can help you think up new ideas for meals.

Begin by planning dinner menus for the week. Lunches can be thrown together from the previous night's leftovers, with the addition of some fresh greens or salad. Breakfasts can be quick, or complicated, depending on your lifestyle, but they generally consist of some kind of leftover whole grain, and either leafy greens or fruit, and maybe some nuts, seeds, or their butters.

Begin each menu by choosing your grain: rice, wild rice, millet, barley, quinoa, buckwheat, spelt, rye, oats, or some combination thereof. Do your grains need soaking? Roasting? You can also round them out with whole-grain pasta or bread.

Then choose your vegetable dishes. Make sure to have at least one lightly cooked or raw leafy green dish at each meal. The second vegetable dish may be cooked longer and include more round and root vegetables. Sometimes the second vegetable is incorporated into a veggie-rich grain or bean dish, like adzuki with winter squash, or fried rice.

Choose your bean dish or other protein. Whether it's adzuki beans, garbanzos, tofu, tempeh, or seitan, or even small amounts of animal protein, figure out your protein dish and plan accordingly; most beans need soaking the night before.

From there, select your other dishes. Which night of the week will you make a nice sea vegetable dish? How many times do you plan to make soup? And which nights of the week will be graced with dessert?

And make sure to get a little bit of pickle every day. . . . That's it.

Here are some examples of nice, balanced meals for different times of the year. This meal is nice and light, great for spring:

Grain: Spelt Salad (page 112)

Bean, lightly cooked vegetable, and pickle: Tempeh-Collard Wraps with Peanut Sauce (page 154)

Root vegetable: Steamed daikon rounds

Dessert: Fresh green apple slices with a squeeze of lemon juice

Beverage: Roasted Barley Tea (page 245)

This is a great meal for summer because it includes cooling foods and yet has a little oil and salt to keep you energized in the heat:

Soup: Watermelon Soup (page 189)

Grain: Lemony Quinoa Salad (page 119)

Bean and pickle: Garbanzo Bean Burgers (page 166)

Long-cooked vegetable: Sweet Stewed Carrots with Corn Sauce (page 128)

Lightly cooked vegetable: Steamed greens

Beverage: Peppermint Tea (page 245), cooled

More warming, and with stronger cooking styles, this is a balanced meal for fall:

Soup and bean: Tuscan White Bean Soup (page 185)

Grain: Millet Croquettes with Sauce (page 109)

Lightly cooked vegetable and sea vegetable dish: Hijiki, Fresh Corn, and Tofu Salad on Arugula with Toasted Sesame Dressing (page 172)

Long-cooked vegetable: Oven-Roasted Root Vegetables with Garlic, Cumin, and Herbs (page 133)

Pickle: Miso Pickles (page 149)

Dessert: Fresh fruit

Beverage: Kukicha Tea (page 244)

This winter meal has foods that are strongly seasoned, rich, and satisfying, while keeping its lightness in the blanched vegetables:

Grain: Fried Rice (page 111)

Bean and long-cooked vegetable: Adzuki Beans with Winter Squash (page 159)

Lightly cooked vegetable: Brad Pitt Vegetables (page 126) with Carrot-Ginger Dressing (page 240)
Pickle: Umeboshi Pickles (page 148)
Dessert: Peanut Butter Cookies (page 201)
Beverage: Kukicha Tea (page 244)

The nice thing about planning is that it's literally the hardest part. Once the plan is done, your subconscious mind goes into action mode and starts figuring out exactly how it's all going to happen. You'll be amazed, as you become a more experienced MILF diet cook, at how good you get at this.

Here We Go Again

I wish I could tell you that you can cook like a maniac on Sunday and then freeze stuff for the week. But most MILFy foods don't freeze very well, and even if they did, their vital freshness would be lost. Luckily for us, most MILFy dishes are good the next day, or even the next. Here's how long each food stays fresh and energized after cooking:

7 days or more: Pickles
3 days: Bean dishes, desserts
2 days: Whole-grain dishes, hearty vegetable dishes, sea vegetable dishes, soups
1 day: Leafy greens and lightly cooked vegetable dishes

So with the exception of lightly cooked green veggies, you don't need to cook much at every single meal. You can get into a rhythm of cooking a lot one night and then taking it easier the next. However, freshly prepared food generally is the best-tasting and has the most energy, so many MILFs, once they get up to speed in the kitchen, get into a rhythm of making a fresh dinner every night.

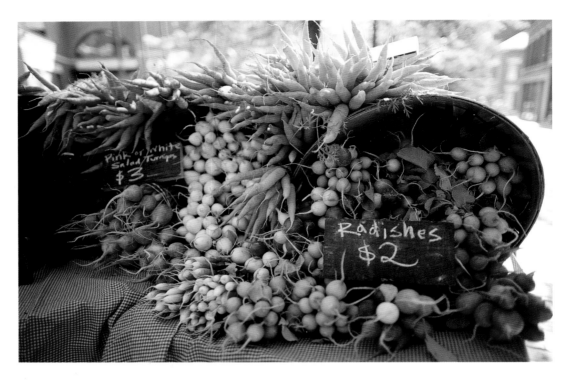

Variety

Many of us like to keep our food choices simple; we find that one perfect smoothie recipe and then repeat it every morning for a year. We have our one go-to dish at the cafeteria. When it comes to food, ruts are very easy to get into.

But that's a problem. Your body has millions of different internal jobs to do every day to keep your vitality at its peak, and every natural food pitches in, in its own unique way, to help your body out. Some foods bring warmth; others cool things down. Some benefit the nerves, while others go straight to the heart. Even among whole grains, there are those that produce more contraction and others more expansion. Nature has designed a plethora of choices to fulfill all our needs and yet we still organize our food the way we do our lives, making it regimented and scheduled and repeated.

But as my MILFy friend Sanae would say, "You change your clothes every day, why not your food?" Now, I understand that just acquainting yourself with MILFy foods might be a huge leap in lifestyle, so I'm not trying to pile your plate too high. I just want to discourage the idea that after a few months or so, you will have found the perfect seven-day menu and you can just repeat it until your kids go off to college. That kind of rigidity doesn't work for the human body and it won't support the overall health of your family.

Don't worry. You don't have to have a degree in food energetics to make the right choices. As natural foods relax you and open you up, you will actually feel the urge to seek variety. Your intuition will prompt you to buy that new vegetable, or sauté the greens tonight, or take it easy on the seasoning. You will be moved in different ways as the seasons change, as your life shifts gears, and at different times of day. Just as nature is changing all the time, so are you. Go with it.

The Dos and Don'ts of MILFy Cooking

DO: Get a buddy. If you've got a MILFy friend who'd like to make this simple change as well, agree to phone, text, or e-mail each other every day. If you have a hard time with follow-through, talking about your plan with a buddy really helps. Share insights, inspiration, and challenges. If you live near each other, share some of the cooking. According to Louann Brizendine, author of *The Female Brain*, connecting with other women through talking activates pleasure centers in our brains and can set off a big rush of dopamine and oxytocin that makes us feel amazing. MILFs need MILFs!

DO: Have a one-pot-meal night. Once a week, make a soupy stew that includes a grain, beans, some wakame sea vegetable, and some up, down, and round vegetables. This brings all the elements into one pot. It's very easy and delicious, and you can hang out with your kids or watch the news while it's cooking. Round it out with some freshly steamed greens and a piece of fruit for dessert. Voilà!

DO: Take a night off. This is a night when you eat out, get something delivered, or serve up a vegan frozen pizza and soy ice cream. You need at least one night off per week. Maybe two.

DO: Change with the seasons. During the year, we go through a big expansion (spring through summer) and a big contraction (autumn through winter). Our bodies feel this shift on every level, and yet we've gotten so "modern," our food choices rarely reflect what's going on around us. We can—and do—eat ice cream in the dead of winter and juicy steaks at the height of summer. This makes no sense to the body. Charged with keeping heat in the winter and dispersing it in the summer, our food and cooking choices need to shift with the seasons.

Spring and Summer

- Emphasize lighter, quicker cooking styles: e.g., juicing, raw salads, steaming, blanching, grilling, and stir-fries.
- Use less salt and less oil as you lighten up in the spring. As summer heats up and you become more physically active, increase them as needed. When in doubt, follow your intuition.
- Emphasize upward-growing and expanded vegetables (but don't skip the downward-growing and round).
- Mix grains, beans, and vegetables in salads; this lightens the energy of the dish.

Autumn and Winter

- Use more slow- and long-cooking styles: long sautés, baking, pressure-cooking, and deep-frying.
- Use more seasoning and more oil.
- Emphasize round and root vegetables (but don't skip your greens!).

DO: Shop intelligently. Make your life easy by stocking your kitchen with the essentials. A well-stocked kitchen sparks creativity and discourages excuses for not cooking. See the list on page 62. Personally, I don't like shopping, so I try to plan well enough so that I don't have to go to the store more than once a week. It doesn't always work, but I try.

If you live off the beaten track, you can order lots of the strange foods I'm suggesting online. Check out milfdietbook.com for resources.

DO: Join a CSA. If you live in a groovy area, you may have Community Supported Agriculture farms near you. Google "CSA" and the name of your state to find out. During the growing season, you can have a delivery of freshly picked vegetables brought right to your door for a very reasonable price. You can't get fresher, more delicious produce without growing it yourself.

Is the MILF Diet Expensive?

Good question. I'll start with the bad news: some of the most powerful elements of the MILF diet—like miso, umeboshi pickles, and sea vegetables—are expensive. But, in general, they're used only in moderation, so it's not like you're buying them new every day, or even every week.

The great news is that whole grains and beans give you a major bang for your buck. I always thought it was crazy that rice is $1.50 a pound. For what it delivers to the body, mind, and spirit, rice should be a hundred bucks a pound! Ditto beans. They are stupidly cheap.

In terms of fresh vegetables and fruit, well, you have a lot of choices. Organic produce is definitely more expensive than the chemical-laced stuff, and it may represent a hike in your current grocery bill. However, you can also get fresh, organic veggies in season through local CSAs or at a local farmers' market, or even grow your own when you can. Plus, organic food is the largest-growing segment of the food industry, so it should be getting cheaper and cheaper as time goes on. You can also mix and match, buying organic whenever possible, but getting conventional produce when that's what you need to do. Better that than a candy bar. Don't let your wallet stop you from eating decent food.

The MILFs I interviewed for this book are not particularly wealthy, but they make feeding themselves and their kids a total priority, and they find ways to make it work. They use leftovers creatively and avoid unnecessary waste, and they also consciously put a price tag on all the benefits they're getting: tons of energy, healthy kids, peaceful families, natural beauty, sparky sexuality, a real sense of personal power, and freedom from disease and from aches and pains. And that price tag reads "Priceless."

DO: Eat locally. This will help you to harmonize with your natural environment. It's most important that drinking water, fruit, and vegetables come from within your region or climate. An avocado in Akron once in a while is fine, but a daily banana/mango smoothie in a four-season climate will make you feel cool, weak, and out of balance over time.

Although rice may not grow in your immediate area, grains, beans, and sea vegetables are very adaptable and tend to have larger growing regions. You can choose from a wider area with these foods.

DO: Explore balance in every meal. As you continue to eat whole foods, you will naturally begin to sense balance within your cooking and meal planning. This is when the MILF diet gets really fun and dynamic. For instance, upward-growing vegetables naturally complement downward-growing vegetables; cool complements hot; cooked feels good with raw; soft goes with crunchy; simple dishes balance more complicated ones . . . you get my drift.

Try to incorporate all five tastes (salty, sour, sweet, pungent, and bitter) in a day—or, when you get really good, in one meal. Play with color as well; a meal of many colors is usually more satisfying, nutritious, and balanced.

Balance Isn't Always 50/50

We tend to think of balance as equality—the scales of justice balancing perfectly, or the black and white yin/yang symbol—but those images aren't helpful when it comes to nourishing our MILFy bodies. You don't need equal volumes of yin and yang foods.

You see, yang force (tight, dense, and compact) tends to manifest itself in more concentrated forms, and yin force (more expanded, loose, and releasing) takes up more space to do its job. For instance, if you were to eat one teaspoon of salt (ugh), you would not feel balanced by drinking one teaspoon of fruit juice; you might crave a whole quart!

In order to feel balanced with nature—and to develop our yin qualities—we need to lighten up a little. Eating too much yang food, like meat, salt, baked flour products, or even long-cooked root vegetable dishes, can make us feel too hot, intense, hyperactive, or—taken to an extreme—stuck and rigid.

You're already lightening your vibe considerably by eating the plant-based foods of the MILF diet, but even within it, your personal "balance" will never be one bite of yang food to one bite of yin.* In fact, what feels "balanced" to you will change throughout the day, throughout the seasons, and over your lifetime. That's why nature gave you intuition—an inner bullhorn that only you can hear. And if you don't feel you can hear it yet, rest assured that by making vegetables and grains your principal foods, you will. The MILF diet will help you learn your body's secret language and recover its original childlike buoyancy.

Finally, don't feel you need to understand this stuff like an expert. Yin and yang can be studied for a lifetime and—because of their paradoxical nature—they have a tendency to boggle the mind. Just continue to put grains and vegetables at the center of your diet and your inner compass will direct you.

* In fact, the ratio is more like 1:5, or even 1:7, depending on the climate you live in, but don't get all caught up in the numbers. It simply means we need to keep our food lighter, plant-based, and less seasoned rather than heavy, meaty, and salt-laden.

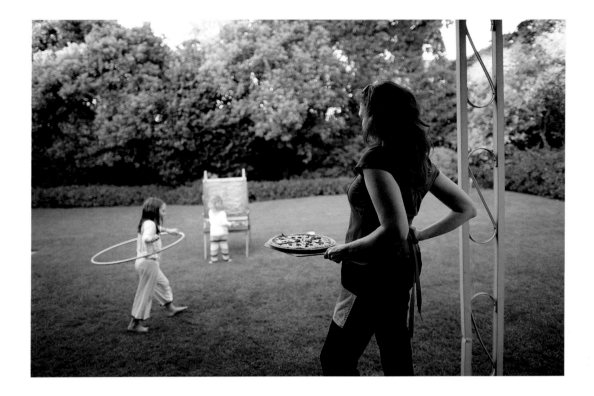

Ideas for Kids' Lunches

- Brown rice sushi
- Whole-grain noodles with tahini sauce
- Fried rice
- Avocado
- PBJ on whole wheat sourdough
- Bean dips with veggies and pita bread
- Whole wheat bagel with fake cream cheese
- Burritos
- Corn muffins
- Tofu hot dogs
- Leftover chili

- Tempeh "tuna"
- Fresh fruit
- Greens rolls
- Dried fruit
- Gardein "chicken" strips made into chicken salad
- Fruit juice
- Organic applesauce
- Desserts from this book
- Homemade cookies
- Whole-grain or rice crackers with nut butter

MILF Shopping List (all organic, whenever possible)

Grains
- Rice (long-grain, medium-grain, and short-grain)
- Millet
- Hulled barley
- Quinoa (red or yellow)
- Roasted buckwheat
- Rye berries
- Spelt berries
- Whole wheat berries
- Whole oats

Beans (Dried and Canned) and Other Bean Products
- Black-eyed peas
- Adzuki beans
- Pinto beans
- Black beans
- Garbanzo beans
- Kidney beans
- Red and green lentils
- Split peas
- Great Northern beans
- Tofu (soft, firm, or extra firm)
- Silken tofu (for sauces and dressings)
- Tempeh

Vegetables
- Leafy greens
- Round vegetables
- Root vegetables
- Pickles

Seasonings
- Sea salt (unrefined, fine grain)
- Soy sauce (Nama shoyu is best)
- Miso (South River, Miso Master, American Miso Co.)
- Umeboshi vinegar
- Mirin
- Brown rice vinegar
- Balsamic vinegar

Oils
- Extra virgin olive oil
- Sesame oil
- Toasted sesame oil
- Safflower oil
- Coconut oil

Fruits
- A selection from your climate, fresh and dried

Grain Products
- Whole wheat flour
- Whole wheat pastry flour
- Corn flour
- Whole wheat couscous
- Whole wheat noodles
- Mochi
- Rolled oats
- Whole wheat sourdough bread
- Polenta

Sea Vegetables
- Nori
- Hijiki
- Arame

- Kombu
- Wakame
- Agar agar
- Dulse

Nuts and Seeds
- Sesame seeds
- Sunflower seeds
- Pumpkin seeds
- Almonds
- Walnuts
- Peanuts
- Hazelnuts

Sandwich Fixin's
- Tahini
- Peanut butter
- Almond butter
- All-fruit jams

Fake Meat
- Yves luncheon meat alternatives
- Gardein "chicken"
- Seitan (WestSoy)

Fake Dairy
- Cream cheese alternative
- Daiya shredded cheese
- Soy yogurt
- Rice milk
- Almond milk
- Soy margarine
- Vegenaise
- Fruit-sweetened soy ice cream
- Rice Dream ice cream

Sweeteners
- Rice syrup
- Barley malt
- Maple syrup

Herbs and Spices
- Rosemary
- Oregano
- Paprika
- Cayenne pepper
- Black pepper
- Thyme
- Other favorites

Cereals
- Crispy rice cereal
- Fruit- or maple-sweetened granola

Beverages
- Kukicha tea
- Roasted barley tea
- Apple juice
- Carrot juice
- Amazake
- Spring water

Miscellaneous
- Kuzu root starch or arrowroot starch

DO: Set a timer. I suggest you develop time boundaries around cooking. Getting into whole foods can feel overwhelming for some people—especially those who aren't used to cooking—so it's important that you have very real limits around the time you ask of yourself on this project. It needs to feel easy, interesting, and doable.

That said, cooking whole foods in a variety of ways takes some time. I'm not going to lie to you about that. You are making a very real investment in yourself, your family, and everyone's health. It will have *huge* benefits, but you must put in some time and some elbow grease. Make it your goal to put aside ninety minutes, two nights a week, to just let yourself dive into the cooking. When you set an actual timer—on the stove, or on your alarm clock—the chatterbox part of your mind will relax and quiet down. You will be more in the moment and pay closer attention than if you are fretting about what's next or feeling the pressure to get everything done in twenty minutes.[2]

On that note, I realize it's all the rage these days to get a meal done in, like, four minutes. That seems to be what society is aiming at: *no* time in the kitchen. But not only is that a radical departure from the history of human development, it's a big part of why we have the health problems that we do, and it cheats you of the very real experience of strengthening your life force through cooking. Spending no time in the kitchen is weakening you, whether you know it or not. Cooking whole foods is profoundly powerful and will stir up your vital energy. You will feel that very quickly.

So you have your two evenings when you put in ninety minutes . . . maybe shave off some computer time, or TV time, or skip that class this once. In this ninety minutes, you make a meal that contains some more-complicated or fun dishes—dessert, a long-cooked bean dish, roasted seeds, maybe a yummy sauce—always making enough to create leftovers for the next few days. And then all the other meals for the week take about forty-five minutes (or less) and are brought together relatively easily through the use of leftovers and more-quickly cooked dishes.

---

2. By the way, setting a timer helps for almost everything—work, housework, even creating forced downtime if you're a relentless doer. Try it.

DON'T freak out about all of this. The information in this book is powerful and it should quietly inform your choices for the rest of your life. However, it may take some time for your body, mind, and spirit to all agree to eat MILFy food three times a day, every day. It took mine a while. Remember that this is not a race, and there is no such thing as perfection. Think of the MILF diet as a practice and do your best. When in doubt, pick up this book and eat some whole grains and vegetables. They will always propel you in the right direction.

Shortcuts

Here are some shortcuts that can save you a little time. I don't recommend them for everyday use, forever, but if the difference between your eating well and eating badly comes down to a couple of shortcuts, then go for the shortcut:

- Use an electric rice cooker that cooks your rice while you're at work.
- Use canned beans once in a while.
- Use store-bought unpasteurized pickles, but be sure to rinse them well—they're salty.
- Use store-bought snacks and desserts (as long as they don't have white sugar or dairy or tons of chemicals).
- Use store-bought salad dressings like Annie's (avoid sugar and dairy).
- Get takeout from Whole Foods Markets' deli or another good-quality deli in your area.
- Have store-bought hummus or guacamole on hand for snackers.
- Buy unsalted, pre-roasted nuts.
- Get premade pizza crusts and pie crusts.

DON'T USE THESE SHORTCUTS
- Powdered miso or miso soup from Japanese restaurants
- Pre-salted nuts or seeds (too salty and made with bad-quality salt)
- Store-bought sesame salt (it can sit on the shelf and get rancid)

Weight Loss

Many a MILF wants to lose some weight. And for the majority of MILFs, just letting go of white sugar, dairy, and processed foods helps their bodies to let go of lots of excess baggage. Add whole grains and veggies to the mix, and the average MILF stays nice and thin. However, for some of us, a little more attention needs to be paid to drop that last ten pounds or so. Here are some tips for squeezing into that old prom dress:

• **Be consistent:** Crazy behaviors like skipping meals or just generally starving yourself actually freak your body out and it starts to hold on to fat, instead of letting it go. Eat three meals, at consistent times, to give your body the message that all is well—the universe is abundant—and it will start to heave a sigh of relief and drop five pounds while you're not looking.

• **Chew:** I cannot stress enough how effective chewing is for losing weight. Proper mastication is not about taking more time to eat your food; it's about absorbing all of its nutrients. Your body actually uses the food you're giving it, feels total satisfaction, and gives you amazing energy. You can't go wrong with good chewing. No matter what you're eating! For a reminder of the technique, go to page 23.

• **Get rid of flour:** Eliminate flour products and lean on whole grains, veggies, beans, and fruit for your carbs. And chew them well, so you feel satisfied. Whenever I do this, I am amazed by how quickly my body drops the excess. When you've lost the weight, have whole-grain noodles just two times a week and whole wheat bread two times a week. Don't go crazy.

• **Carrot-Daikon Drink:** This drink (page 248) is great for quick weight loss, but you should drink it only once a day—a half hour before breakfast—for ten days. After that, it's okay to have it two times a week forever, but don't do it day after day after day. You will find that the daikon's diuretic power makes you feel "fantabulous," but too much carrot-daikon drink can make you release minerals and make you feel weak.

• **Get consistent exercise:** You don't need to run the New York marathon. Just as with healthy eating, it is consistency that the body loves when it comes to exercise. Yoga one or two times a week and three cardio workouts of about twenty minutes each should give your body the signal to burn excess fat.

• **Don't eat for three hours before bed:** If you go to bed on a full stomach, your body spends the night working instead of resting. This is not only bad for your beauty sleep, but also bad for your metabolism. You will lose weight much faster if you go to bed on an empty stomach.

- **Do the body scrub:** The body scrub (it's coming up on page 76) is really good for just about everything, not just your skin. By stimulating your skin, you're stimulating all your internal organs, and your overall chi will pick up speed.

- **Meditation:** Meditating for five to twenty minutes a day is great for keeping your mind clear and your body relaxed. It also helps enormously with impulse control, so you can pursue your deeper dreams instead of candy-bowl hopping at work. See page 97 for a primer on meditation.

- **Get variety in food:** If your eating becomes too simple (miso soup, rice, broccoli . . . miso soup, rice, broccoli), you'll get contracted and start craving strong expansion, i.e., a binge. Vary your grains, your veggies, and your beans regularly, so your body feels nice and abundantly nourished.

- **Don't skip the sweets:** Make sure you get a nice fruit dessert or something made with brown rice syrup at least once a day to satisfy your sweet tooth. In the old days, dieting meant not having anything sweet or fun, but that's not the case anymore. Make sure you feel like a secure, satisfied, smirking little princess. That way, it's easy to continue.

- **Go easy on salt and salty condiments:** Your body needs salt, but not too much. The more salt you eat, the more you will crave sweets, or simply more food. Go easy on the miso, shoyu, salt, and pickles, and you will not feel the need to eat too much.

Feeding DILFs and Kids

My MILFy friends are full of suggestions for feeding DILFs and kids. All together, the MILFs I've spoken to for this book have practiced the MILFy way for a total of over *four hundred years* and have thirty-seven kids among them, so they know a thing or two:

DILFs

Remember that men are naturally more yang than we are. This means that they crave—and can tolerate—more protein, more salty seasoning, and denser foods. Here are some practical tips for feeding men well on the MILF (or, should we say, DILF) diet:

Do: Offer him plenty of beans and protein dishes. Men generally need more protein than women do (unless the woman is pregnant or an athlete). Some men also enjoy a certain density and richness in their protein dishes, like those qualities found in seitan and tempeh. *Mmmm . . .* Make a nice, rich protein dish and just let your DILF attack it. If he's a die-hard meat eater, cook beans with chunks of meat so he gets a taste for the beans at the same time.

Do: Give him stronger seasoning. Because men have more muscle mass, and denser blood, they can tolerate a little more salt than we can. Olives and pickles are great to serve as side dishes. Now, this isn't an excuse for him to drown the rice in shoyu (soy sauce) or to bury the kale in sesame salt. Too much salt can lead to grouchiness, muscle tightness, cravings for sweets, and an overall too-yang condition. But because men are naturally more yang, they can handle a little contracting.

Do: Take out your serving (and the kids' servings) when making family whole-grain dishes like fried rice and then season his a little more before the end of cooking. You don't need to do this every time, but once in a while it's a nice way to serve him a manly, macho dish.

Do: Keep the sesame salt handy for him. However, don't have shoyu, raw sea salt, or raw miso at the table. Uncooked, they are too hard to assimilate properly into the body, and salting habits are easy to form and hard to break. Keep freshly made sesame salt (page 253) instead. It's got calcium and it's good for his heart. But go easy here, too; MILFs and kids should have only about 1 teaspoon per *day* and DILFs can do 2 teaspoons.

Do: Go for grains. Because they are more yang, DILFs generally like more grains and fewer vegetables. That's okay. You will keep a nice spark between the two of you in the bedroom if you gorge on the veggies and go a little easier on the grains while he gorges on the grains and goes easy on the veg. However, if he loves his veg, don't discourage him. Let his intuition do the choosing.

DO: Cater to his tastes. Remember, you are in this for the long haul and you are performing nothing less than magic. MILF Meredith McCarty suggests adding herbs, spices, and moderate amounts of oil to make things interesting. Make a kick-ass dessert every once in a while to keep his sweet tooth satisfied. Appeal to his tastes, and if he's picky, don't change things too quickly. Every MILF warns not to take lack of interest in the food personally; these things take time. There is a chapter in the recipe section exclusively for DILFs, so start there. If you can find one or two recipes he likes, you've done a great job and he will begin to feel the results, and he may never associate them with the food. But you know the truth. If you have a DILF who simply sits down and eats whatever is placed in front of him, that's great. After that short period of detox, he will feel wonderful.

DON'T micromanage your DILF or his eating choices. Set him free: when he's at work, he will go out and eat with colleagues at various restaurants, and that's okay. Men, because they are more yang, tend to be less sensitive, and that steak won't make him feel quite as funky as it would you. When men feel they are free to expand out into the world, they return home much more happily. Yin and yang.

Feeding a DILF can have great results. Amy Rohlnick, mother of three, married a man on meds for high cholesterol and allergies. After she worked her MILF magic, his cholesterol went from 230 down to the 170s and he threw away his allergy medication. Recently she woke up, looked out her window, and saw him—in his skivvies—picking kale from the garden for their breakfast.

Kids

When it comes to helping kids transition to better-quality foods, MILFs have developed all sorts of practical—and sometimes stealthy—tips for feeding kids. Take a look:

DO: Add before you subtract. Do not yank favorite foods from the table. You're not here to start a family earthquake. Cook meat with beans. Add more vegetables to soups and sauces. Put sea vegetables into soup stock. Introduce delicious healthy desserts. Make tempura!

Sarah Loring, mother of four, suggests offering transitions: "from doughnuts to whole-grain muffins . . . to whole-grain cereal . . . to soft-cooked whole-grain porridge." She adds: "It doesn't always have to be obvious: mix a little wild rice into white rice, then add brown to the wild and white. Then increase the proportion of brown. Give everyone a chance to get used to it. Keep the joy in food."

DO: Go easy on salt and salty seasonings. Because children are small—with less blood volume and muscle mass than adults—a little salt goes a long way in their little bodies. Too much salt, in the form of miso, shoyu, or sea salt, can make kids cranky and irritable, and cause them to crave extreme yin foods. Make sure your kids have a wide selection of good-quality sweets, like desserts made from brown rice syrup, maple syrup, and fruit, and be sure to go easy on the salt. Babies under one should have no added salt at all.

DO: Eat together. A family is like a battery that needs to be recharged regularly. Eating together is one of the best ways to renew your connection to and love for one another. MILFs stressed that eating at least one meal a day together, enjoying food and exchanging daily events, makes a big difference in the health of their families. Even if you can manage it only on the weekends, make it happen.

DO: Be a supermodel. Kids love to emulate their parents, at least until puberty hits. Take advantage of this natural mimicking and eat well yourself. You can't expect your kid to chomp down on a carrot when you're savoring a candy bar. So get rid of that chip stash. It will be discovered. Eating well is a family affair.

DON'T take it personally when a dish is rejected. You're in this for the long haul, and if you feel discouraged by the family's rejection of one dish, or one meal, it's going to be a challenge to stay the course. Say a little prayer before you serve dinner ("Hey, Universe, help me to turn the results of this meal over to *you*") and detach. You will have your big hits and your big misses. It's okay. Every MILF does. Just keep on truckin'. Over time, the food will win.

MILFs also said they sometimes made two separate meals in the beginning—or a variety of dishes—to keep various family members satisfied. Forcing people to eat things they don't like rarely works in the long run. Family members change and grow constantly, so staying flexible in the kitchen is a must.

Stealth Health

You need to shut up about this. Zip it, girls. I mean it.

Yes, of course, share with your MILFy friends. But when it comes to your family, this is a stealth health mission. Shut the freak up.

Let the food do the talking.

Over time, your nine-year-old will notice that she has a headache, or bad dreams, after eating birthday cake at Emma's house. All you have to ask is "What happened? What did you eat?" Let *her* figure it out. Not you. If you are doing all the figuring out, you interfere with her listening to her own internal signals. Over time, she will start to put two and two together. It doesn't mean she'll have the perspective or discipline to stop eating crappy stuff at nine years old, but she's building an archive of experiences that will serve her the rest of her life. She is finding her balance.

Ditto your DILF. Let him proudly declare that he's pooping more easily. That he's playing a better game of tennis. Greet it with a ho-hum "That's nice, sweetheart." Let *him* realize how sluggish he feels after eating the roast beef at the wedding. You don't have to warn him before he takes that first bite.

And all the changes you're noticing in yourself and your own burgeoning MILFiness? No need to enumerate them at the dinner table. Your family will *feel* that your mood is more stable. They will hear you laughing more. Your DILF will notice that your skin is glowing. Let them put two and two together. The more they discover for themselves, the better.

But you must be patient. This doesn't happen overnight. And I *know* you want to talk about it. Hell, you're a woman . . . and you've discovered something that helps your nearest and dearest. . . . *You want to shout this from the roof of a Walmart!* As I said, that's what your MILF friends are for. Pick up the phone and tell them that your teenage son's back acne is clearing up, but do not . . . and I mean *do not* . . . post a photo of it on Facebook.

Everyone runs from a zealot. And, believe me, this information is powerful enough that people get downright religious about it. But you must curb yourself at home. Every MILF who contributed to this book agrees with me. There will come a time when your family naturally starts asking questions or bringing up the changes they're feeling, and then you can add your two cents. But be careful to speak only from your own perspective and experience. Never preach. As long as Mommy is pontificating about brown rice and curly kale, it becomes something that you own . . . something associated with *you* . . . and that invites others to rebel against it. Kale will no longer just be kale. It will have your personality attached to it, and that's not fair to Mother Nature.

She's sent you on a secret mission. It's called stealth health. So zip it.

DO: Sneak stuff in. There's no reason to hit them over the head with what they're eating; just serve it and make it look similar to things they have had in the past. MILFs have learned some very skillful ways to get healthier foods into their families' bodies.

- Use eggs and tofu together to camouflage tofu.
- Serve your bean dishes with chunks of organic meat.
- Put seaweed into soups.
- Put seaweeds like dulse, wakame, and kombu into the cooking water of your oatmeal or pasta.
- Grate carrots into pancake batter, muffins, spaghetti sauce, or anything else you can get away with.

DO: Keep the house stocked. Be prepared for after-school blood sugar crashes and midnight noshing. Have the fridge and cupboards stocked with good-quality snacks like hummus, guacamole, raw vegetables, fresh fruit, dried fruit, nuts, puddings, cookies, popcorn, bread, nut butters and all-fruit jams, soy cheese pizza, corn chips, and any other MILFy treats you can dream up or find at the health food store.

DO: Get the kids to help. With seven children, MILFy Melanie Brown Waxman understands the power of a team effort: "There are lots of jobs in the kitchen that kids can do without getting into trouble: shucking corn, washing vegetables, setting the table, and cutting soft foods with a plastic knife. When kids get involved, they are more likely to taste and enjoy the food."

DO: Give them choices and boundaries. Kids shouldn't be allowed to run roughshod over the kitchen, but their desires should also be respected.

Sarah Loring had her kids make a list of their favorite foods and post it on the fridge, then she tries to include those foods as often as she can. Each child is also allowed to choose one food that he or she never has to eat, and if it shows up in a dish, that kid can take a pass. The child does, however, have to eat everything else.

Special occasions and birthdays are the perfect time for children to choose their meals and pick their favorite dishes, but MILFs warn against letting small kids hijack the menu the rest of the year.

DO: Let them roam outside the home. All my MILFy friends agree that kids should be free to experiment outside the home. In fact, they suggest that this is good for kids, as it hones their relationships to their own bodies and intuitions. When kids go out and eat pizza and ice cream with their friends and feel cranky the next morning, they start to learn the power of food.

DO: Stay in control of the kitchen. Be a strong and steady presence in the kitchen. Unless you have a DILF who loves to cook (hallelujah!), you need to hold a space in the kitchen, or no one will. This doesn't mean that you have to be married to the kitchen, but you should be the one in charge. Throw out the junk and don't let it creep back into the cupboards. If you want something extreme, get it out at a restaurant. Cook regularly, so that you support your family on a biological level consistently. Learn how to say no when you need to. This is your magical space and the more you step into it, the more it will be respected and do its lovely work.

DO: Enjoy the results. By feeding your family MILFy foods, you are changing their lives from the cells on up. Make sure you take a moment to appreciate the magnitude of what you're accomplishing. Call a MILFy friend and celebrate.

DON'T forget the love. Every MILF I spoke to expressed how important it was to keep love in the kitchen and at the dinner table. This isn't about eating perfectly or being in total control. Life is an ever-changing, flowing, and (hopefully) fun journey. If you get too uptight about what's going into everyone's mouth, you lose the good-quality yin you're bringing to their lives. Eating is meant to be enjoyable.

And some final words of wisdom from MILFy Melanie Brown Waxman: "Parenting is not something that can be ruined or created in one day. This makes preparing nourishing meals for our children an exciting adventure. Often we try to be the perfect parent, but accepting our mistakes is really part of good parenting and learning as we go along."

Eating Out

Eating out can be downright easy on the MILF diet. All you have to do is look for the VCP—veggies, carbs, protein.

All restaurants have vegetables. In order to remain MILFy, ask for your veg to be sautéed in olive oil, or steamed, or blanched. These days, many restaurants pride themselves on making sophisticated vegetable side dishes as their plant-based patrons grow in number. A couple of veggie side dishes can be very satisfying.

Carbs are a little trickier, but far from difficult. Many Chinese and Japanese restaurants (and health food restaurants, of course) have brown rice, but other places may have just white noodles, white bread, or potatoes for your carb. If you don't eat out very often, indulge and enjoy yourself. Why not? Life is short. If you do eat out a lot, you might want to double down on the vegetables, or even bring your own whole grain.

Plant-based proteins are also easy to find in many ethnic restaurants; there are great bean dishes in Indian, Mexican, Middle Eastern, and all Asian cuisines. At an Italian restaurant, you might find a lovely bean soup. Ditto the French places. If you're not a vegan MILF, choose a fish dish. Protein selection might be tricky at some of the more conventional American restaurants, but if you look hard enough, you'll find something to fill you up. . . . Believe it or not, Denny's has a veggie burger and even T.G.I. Friday's serves deep-fried green beans, nacho chips (no cheese, please), and guacamole, so no family power struggles need ensue.

Dessert: I've gotten used to skipping desserts in restaurants, unless it's a health food place or they're willing to whip up a fresh-fruit plate. Even if a fruit plate is not on the menu, ask for one; many restaurants are happy to accommodate with a lovely platter of fruit. Remember: You pay their bills.

My biggest rule of thumb for eating out is that I avoid white sugar, meat, and dairy. I find that all of those foods have a way of taking themselves home with me and haunting me for a couple of days. I don't like that. But beyond those three no-nos, I just enjoy myself.

Finally, go out and explore the world of restaurants, using the MILF diet guidelines as good friends. MILFs live fully.

MILF Beauty

> Many people think I am in my **twenties** and are surprised that I am twenty-plus years older than that. They are amazed at my skin, my hair, and my "shine." —Amy Rolnick, MILF

Whoever said "beauty is only skin deep" didn't hang out with enough MILFs. If he had, he would have known that, because the body's skin is a direct reflection of the health of your internal organs, beauty is decidedly *not* skin deep. Your skin is your report card.

We could all get away with murder in our twenties: staying out all night, dancing like fools, drinking with gusto, and finishing the night with a cheeseburger, we still woke up every morning looking dewy. But, let's face it, those days are over.

More mature ladies need a more mature, and comprehensive, beauty plan; one that not only makes us look our best, but supports our beauty on every level. Luckily for us, the MILF diet does just that.

By abstaining from meat, dairy, and sugar, you are enhancing not only your health, but also your appearance. Sugar causes wrinkles, while meat and dairy inhibit good circulation to the skin and introduce lots of toxins. Saying bye-bye to coffee is also a smart move, as it dehydrates. Processed foods are a big beauty no-no, since they contain zillions of chemical stabilizers and preservatives. Remember, if it's not good for your insides, it's not good for your outside.

And by eating whole grains, vegetables, sea vegetables, and plant-based proteins, you will have a glamorous poise, lose weight easily, and have gorgeous skin, hair, and nails. Even your eyes will become brighter and whiter—you'll see. Remember, whole natural foods are designed to support you as a part of the natural world, and nature is beautiful, no? Mother Nature wants you looking your best.

And this stuff works: Amy is not the only MILF who looks five, ten, or even twenty years younger than her actual years. And it's not just that time slows down. Eating well and following these tips can actually make it go backward. Whole foods, full of natural life force, actually help your cells to regenerate and rejuvenate. Stick with the MILF diet and you'll see what I mean.

In terms of products and makeup, I'm not going to furnish a list. Most MILFs don't go crazy with products, but when they do use a cream or a powder, they choose from the most natural ones possible. The fewer chemicals and perfumes, the better.

So here are my two big beauty tips for you:

1. Don't use soap on your face.

2. Do a body scrub every day.

Let's look at these:

1. Don't use soap on your face. I stopped using soap on my face in my early twenties, when I learned the magic of the body scrub. By doing it (see instructions below), I slough off dead skin cells, increase the circulation to all the new skin I uncover, and increase my overall chi flow.

The results are clear: in the last twenty years, I have been complimented on my skin hundreds of times. In fact, it's the compliment I get most, even from perfect strangers. No doubt, the MILF diet, which includes lots of whole grains, veggies, and sea vegetables, is the underlying cause of all this glow, but how I treat my face topically makes a huge difference, too.

We all know that soap dries the skin. So because I don't use soap—and my diet keeps me juicy and hydrated—I don't tend to need moisturizer. In fact, with the exception of a little powder when I go out, I never put anything on my skin. I also wear a hat when I'm out in the sun—as a redhead made of Scottish genes, that just makes sense.

But that's it. That's my beauty regimen, at least for my face.

I don't think I appreciated the power of my habits until I looked down at my hands one day and was greeted by the claws of a lizard—dry, cracked, and downright old-looking. I was bummed out! And guess what? While I haven't been putting soap on my face, I have most *definitely* been washing dishes with dish soap. Dunking my hands in soapy water thousands of times over the last twenty-odd years, without gloves. Stupid Jessica. And my lizard hands are proof. Soap kills!

2. Do a body scrub every day. The body scrub is a quick routine that will make your skin amazing. Because we are constantly changing, our skin is always being sloughed off. But if we don't actively help our skin to shed, it hangs around too long, making everything less than sexy. The body scrub will keep your skin constantly renewed and glowing. But that's not all: the body scrub will stimulate your circulation, energize your whole body, and help to break up fat under your skin. You'll quickly get addicted to it.

Here's how you do it:

Either before or after you shower, fill your bathroom sink with hot, hot water. Dunk a washcloth in it and let the cloth get completely wet. Take it out, wring it out, and bring it to your forehead. Scrub. Hard enough to make your forehead skin go pink. Continue with your cheeks, nose, chin . . . everything except your eyes and the delicate skin around them. Even do your ears and behind your ears. Scrub until the skin turns pink.

When the washcloth cools off, redunk it. Continue with your neck, chest, and armpits. Avoid your breasts, but go around and between them. Now down your arms all the way to your hands and fingers. Do every finger individually and carefully, redunking when the washcloth loses its heat. Your body will start to look reddish-pink, in patches. Reach around to do as much of your back as possible or get your DILF to do your back.

Continue with your belly, lower back, and groin area, avoiding direct scrubbing of your privates. Go down your legs, covering all 360 degrees, and finish with your feet and toes, being careful to get the bottoms of your feet. Scrub each toe individually.

Yowza!!!! You will feel so alive.

Note: Make sure you do the body scrub out of the shower. It's important that the part of your body getting scrubbed is experiencing a warmer temperature than the rest of your body. This will force your blood to be stimulated and circulate to that area. In the shower, your whole body temperature is raised at once and the area being scrubbed doesn't get stimulated as strongly.

A Word on Aging

Let's face it: our culture's view of aging is pretty crappy—especially for us women. We are encouraged to associate our golden years with disease, brittle bones, and the loss of our ability to function like regular human beings. Getting older brings prescriptions, operations, and the aches and pains we accrue like little badges of maturity. We believe that if we are genetically lucky, we can skirt the real bad stuff, but the cruel passage of time still spells misery of some sort. At least that's what we tell ourselves.

This horror movie version of aging makes perfect sense for a culture stuffing itself with foods that destroy our bodies: between meat, sugar, dairy, and processed foods, we feed an ever-growing garbage dump inside our bodies called "suffering." Of course, it can take years for accumulations to build, for symptoms to appear, so we rarely connect the dots between what's going into our mouths and what's showing up in our blood work. And most doctors are trained to rescue us (from ourselves!) with a pill. A pill that makes us need another pill. And then another one.

In the last fifty years or so, this model has become so ingrained in our collective psyche that it's hard to imagine aging as anything other than an awful, pathetic, and slippery slide into oblivion.

But your future will be different. And it begins, right now, with changing your beliefs about aging. So let's toss out North America's profit-driven Pathetic Decline Model and borrow a new one from the people of Okinawa, or the Seventh-day Adventists in Loma Linda, California, or the MILFs of Sardinia, Italy. All of these cultures are well documented as some of the longest-lived on the planet, and all of them eat less meat, less dairy, fewer refined carbohydrates, and practically no processed foods. Instead, they go crazy on grains, fresh vegetables, and other natural goodies. Hello, MILF diet!

And their diets seem to be working on their minds, as well. These healthy societies not only live longer than the rest of us, they have a different perspective on aging: elders are honored, respected, even venerated. Whereas our society considers thirty-five our "sell by" date, more traditional cultures understand that one can get stronger, more loving, and more spiritually powerful over time. In fact, Dan Buettner, author of *Blue Zones: Lessons for Living Longer from the People Who've Lived the Longest*, says that, between ages eighty and one hundred, we are meant to make "an evolutionary leap" as we continue to develop.*

That's *your* future, MILF. By eating the MILF diet, you will get healthier as you get older. Instead of adding to your suffering pile, you are tossing logs onto the fire of your vitality. And you're nourishing not only your body but your mind and soul as well—making yourself wiser, smarter, and MILFier with every day that passes.

It can be difficult to find models for this in our culture, but they do exist. Amy Rolnick, the forty-six-year-old MILF you see on page 351, took up competitive swimming after starting the MILF diet. MILFy Jane Stanchich—who cured herself of osteoarthritis using the MILF diet—reported in her early fifties, "My life gets better and better with every passing year." Sanae Suzuki, who used the MILF diet to fuel her recovery from ovarian cancer over eighteen years ago, claims, "My mental clarity, memory, and ability to focus are so much better than what I imagined they would be at this age."

Just think of these ladies next time you see a commercial for a prescription drug.

And in case you assume your MILFy enjoyment of sex will weaken over time, fear not. Dr. Martha Cottrell, an eighty-three-year-old MILF and physician who has been eating this way for more than thirty years, gives us a peek into her sex life: "There has been no waning of interest or enjoyment in this part of my life. I continue to be a curious and playful romantic fool!"

And this makes perfect sense. You see, nature has a perennial and potent oomph: the earth keeps spinning around the sun. Flowers keep blooming. Volcanoes keep blowing. And whole grains contain a strong and steady vitality that will move through you, no matter what age you are. It's that simple.

But does that mean you'll never die? Of course not. Every MILF will eventually take her final curtain call. But instead of a frenzied, scary, and anxiety-filled drama, a MILF's passage can be smoother, more relaxed, and more natural—for death, we must remind ourselves, is as natural as birth. And get this: the vitality of whole foods can *propel* a MILF's unfettered spirit into the great expanse of the vibrational world—The Big Yin. And in that sense, death is simply the closing of one spiral and the opening of the next. Instead of fearing this last great release, a MILF surrenders to it with a satisfied wink and a sigh.

Now, *that's* MILFy.

* http://health.usnews.com/health-news/family-health/articles/2008/03/25/from-4-long-lived-cultures-9-tips-for -longevity?PageNr=1.

5

· · · · · · · · · ·

MILF Sex

Health is sexy.
—Sarah Loring, Connecticut MILF

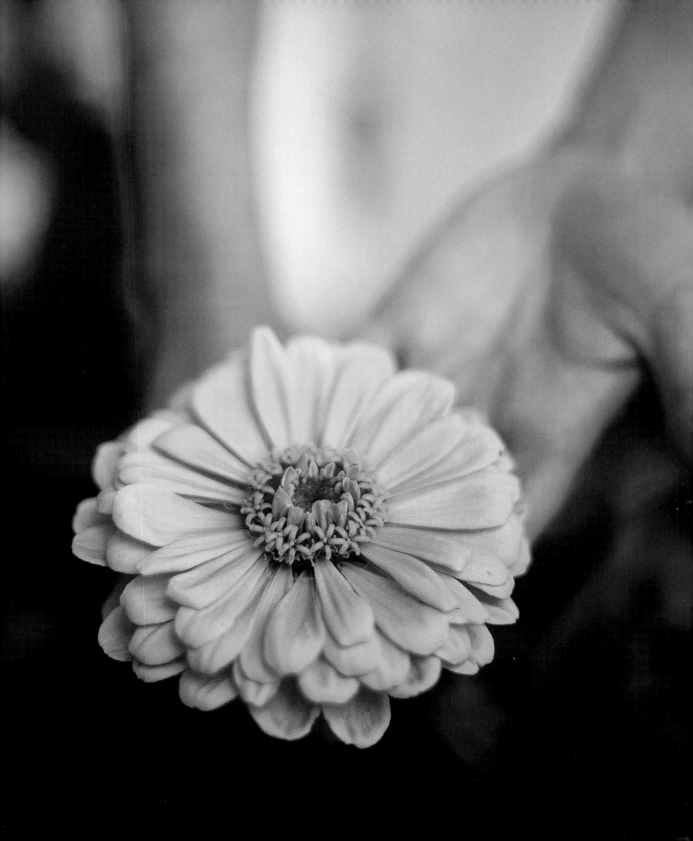

Let's not forget what the "F" in MILF stands for; a true MILF is sexy in a deep and powerful way. Because she eats whole and balanced foods, *she* is whole, and her chi runs through her unimpeded. She is fully present in her body. That natural yin energy—which men go crazy for—is her calling card. MILFiness is about more than image; it's a force.

There are lots of ways the MILF diet is going to improve your love life. First, you will lose weight. If those extra ten, twenty, or hundred pounds are making you feel less than sexy, don't worry, they're on their way out. By losing weight, you will become more sensitive and feel more attractive. You'll also get more attention.

But more than offering you thinness, the MILF diet will give you a sparkly vitality. Energy moves easily and efficiently through nature, and your body is a part of that. Where there have been energy blocks, there will be movement. Where there has been tension, you will be able to relax. This won't happen overnight—some blocks may be deep and even require some emotional work—but fear not: they will move and your chi will flow where it's supposed to. I think this is what's most attractive about the MILFs I know; they are fully alive and present in their bodies.

Finally, MILFs are sexy because they are more yin. MILFs also know the power of female energy and they enjoy the force field between a man and a woman. Because she is eating whole grains and vegetables, a MILF experiences sex from a more vibrational and spiritual plane. She loves the manliness of her DILF, while she enjoys her womanhood fully.

To review, men are governed by a downward, contracting, and focused force. Women are governed by an upward, expansive, and dispersing force. Because yin and yang are constantly seeking to connect, sex is about allowing these forces to come together.

Hopefully, when you and your DILF met—or on the day you realized you were attracted to him—you felt a magnetic pull toward his being. Some couples experience this as a thunderbolt, while for others it grows slowly out of communication and trust. Either way, there is a natural electricity between you that keeps you coming back to the same house every night.

This electricity may have dominated your relationship at first—keeping you in bed at all hours, making you do it in weird places at weird times, and generally making you gaga for each other. That's great. This electricity, especially in the first couple of years, causes you to secrete lots of happy and exciting chemicals.

But as time wears on, the electricity seems to fizzle a bit. You get used to it. You take it for granted. You sometimes have fights that seem to flip your attraction into its opposite— repulsion. In a mature relationship, nonsexual factors like love, trust, and a mutual bond keep you committed as much as the electricity once did.

But you can have both. The MILF diet is all about feeling that electricity again. Okay, maybe not the one you felt before you saw him clip his toenails over the rug; but the fundamental electricity that brings you together is still there and can be strengthened.

Exercise: Feel the Circuit

Stand about a foot from your DILF, face-to-face. Now put your hands out, left palm down and right palm up, and have him do the same. Let your palms hover over each other's—not touching. Just relax your body, and your gaze, and feel what you feel. There should be some kind of natural charge between you. Together you make a circuit of energy and you should be able to feel it—a little or a lot.

It may be most obvious at your hands, but relax a bit more and see if you can feel any sense of energy created between the two of you that registers in your body. Your chest may feel as if it expands or shuts off a little. Your pelvis may want to move forward or retreat. You may feel anxiety or you may feel blissfully relaxed. Your mind might slow down or speed up. These are all indicators of the energy between you—where it's flowing and where it's blocked. Don't judge whatever constriction you may feel; when you eat whole grains and vegetables, it will begin to flow more smoothly.

Step away from each other and just go back into yourself. Go back to what feels like your individual state of "normal." In a few minutes, do the exercise again. You'll begin to recognize that very real force between you.

One of the great benefits of sex is letting this circuit of energy move in its deepest, most primitive way. When this energy lets loose, it's very healing to your body and to your relationship. By entering into this circuit, the two of you become greater than the sum of your parts and balance each other's imbalances.

Let's imagine the energy that occurs between you during sex: it enters through the top of his head, courses down his midline, exits his penis, moves up your vagina, where it connects with your yin force, and travels all the way up your midline and out the top of your head. In this way, sex connects you not only to each other, but to the universe.

Intercourse is intensely powerful. If you are relaxed and open to it, all this rhythmic energy moves up your spine, literally pushing your chi to flow out of your heart toward your partner (as feelings of love and connectedness), stimulating your vocal cords (hard not to make noise when it's happening), and out the top of your head, where you naturally release this force back into the ether.[1] Because you are governed by yin, your role is to receive and transmute this strong energy.

As this happens, his excess energy gets released, and when he's done, he relaxes and his upper chakras can open. He becomes more available to the love between you and to a feeling of connectedness to the universe. He goes from yang to yin.

You, on the other hand, gain in energy—getting strongly charged at your base, like a battery—as all that yang energy moves through you. Feeling more positive, strong, and secure, you go from yin to yang. In this way, you both become more balanced—feeling satisfied and whole—until the polarity builds once more and you want to do it again!

A true MILF, eating grains and vegetables as her principal foods, knows how to work with these energies; she brings a soft, open receptivity to the bedroom that not only allows her DILF to feel powerful, but she receives his yang force, transmutes it, and releases it back into the universe. A MILF is a bedroom witch.

---

1. When the upward energy is strong, it moves through the brain, and it's quite impossible to hold a thought. I think this is what is meant by "f*#king her brains out."

Exercise: Be the Fountain

I remember that when I learned about female energy moving up and out, it seemed like a pretty woo-woo concept to me. I had only ever perceived my body as . . . well, a *body*. A dense collection of matter. I had never considered that there might be a powerful energetic template behind it.

But since my awesome hairdos and scintillating personality weren't winning me any gold medals in the dating Olympics, I decided to try imagining this fountain of energy flowing inside of me. Whenever I was in the presence of a man I found attractive, I would take a deep breath, relax, and simply imagine a fountain flowing up my midline, out the crown of my head, and connecting me with the beautiful and vast yin universe—my true home. As I continued to eat MILFy plant-based foods, I would actually *feel* my life force moving up, and instead of sending out energy tentacles to the attractive guy, I sent them up into the ether. Whereas in the past I would have tried to create a connection, I now imagined guiding both our energies back up to the universe.

And it worked. The fountain actually allowed me to release my ego, connect with my source, and create the yin space for a nice yang man to enter my energy field. And he did. The fountain become my secret weapon.

I thought I had made this stuff up until MILFy Meredith McCarty told me her story: A friend suggested that the next time she saw someone she was attracted to, she should do nothing, stand still, and pull her forces inward, letting him come to her. One day, during a yoga training with two hundred other participants, she saw an appealing guy all the way across the gym. When everyone was instructed to find a partner, she did her version of the fountain trick: "I stayed still, looked down, and in a couple of minutes, he came and stood next to me." She remained still, letting him do the yang work: "He asked me if I'd like to be his partner."

They remained together for the next nineteen years.

Of course, this upward force comes out of all your chakras, especially your big MILFy heart, but for the purposes of meeting a new and intriguing man, just pull it in and send it up the heavens until he's proved himself worthy of your love.

But in a world of extreme foods, this soft receptivity can get stomped on or be blown out of the water completely. Here are some common problems that arise from imbalanced eating.

When a man becomes too yin: These days, men are ingesting tons of yin foods and substances. Between alcohol, marijuana, prescription meds, ice cream, soda pop, iced and cold beverages, chocolate, and other sugary foods, the yang force of a man can get severely weakened.

Male sexuality depends on good-quality yang force. Blood needs to move down into the penis to create an erection. In order to maintain that erection, the veins on the underside of the penis need to clamp shut, trapping all the blood in the shaft. This also requires strong contracting force. When the man's diet is too yin and expanded, he doesn't have enough downward yang force to keep blood concentrated in his genitals. Plus, the clamps on the underside of the penis become weak and cannot shut completely, preventing the erection or causing it to wither.

This can lead to anxiety about the issue, which just makes the problem worse. Men who eat too much yin food may be really great to talk to, and be quite emotionally open, but the yang force necessary for a manly roll in the hay just isn't there.

When a man becomes too yang: Yes, men can become too yang. Just because that is their dominant mode doesn't mean the energy can't tip overboard. When a man eats tons of meat, lots of salt, and hardly any vegetables or fiber, he can have too much downward, constricting energy, which brings about a whole different set of problems:

First of all, the contracted nature of yang foods like meat can make his energy tight and too intense. Arteries that feed blood to the penis can become constricted, just like arteries to the heart or brain. This can produce a whole different kind of erectile dysfunction from blocked arteries.

If he *can* get it up, the pressure from all the excess yang force, including the extra testosterone he's getting from his diet, can cause premature ejaculation. All this animal food can also give a man an animalistic quality in the bedroom. This might be fun every once in a while, but his energy is concentrated so low in his body that he can't open to an emotional exchange. The saturated fat of meat can also give him a layer of insulation that reduces his sensitivity to his partner and the circuit of energy he is creating with her. Plus, all the contraction of the yang force can keep him arrogant and self-centered. It's as if he's trapped in a shell or behind a shield—cut off. Worst-case scenario: all this yang force can make him hard, obsessed, critical, habit-driven, or even violent. Extra-strong yang can also lead to sexual compulsivity or addiction because the downward force is so strong that his penis becomes his only portal of energy release.

When a woman becomes too yang: When she eats lots and lots of animal food, a woman becomes a bit of a man in the bedroom. And I don't mean she likes to be on top every once in a while. This cowgirl focuses downward as well, concentrating exclusively on her orgasm, and is not terribly open to the energetic circuit she's a part of. She is often dominant in the bedroom, having no inkling of what it means to relax, let go, and receive. She may also be critical of her partner and point out his flaws. Henpecking is the sign of a woman who's gotten too yang.

When a woman becomes too yin: Between high fructose corn syrup, sugar, ice cream, chocolate, iced and cold drinks, tropical fruit juices, alcohol, and drugs, becoming too yin is very easy these days. A woman who is too yin shows little interest in sex or just submits to it without relish. Her container is weak and she can't receive and enjoy the yang energy before it dissipates. She has a hard time getting hot blood to move down into her pelvis and sustaining arousal. Even though women are on the yin side of things, yang force is needed to experience an orgasm, and some women just can't gather enough good-quality yang to make that happen. For such a woman—unable to maintain a charge in her pelvis—all her energy is released from her upper chakras, spilling exclusively out of her heart, her mouth, and her mind. She cries a lot, worries, and talks excessively. She may have difficulty conceiving or carrying a pregnancy to term. It's not uncommon for a woman who is too yin to have severe self-consciousness about her body and to find it hard to relax while naked. She is self-centered, too, but in a yin way.

Of course, in reality, everyone's a bit of a mixed bag. Because both genders ingest all sorts of extreme yin and yang substances these days, a woman can be both dominant *and* secretly fragile, while a man can be both aggressive *and* passive. It's only when both parties start experiencing inner balance that their energy can flow easily between them in a healing and loving way.

Obsession with orgasms: This is a general problem in our super-yang culture. Ever since the female orgasm came out of the closet, mutual orgasms have become the standard of sexual equality and the definition of sexual satisfaction; everyone enters the bedroom with his and her skills and desires, and a mutual transaction is made: "You make me come and I'll make you come." Unless a woman climaxes every time she has sex, there's something askew.

But this is looking at sex through a male lens. To a man—whose sexuality is all about contracting down to a point—sex isn't *sex* without an orgasm. His spiral is contracting and yang. But to a MILF—whose spiral is expanding—orgasms are great, but they're just one color in a much bigger sexual rainbow.

The truth is, women are extremely variable; no two women are alike and each woman experiences a grand hormonal roller-coaster ride every month, giving her different sensitivities and desires on different days. We don't always *want* to have an orgasm—sometimes it's not even on the radar. But that doesn't mean we're not enjoying ourselves.

And I'll bet you didn't know that women experience a different type of satisfaction from "coming" than men do. A study conducted in the Netherlands showed that orgasms mean quite different things to men's and women's brains; in ours, an orgasm means that the anxiety and fear center (the amygdala) basically shuts off. We go into a lovely trance, freed from all worldly troubles. Although the physical sensation of the orgasm certainly registers in our brains—and feels good—it is the total release from stress that is our biggest payoff. (And, by the way, this reduction in stress occurs—to some extent—during all female sexual arousal, whether at the beginning of foreplay or during a climax. So we don't always need to "come" to get our goodies. Ask any woman if there are times of the month when she'd rather have a good foot rub than an orgasm.)

For your DILF, the fireworks occur in a different part of his brain and he reacts very strongly to the sensation of pleasure being generated by his penis. Although his fear center is subdued as well, it happens less than it does in the brain of the female, and his focus remains squarely on the sensation of the act.[2]

But we MILFs are sensitive all over, so the nibbling of an earlobe or gentle kisses on the shoulders can send electrical storms through our nervous systems, while releasing the stresses of an entire week. We are sensitive and tactile, and our chi likes to move outward, opening our hearts as much as our vaginas.

Even now, studies about sexual "dysfunction" often point to a woman's consistent ability to orgasm as the single benchmark of healthy sexuality. . . . Argh. As if women don't experience any pleasure unless they climax . . . as if our bodies are flawed . . . as if women don't play a holy, healing role in the spiral created between two lovers! It's a limited, myopic, yang view of sex that holds us up to a male model and finds us wanting.

And just as our hormones climb up and down little mountains throughout our cycles, and throughout pregnancy, any MILF can tell you that there are hormonal hills and valleys over the course of one's lifetime. We may be randy little Ritas from twenty-five to thirty-five, but as our testosterone levels fall after our mid-thirties, so does the male side of our libido.

---

2. http://www.timesonline.co.uk/tol/life_and_style/health/article535521.ece.

You see, you have a yin and a yang side of your sexuality. Your yang side is like a man's; it wants to get all contracted and is focused on "coming." And that's great. Enjoy it. But to become obsessed with having an orgasm every time you have sex will blind you to the yin side of your sexuality, which is about receptivity, sensitivity, connection, channeling energy, and transmuting yang force. Your yin side is very powerful. You are uniquely able to channel your DILF's contracting energy up into the heavens or to capture it to start a new life. That's pretty cool.

Maybe because men have a whopping *ten to one hundred times* more testosterone than we do, they can't even imagine sex without an orgasm. To the goal-oriented male mind, orgasm-less sex spells failure. And, of course, the more they project their orgasmic agenda onto us, the more pressure we feel, which, as every MILF knows, can put the kibosh on "coming." Ironic, no?

Let your DILF worry about "coming." You are governed by a relaxing, releasing force. You receive and liberate energy, sending it back to your partner and up to the heavens; this is your womanly power. One of the great pleasures of sex is to receive all that energy, let it pass through you, and surrender it to the ether. And surrender can feel delicious.

Forget "coming." You're *leaving.*

Getting all focused on an orgasm when the universe is pushing you to melt into transcendence just doesn't work. It's like inhaling and exhaling at the same time. If you're meant to climax, you will want to help make it happen. But if you don't, let yourself off the orgasmic hook and enjoy the powerful energy moving through you, the love being exchanged with your partner, and the vibrant electricity of the spiral you create together.

And remember, we will never be able to adequately explain to men what intercourse feels like for us. Even funky toys inserted into funky places can't replicate the experience of vaginal penetration. So in the bedroom, you are experiencing something he has never felt and never will. You are on a private, secret mission given to you by the infinite universe. Enjoy.

Warning: It's not unusual when people begin the MILF diet to feel their libidos wane for a bit.

You see, MILFy foods are designed to make your body stronger and healthier on every level, and they start their work by strengthening your blood. And then your blood gets to work on your vital organs: your kidneys, liver, spleen, etc. It is only after your basic survival functions are strengthened that your blood rebuilds your reproductive organs. Because, let's face it: reproductive organs are luxury items on the car; unlike your heart, liver, and bladder, you could survive without them. So they are last on the list of nature's healing schedule.

When I started the MILF diet, I lost my menstrual period for quite a while, and it's not uncommon to experience diet-induced amenorrhea for a few months. If it lasts more than six months, you may want to get checked by a doctor to make sure everything is okay, but if you feel fine in every other way and show no other symptoms, please don't panic. Your body is doing some deep healing and your reproductive organs are taking a rest. If you're eating quite strictly, open up a bit, going easy with salt (shoyu and miso) and making sure to get natural sweeteners, fruit, and good-quality yin foods. Instead of taking any hormones or supplements, I started making my diet more yin, and my period came back when I fell in love with a new man.

Your DILF may also lose his mojo for a bit, but it will come back. If he's changed his diet quickly and is eating very cleanly or rigidly, his body is also healing, and he simply doesn't have the excess energy to put toward sexuality. He will, and when he does, it will be lovely, good-quality yang. Have fun.

Finally, by embracing the MILF diet, the connection between you and your DILF will be supported on all levels. You'll find that you communicate better, feel more at peace together, and enjoy that lovely polarity in the bedroom.

Sex and Your Dinner Plate

Although the majority of the MILF diet is the same for both partners, MILFs and DILFs can each indulge a little on their respective ends of the energy spectrum. DILFs can eat a little more yang food than women do (more grain, denser protein dishes, slightly more salty seasoning and condiments, more long-cooked dishes), while MILFs should hang out on the yin side of town (more vegetables, less seasoning, lighter cooking styles, more sweet and soft food). This doesn't mean DILFs shouldn't eat any greens, or salads, or desserts—or that MILFs should skip the yang foods. It's just that each gender should emphasize its own end of the spectrum. In fact, it's very good for MILFs and DILFs to eat slightly differently in order to feed the spark between them and to keep their spiral strong.

You don't need to go crazy with this difference; in fact, many couples simply choose their foods like this intuitively, but if you're aiming to consciously increase your bedroom magnetism, follow the rules of yin and yang.

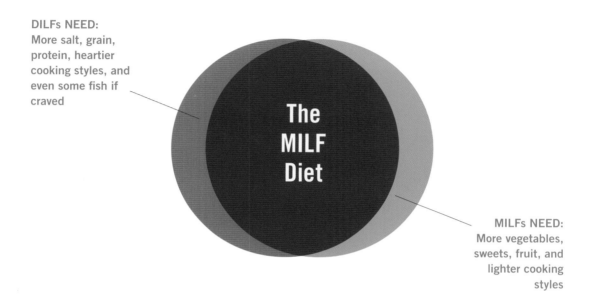

DILFs NEED:
More salt, grain, protein, heartier cooking styles, and even some fish if craved

The MILF Diet

MILFs NEED:
More vegetables, sweets, fruit, and lighter cooking styles

6

Ch-ch-
ch-ch-ch-
changes

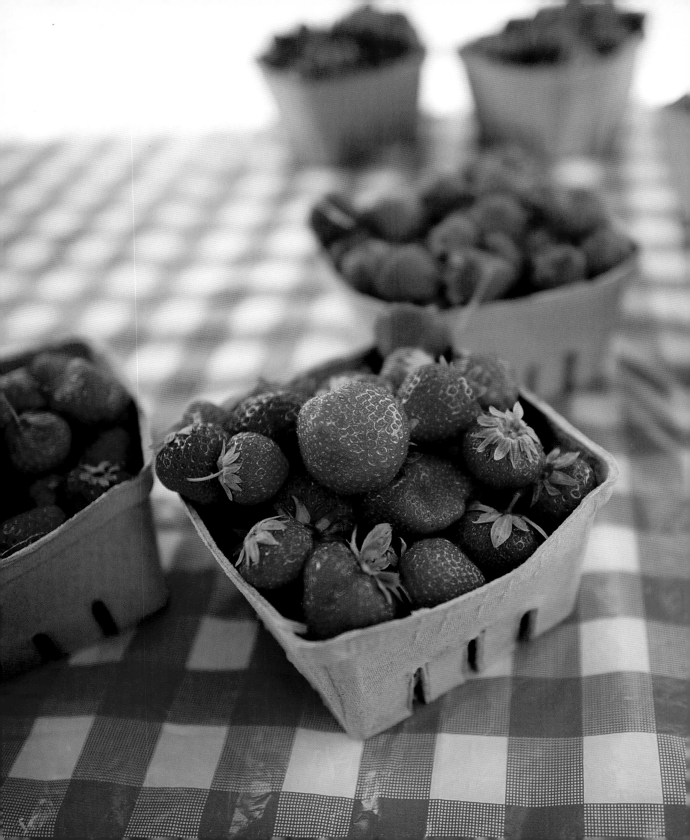

The MILF diet will change you from the inside out. I promise. Some of the changes will be obvious and physical, while others will take place on more subtle planes of perception. Get ready for the following shifts.

Detox: No matter the rate at which you introduce the MILFy foods, they will cause your body to detox. Remember, these are nature's foods; they have actual *power,* and their sole agenda is to make you stronger. In order to do this, they have to chuck out all the gunk sitting around in your body.

The faster you adopt the MILFy foods, the stronger your detox experience will be. And by "stronger," I *kinda* mean "more uncomfortable." It is not unusual for people who give up meat, dairy, white sugar, caffeine, and processed foods—and replace them with powerful MILFy foods—to experience some lovely cocktail of the following: headaches, nausea, depression, fatigue, diarrhea, constipation, weird body odors, phlegm, aches and pains, strange dreams, irritability, and any number of other funky things. If you let go of everything at once and dive into the MILF diet full-force, you will feel big changes quickly.[1]

Remember, your body is cleaning itself out at Mother Nature's bidding, and as a bad food exits, it likes to say, "Hi there, remember *me?*" As your chi gets stronger, your body may also rewire its inner systems in mysterious ways. For example, about a year after I started the MILF diet, I had odd shooting pains down my shins. They lasted for about a week. I had no idea what they were from—I hadn't run the marathon the week before or even walked too strenuously. And then they left—as mysteriously as they came—never to return. Another time, I had strange issues with coordination and physical balance that lasted a couple of weeks. Again, they passed and never came back. Rashes, twitches, flashbacks . . . you name it. The body has many ways of clearing its decks.

---

1. For more information on what you may experience letting go of one food at a time, go to the chapter on individual foods starting on page 254. At the end of each segment, there are tips on letting go of each food.

The thing to remember is that these things pass. And, in their stead, you will discover amazing new goodies like balance, peace, sensitivity, renewed flexibility, energy, joy, and an inner drive to feel even better. If any symptom of discharge persists—without cease—for more than ten days, go see your care provider to make sure everything is okay. And when you find out you're fine, I encourage you to continue to eat well and just let the discharge continue. Rest, relaxation, patience, and continual healthy eating will see you through to the other side.

For some people, the MILF diet is modified to help them recover from serious—even life-threatening—illnesses. By consulting with a macrobiotic counselor (see Resources on my website), many people have received dietary recommendations that have fueled their healing.

Clarity: Now, change is good, but it can also be a little scary. Eating whole, natural foods brings—among other things—clarity, and clarity can be intense.

Your senses will become clearer: Don't be surprised when you start to see, smell, taste, and feel things with more clarity. Meat, dairy, sugar, and other extreme foods have kept you in a bit of a fog, and whole foods will bring back your God-given sensitivity. Many MILFs found that nature erupted into Technicolor as their senses came alive.

Suddenly your feelings will be clear: Whereas that candy bar made you feel spacey and vague, whole grains are making you crystal clear about how you *actually* feel. Sometimes you feel sad, sometimes you feel angry, sometimes you feel ridiculously happy, but the only thing you truly know is that these feelings are becoming really, really *clear*.

That's okay. Share them with your DILF or a warm MILFy friend. Or a therapist. Feelings are natural and they are meant to carve you deeply—and beautifully—earning you the gift of compassion for others. And when they're hard, remember that feelings always pass, especially when you're eating clean food.

Eating nature's food will also make you clear about what you want. If you've been repressing your true desires, whole grains and vegetables will help you to express them. Maybe you want a new job. Maybe you want a regular date night with your DILF. Hell, maybe you want a divorce. Don't panic. You don't have to take action on every desire. There is always time for communication, counsel, and divine guidance. Let your thoughts, feelings, and desires ferment a little, trusting the alchemical magic of nature. If the desire is meant to be fulfilled, it will get stronger over time and you will act on it. The food will push you to do it. If it's just an emotional hissy fit, it should pass.

You'll get clarity on your limits: eating well will make you clear about what you're capable of. Because whole grains will help you to find your inner balance, you'll meet your healthy limits. Maybe you *can't* do everything for your daughter's bake sale this Saturday. Maybe you *don't* actually enjoy listening to your cousin complain 24/7. Maybe you just need to sit in peace for ten minutes and gather yourself.

It's okay to say no and to nourish yourself. In fact, it is only by being nourished that you can remain the fertile, flowing fountain at the center of your family. Nourishment includes good food, warm hearts, being heard, and being respected. It can also mean a leisurely read of the Sunday paper or a lively debate over dinner. Being nourished also means getting rest, spiritual support, and having some fun. Don't be a martyr. Get nourishment.

Creativity: The universe is always creating things—that's its shtick—so as you eat food with strong chi, you may find yourself blooming in many directions. It's not unusual for MILFs to be veritable Renaissance women. Melanie Brown Waxman, MILF from Philadelphia and mother of seven, is a great example: "My creativity opened up when I changed my diet. . . . There was one occasion where I was cooking dinner, painting a piece of furniture, and writing a book all at the same time. A friend stopped by and saw me by the stove with the paintbrush still in hand and said, 'That is a novel way to cook!'"

Intuition: That little voice inside will get stronger, so listen to it: "Hug that child." "Take that class." "Topple that government." The book you hold in your hands is a product of continual gut-level promptings from the universe. Clarity makes room for divine guidance and instruction, so start to listen. You have a mission. And if you're afraid of what it's saying and you have to eat a candy bar to shut it up, don't worry. The universe is patient. It'll come back when you're ready.

Ego deflation: As you continue to eat whole grains and vegetables as your primary food, you'll notice something funky happening: the old "you" will begin to disappear.

Mood swings will dissipate. Strong opinions won't seem so important anymore. As natural foods nourish your spirit and your true self, layers of personality will soften and actually begin to dissolve. Self-centeredness naturally lessens.

We live in a world that's all "HeyLookAtME!!," so detaching from your ego can feel a little scary. But you'll soon find that it's a relief to just relax and let your big old personality rest. Or even space out. By letting go of the chattering self, you can tune in to deeper and more powerful parts of yourself. You are much more than a personality.

Spiritual growth: The parts of you that remain will long to connect with the universe. Or God. Or whatever you choose to call it. This is natural, for you are a part of it. Feed this hunger with spiritual literature, or a religious community, or meditation. Your soul has its own needs and its own path, so listen to its promptings. When you feel a tug on your spirit to connect with something bigger than yourself, surrender.

Whole foods will bring you to a quiet, centered peace inside, and many MILFs find that practicing meditation or yoga—or some other spiritual pursuit—helps them to come back to their peaceful center and bring that peaceful energy more easily to the world.

MILFy Mind

Meditation is one of the most practical things we can do—up there with online banking and a cardio workout.

You are an ever-changing and ever-growing energy *event*, so just as you scrub off daily layers of skin, it's important to have a practice that allows layers of desires, attachments, and identity to be sloughed off. Meditation creates the quiet space inside you from which this mental and emotional buildup can be released.

Don't worry. There's a "you" behind all that stuff. In fact, you have a warm, blue Caribbean Sea of MILFiness inside you. It's about time you found it.

Here's how to meditate: Set a timer for ten minutes. Sit in a comfortable position with your spine erect. No need to cross your legs in crazy ways, and it's fine to sit in a chair, or on a couch. Close your eyes and bring your awareness to the sensation of your breath going into and out of your nose. It's a very subtle sensation . . .

That's it. Every time your mind wanders, just bring it back to the feeling of your breath going into and out of your nostrils. Not the *idea* of your breath, but the feeling of it.

And when your mind rebels, and begins to wander (and it will . . . even the Dalai Lama's mind wanders), just bring it back to the sensation of the breath. And bring it back again. And again.

FYI: Your mind will never stop wandering completely. There is no place where meditators flatline into a totally thought-free state. The best meditators in the world still have thoughts passing through their noggins. The difference is that, as they continue to practice meditation, they are less attached to those thoughts. Thoughts float by like clouds instead of grabbing the monk by the throat. A practiced meditator can relax within the swirling spiral of the mind and watch it slowly settle down, but thinking never goes away completely. You need to know that. The gaps between thoughts get longer—and fill with a delicious, expansive peace—but thinking never dies completely. Lots of people I know think they can't meditate because they carry the misconception that their minds should disappear. Not so.

Meditation will bring forth your yin power: By continuing to focus on sensation instead of thought, you are detaching from the active, goal-driven (yang) conscious mind and sinking into the more powerful (and more yin) subconscious mind. After you meditate for twenty minutes or so, your body will flip from its sympathetic nervous system mode into its parasympathetic one. Yang to yin.

As you continue meditating, you will feel more connected to your body and more present for the adventure of your life. Instead of spinning around in your mental dramas, you will be tuned in to the deep promptings of your soul. And your personal power will grow; when you tune in to yourself on this deeper level, your ability to affect your worlds grows, too. I mean, hey, what's the point of eating all this good food and having a MILFy body if you don't enjoy your experience fully?

When you've done ten minutes for two weeks, go to fifteen, and then twenty. I try to meditate for twenty-five to thirty minutes a day. Most days, my mind slows down, my body relaxes, and my soul expands. And my day rolls out like sweet rice syrup. Once in a while, my mind just won't stop churning, and all the meditation has done is stopped me from throttling someone. But that's good. It's still illegal to throttle people.

P.S.: I realize that for some of you with young kids, even ten minutes of quiet "alone time" is a ridiculous fantasy. If that's the case, just become mindful of your breath in the moments that are available to you: while nursing, waiting in the car for kids to emerge from school, pushing a swing at the playground. Instead of letting your mind churn, bring it back to the breath and train it—like a puppy—to settle.

Love: As your body gets stronger, your spirit will get stronger. You will automatically bring this positive force to your family, to your friends. This spirit—when channeled through the heart and not the ego—is unconditional love. Directing it can bring about profound healing in your life and the lives of others. Remember, we women—governed by expanding yin force—are really good at channeling love, and by doing so, we are liberated. MILFy Meredith McCarty used her soul's energy to heal conflicts in her life:

"Every morning for a month, I pictured people in my mind's eye with whom I had unfinished, unpleasant personal issues. I pictured them, one at a time, and said aloud:

"'I am very sorry for any hurt I may have caused.

'Please forgive me. I forgive you.

'Please be happy. I will be happy.'

"At first I was so angry, I couldn't possibly forgive, but as I said the words every morning, I started crying, softening, and the anger dissipated. After a month, I was a freer person, having let go of the negative attachments and reclaimed my calmer, more positive self."

I hope you can see that the MILF diet is much more than a way of eating; it is a way of strengthening your entire being, on every level. Just as the universe supports the earth, the trees, the oceans, and all the animals, it aches to support you. It's time to open yourself and let it in.

7

· · · · · · · · · ·

Recipes

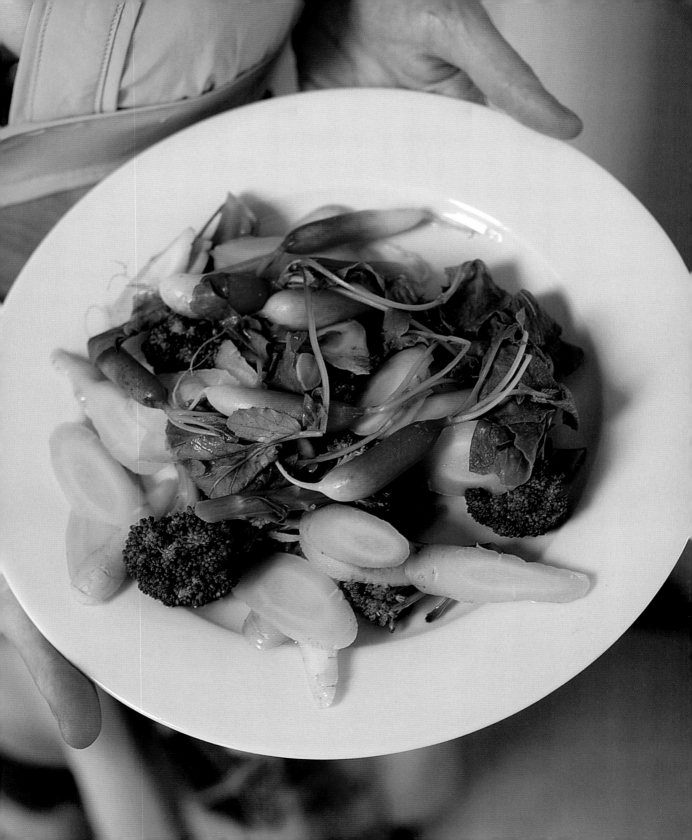

Whole Grains

Rice: There are literally hundreds of varieties of whole-grain rice. Although they are mostly referred to as brown rice, whole-grain varieties include the red Wehani and Black Japonica. There's also brown basmati, which is nice and aromatic; sweet brown rice, which is higher in fat and slightly sticky; and let's not forget wild rice, which is actually a grass, but who cares?

Brown rice—as you'll see it in the store—generally comes in three types: short-grain, medium-grain, and long-grain. Short-grain is more compact and yang, so it's best for fall and winter and when you need a boost of strong energy. Long-grain is more yin and expanded, so it's great for spring and summer and when you want to relax. Medium is in between, so it's good here and there.

Brown rice is very good for the lungs and large intestine because it helps to eliminate toxins from the body. Gluten free, rice is also naturally sweet-tasting when it's well chewed, so people tend to like it. It's easy to get the family to try and generally makes everyone feel peaceful and satisfied. However, too much brown rice—day in and day out for months—can make you too contracted and inhibit your natural yin energy from flowing out. Make sure you get lots of variety in your grains so rice's natural contraction doesn't take over.

Barley: Barley has, over many years, become my favorite grain. It is light and expansive, and I love the clear, buoyant energy it gives me. It, however, is a slightly harder sell for the family because it's a little chewy and even has a subtle sour flavor compared with that of rice. However, rice's contracting nature and barley's expansive nature make them a great combo when cooked together, and Universally Loved Barley Salad, on page 114, will make a barley fan out of any scoffer. Barley's upward energy is more yin, making it cooling and a tonic to the liver and gallbladder. Barley is also great for your skin, keeping it clear and glowing. Eat barley often.

What About Gluten?

If you think you are gluten-intolerant (but don't have full-blown celiac disease), I would encourage you to try gluten-containing grains in their organic whole form, to see if you still find you react to them. Often what appears to be gluten intolerance is really intolerance to refined flour products. You might find the whole grains themselves go down just fine. If not, there are plenty of gluten-free grains to enjoy.

Millet: These tiny yellow pellets are not just for the birds. Millet has a long history in both China and Africa and is the only grain that is naturally alkalizing. Although millet's flavor might seem a little bland at first, it dresses up very nicely, and you'll find millet croquettes, millet mashed "potatoes," and even a "cheese" cake made from millet in the recipes. Millet has a natural settling, centering energy and is a tonic to the stomach, spleen, and pancreas. It is also gluten free.

Quinoa: This wonderful grain, native to the Andes Mountains of South America, is light, delicate, and a total nutritional powerhouse. A complete protein, it is also gluten free and considered a veritable superfood because it is high in iron and calcium and is a good source of manganese, magnesium, and copper. Quinoa has a very distinct nutty flavor, especially when roasted before it's boiled. It's delicious cooled and tossed with vegetables for a salad, cooked into a soup, or combined with other grains. Let quinoa sneak into your life.

Wheat, spelt (farro), and kamut: I'm putting these together because they are cousins and have similar qualities. We are all familiar with wheat, but generally only when it is ground into flour. But have you ever tried a whole wheat berry? Wheat berries are chewy and delicious, especially cooked with rice or barley. Spelt berries are slightly larger than wheat berries, and kamut is the longest of all. They all contain gluten, have light, upward energy, and are good for the liver and gallbladder.

Rye: *Mmmm* . . . I have a little thing for rye. Maybe it's because my people are Scottish, but I just love the slightly sweet, chewy taste of whole rye berries, especially pressure-cooked with rice. Rye is darker in color than wheat, spelt, and kamut, but is also great for the liver and gallbladder. And, yes, it's got gluten.

Buckwheat: Not related to wheat at all, buckwheat, or "kasha," is actually neither a grain nor a grass, but it's commonly thrown in with both because of how it's used. Native to eastern Europe and Russia, buckwheat is very yang and actually delivers real heat to the body. If you live through long winters, cook buckwheat every ten days or so when it's cold outside. For those who live in warmer climes, a light buckwheat salad is fine every once in a while, but for regular use, it's too warming. Buckwheat is gluten free and a tonic to the kidneys, bladder, and reproductive organs.

Oats: We're all familiar with oats, but usually the rolled or steel-cut variety. Those are fine here and there, but it's the whole oats that make horses run so fast. When cooked well, oats produce a wonderful sweet cream that can bring a smile to any face on a cool morning. They are also great cooked with rice. Oats are also good for the liver and gallbladder. Whether oats contain gluten is a little hard to say; they do contain *one* of the compounds that tend to aggravate gluten intolerance, but they lack all the others. Not everyone reacts badly to oats. However, oats are often processed in plants where wheat and other gluten-bearing grains are processed, and that can be a problem. You may have to find out for yourself if oats work for you.

Corn: The corn we eat on the cob is more a starchy vegetable than a grain, but in Mexico and Central and South America, flint corn or dent corn is used. It is the big, hard kernels of dent corn that are known as posole in soup, and that are ground down into grits, polenta, and corn flour for tortillas. Corn is an amazing grain that has a naturally warm energy that radiates to the periphery. It's like eating the sun. Corn is a gluten-free tonic to the heart and small intestine and is perfect for the summer.

Grain Cooking Chart

GRAIN	PREPARATION	BOILING (H_2O:GRAIN)	PRESSURE-COOKING
Rice	Soak	50 min. (2:1)	50 min. (1.5:1)
Barley	Soak	45 min. (2:1)	45 min. (2:1, drain if necessary)
Millet	Rinse and dry-roast	25 min. (3:1)	20 min. (3:1)
Quinoa	Rinse and dry-roast	25 min. (2:1)	Not recommended
Spelt	Soak	50 min. (2:1)	50 min. (2:1, drain if necessary)
Kamut	Soak	50 min. (2:1)	50 min. (2:1, drain if necessary)
Rye	Soak	50 min. (2:1)	50 min. (2:1, drain if necessary)
Wheat berries	Soak	50 min. (2:1)	50 min. (2:1, drain if necessary)
Buckwheat	Do not soak	15–20 min. (2:1)	Not recommended

Mix 'n' match: One way to increase your variety and just generally shake up the energy of your cooking is to cook grains together. You can do a 50/50 mix or add other grains to rice in a 1:3 ratio. *Mmmm* . . . rice with rye . . . rice goes well with everything.

Because spelt, barley, wheat, and rye all cook at about the same rate as rice, they are easy matches, but millet, quinoa, and buckwheat cook faster. In that case, cook for the amount of time the rice needs, not the secondary grain. In other words, go the full fifty minutes even though the second grain is cooked faster.

Pressure-cooking: You'll notice that the pressure-cooking times on the chart above are roughly equivalent to the boiling times, which may seem odd if you've bought your pressure cooker as a time-saver. The MILF diet uses pressure cookers not because they are faster (although they can be), but because they give more yang energy to the grain, contracting it so much that it sort of explodes from the inside out. During autumn and winter, or when you simply need some strong oomph from the inside out, reach for the pressure cooker.

Salting grains: In general, you should use one pinch of sea salt per cup of dry grain. The salt helps the grain to cook better. However, when I say "pinch," I don't mean some Emeril Lagasse "essence" sprinkled into the pot. A pinch is the amount of salt caught between the pads of your dry thumb and index finger. It's not much. Remember, salt is powerful and you don't need a crazy amount.

Soaking grains: There are two reasons to soak grains: First, rice contains a compound called phytic acid that can inhibit the absorption of certain nutrients, so it's best to soak your rice, and discard the soaking water, for that reason. Second, grains like whole barley, wheat berries, spelt, rye, oats, and kamut should be soaked because it softens the grains, making them easier to cook and more digestible. When soaking these grains, you do not need to discard the soaking water and can cook with it.

Before soaking, sort through grains to find and discard hulls and other debris. Rinse the grain twice, draining carefully each time. Add the soaking water and let the grain sit, uncovered, or covered with a sushi mat, for three to twelve hours. If you live in a hot climate, refrigerate soaked grains after a few hours if you're not going to use them immediately. Before cooking, pour off the soaking water or, if using, measure it for use in cooking the grain.

Dry-roasting grains: Millet and quinoa are extra delicious when they are roasted before boiling (ditto buckwheat, but you can buy it pre-roasted). Just rinse them well—especially quinoa, which contains a protective coating that can taste soapy—drain quickly, and toss in a heated saucepan. Stir continuously as the grains dry and then begin to become slightly golden and aromatic. This can take a few minutes. When they are nice and roasted (but not dark), add measured water to the saucepan. If you're roasting in a skillet, pour the grains into a pot of boiling salted water. Reduce the heat immediately and simmer for the required time listed on page 105.

Basic Brown Rice

Serves 6

---

2 cups short- or medium-grain brown rice, soaked for 3 to 12 hours and drained
4 cups spring water
2 pinches sea salt

Place the rice and water in a heavy pot that has a tight-fitting lid and bring to a boil, uncovered, over medium heat. When it is boiling, add the salt, reduce the heat to low, place on a flame deflector,* cover, and simmer for 50 minutes. Turn off the heat and let the rice sit for 5 minutes to unstick from the bottom of the pot. Fluff with a wooden spoon and serve.

*If you are cooking on a gas stove, and if you have a flame deflector. They are also called simmer rings and are available at Amazon.com.

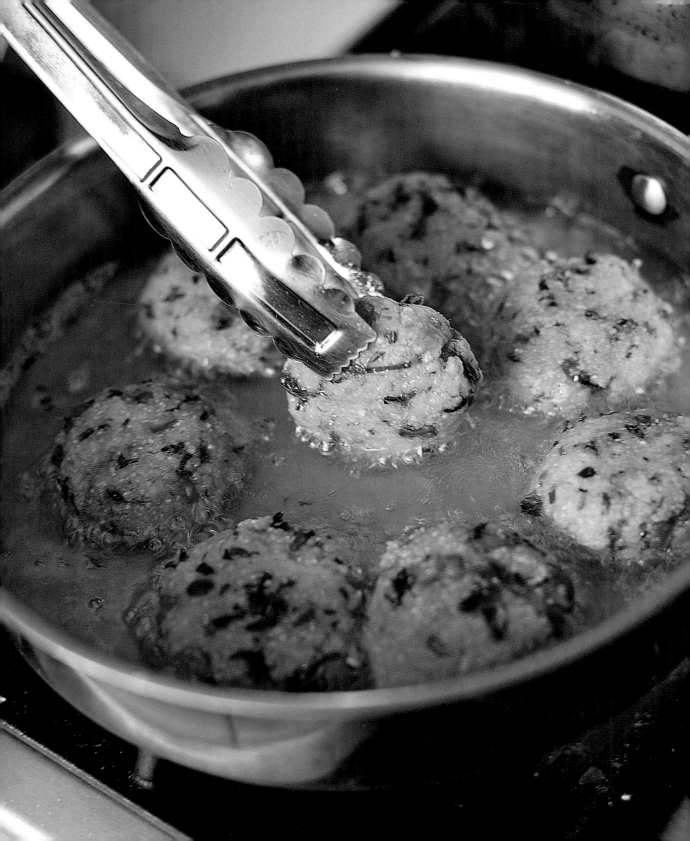

Millet Croquettes

Serves 3 or 4

These little burgers are a bit labor intensive, but worth it. They are warming and satisfying, and the sauces make them a treat. Thanks to Howard Wallen for his help with these.

1 cup millet
3 cups spring water
½ teaspoon sea salt
2 teaspoons olive oil
1 bunch scallions (about 7), finely chopped
½ cup diced carrot
2 teaspoons shoyu

½ cup chopped fresh parsley
½ cup cornmeal, plus extra for coating
Safflower oil, for frying

SAUCES
Sun-Dried Tomato Ketchup (recipe follows)
Apricot-Mustard Sauce (recipe follows)

1. Rinse the millet well and dry-roast in a medium saucepan over medium heat, stirring constantly to avoid burning. The millet is done when it is slightly golden in color and gives off a nutty fragrance.

2. In another saucepan, bring the water and sea salt to a boil. Add to the roasted millet in the hot pan, reduce the heat to low, cover, and simmer for 20 minutes.

3. Meanwhile, in a skillet, heat the olive oil and sauté the scallions for a minute or so. Add the carrot and shoyu and sauté until slightly tender. Remove from the heat and set aside.

4. Make one of the sauces and set aside.

5. When the millet is done, lay the sautéed scallions and carrot on top of the millet, cover, and simmer for 5 more minutes.

6. Remove from the heat and mix in the parsley and cornmeal. Let the mixture sit for 10 to 15 minutes, until it's cool enough to handle with your hands.

7. Form small croquettes, palm-sized balls. Dredge with the extra cornmeal.

8. Heat about half an inch of safflower oil in a skillet over medium heat, making sure it doesn't smoke. Test the oil by dropping in a tiny bit of the millet mixture; if it bubbles and quickly floats to the top, the oil is ready. Carefully place the croquettes in the oil and fry for 3 to 4 minutes on each side. Remove from the oil with tongs and drain on a paper bag.

9. Serve hot with one or both of the following sauces.

Sun-dried Tomato Ketchup

One 8.5-ounce jar sun-dried tomatoes
  in olive oil
1 clove garlic, minced
1 to 1½ cups diced fresh tomatoes

½ cup brown rice syrup
2 tablespoons shoyu
½ cup apple cider vinegar

Blend all the ingredients (including the oil from the sun-dried tomatoes) in a blender. Adjust seasonings to taste. The sauce should be quite tangy—the perfect complement to the millet croquettes. This recipe makes more than you may need (about 3 cups), but it goes really well with lots of things and can even serve as the family ketchup for a week or so.

Apricot-Mustard Sauce

1 cup fruit-sweetened apricot jam
½ cup spring water
1½ tablespoons organic Dijon mustard
1 teaspoon shoyu

Juice of 2 limes
1 knob of ginger, grated and squeezed to
  make 2 teaspoons ginger juice

Whisk all the ingredients in a bowl and serve either on the croquettes or on the side as a dipping sauce.

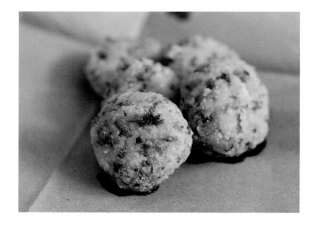

Fried Rice

Serves 6

Fried rice is an excellent way to get the family to eat brown rice. By adding lots of oil, vegetables, and shoyu and—when you're still transitioning—a little meat, you can make it incredibly delicious and satisfying. And remember, it's hard to go wrong with fried rice. Just sauté the heartiest vegetables first, then add the rice, the lighter vegetables, seasoning, and a sprinkling of water to make it steam for a few minutes. Voilà! Mix and serve. The following is a more yin preparation, suitable for spring, and summer and for MILFifying. In the "For DILFs" section, you'll see a fried rice recipe on page 236 that's better for autumn and winter and for when your man wants to DILFify.

---

1 red bell pepper
1 to 2 tablespoons extra virgin olive oil
1 medium onion, diced
Sea salt
Dash of umeboshi vinegar
12 cremini mushrooms, sliced

4 cups cooked basmati rice
$\frac{1}{3}$ cup spring water
Kernels from 2 ears fresh corn,
  or 1 cup frozen corn
1 tablespoon shoyu
Chopped scallions, for garnish

---

1. Roast the red pepper over a medium flame, turning it often to blacken all over. Place it in a paper bag for 10 minutes to let sweat. Remove from the bag and peel off the skin. Cut into slices and then dice.

2. Heat the oil over medium heat in a skillet. Add the onion and a pinch of salt, and sauté until translucent. Add the roasted red pepper and the umeboshi vinegar to preserve the pepper's red color. Add the mushrooms and another pinch of salt and sauté until the mushrooms become soft.

3. Place the rice on top of the vegetables, sprinkle with the water, and place the corn on top of the rice. Sprinkle with the shoyu, cover, and cook over low heat for 5 minutes.

4. Garnish with scallions and serve.

Spelt Salad

Serves 4 to 6

This is a colorful and satisfying grain salad brought to us by MILFy Sarah Loring of Connecticut. Her food has a certain graceful quality. This is wonderful and refreshing served on fresh lettuce leaves and goes with just about everything.

1½ cups spelt, soaked and drained
4 cups spring water
Sea salt
1 small red onion, diced
1 small green bell pepper, diced
1 carrot, finely diced

¼ head red cabbage, diced
¼ cup chopped fresh Italian parsley
1 tablespoon shoyu
1 tablespoon apple cider vinegar
1 tablespoon olive oil
Pinch of freshly ground white pepper

1. Place the spelt in a saucepan with the water and a pinch of sea salt. Bring to a boil, reduce the heat to low, cover, and cook for 1 hour. Pour into a colander, draining any remaining liquid, and set aside to cool.

2. Put the diced vegetables in a large bowl. Add the parsley, shoyu, vinegar, olive oil, and white pepper, and mix. Toss with the cooled spelt. Taste and adjust the seasonings if necessary.

3. If you let the salad sit for an hour or more before serving, the flavor deepens and becomes more complex.

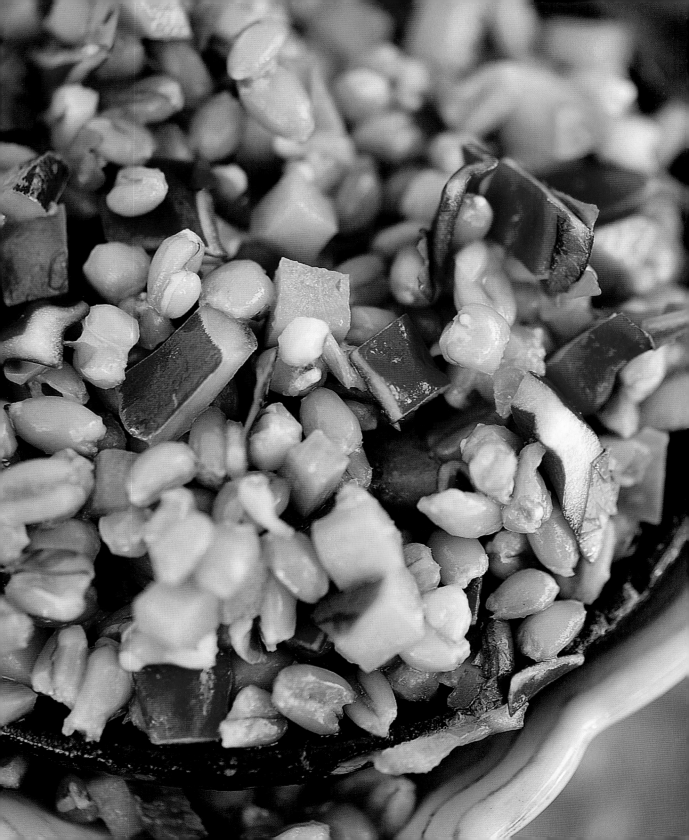

Universally Loved Barley Salad

Serves 6 to 8

I've made this dish for a long time and I've heard only good things about it. My dad totally digs it.

DRESSING
2 tablespoons fresh lemon juice
1 tablespoon Dijon mustard
Pinch of sea salt
2 tablespoons sherry vinegar (or
   1 tablespoon apple cider vinegar and
   1 tablespoon umeboshi vinegar)
1 tablespoon minced shallot
¼ cup olive oil

SALAD
5 cups spring water
2 cups pearl or hulled barley, soaked and
   drained
½ teaspoon sea salt
2 bay leaves
2 tablespoons chopped fresh oregano or
   2 teaspoons dried, crumbled
⅓ cup chopped pitted kalamata olives
⅓ cup drained capers
½ cup pine nuts, toasted
¼ cup finely chopped scallions

1. To make the dressing, combine all the dressing ingredients in a mixing bowl or dressing bottle and set aside.

2. To prepare the salad, bring the water to a boil. Add the barley with the salt and bay leaves. Simmer for 1 hour, or until all the water is absorbed. Let cool.

3. Remove the bay leaves and add the dressing and oregano. Refrigerate for about 2 hours, or until ready to serve.

4. Add the olives, capers, pine nuts, and scallions. Serve.

Buckwheat Pilaf

Serves 4

This dish, concocted by DILFy Howard Wallen, really plays off the strong flavor of the buckwheat by bringing some sourness and spiciness to the mix. The walnuts also give it a crunch. I think you'll like it.

½ cup walnuts
¾ cup spring water
½ cup buckwheat
2 cups diced peeled russet potatoes,
   or cauliflower pieces
2 tablespoons sesame oil
1¼ cups finely diced onions

1 cup halved mushrooms
¼ cup chopped sauerkraut
6 cloves garlic, minced
2 teaspoons dried thyme leaves
2 teaspoons chili powder
¼ teaspoon sea salt
¼ cup finely chopped fresh parsley

1. Preheat the oven to 350°F.

2. Roast the walnuts on a baking sheet for 20 minutes, or until lightly browned. Remove the walnuts to a plate and let cool. Chop the walnuts coarsely and set aside.

3. Meanwhile, in a 1-quart saucepan, combine the water and buckwheat, bring to a low boil, and cover. Remove from the heat and let the buckwheat sit to absorb the water.

4. In a steamer, steam the potatoes for 15 minutes (cauliflower for 10), or until firm but soft, then set aside to cool.

5. In a medium skillet, heat the oil and sauté the onions, mushrooms, sauerkraut, garlic, thyme, chili powder, and salt for about 5 minutes, or until the onions are translucent. Add the potatoes, buckwheat, nuts, and parsley, and mix well. Heat everything together, then remove from the heat and serve immediately.

Garlic-Rosemary Millet with Mushroom Gravy

Serves 4

Millet does a million things. Because it's got a mild taste, it goes really well with vegetables—like carrots, squash, or cauliflower. In this dish, the cauliflower and the millet whizzed together taste like potatoes. Add the rosemary, garlic, and mushroom gravy. . . . OMG.

1 cup millet
3 cups spring water
2 cups cauliflower (in small florets or medium-sized chunks)
Sea salt
1 teaspoon olive oil
4 cloves garlic, minced (more if you're a real garlic fan)
2 teaspoons minced fresh rosemary

GRAVY
1 tablespoon olive oil

2 cups thinly sliced cremini, white button, or shiitake (fresh or dried and reconstituted) mushrooms
Pinch of sea salt
3 cups spring water
¼ cup shoyu
2 teaspoons mirin
Dash of brown rice vinegar
2 tablespoons tahini
2 tablespoons kuzu root starch, dissolved in ½ cup cold water
Scallions, parsley, or chives, for garnish

1. Rinse the millet well and place in a heavy 2-quart pot. Over medium heat, stir the millet continuously until it dries and becomes aromatic and ever so slightly golden in color. This can take 5 to 8 minutes. Add the water and cauliflower. Bring to a boil and add a pinch of salt. Cover and simmer over a flame deflector for 30 minutes. Remove from the heat. Put the millet through a hand food mill, blend in a food processor, or blend in the pot with an immersion blender. Blend to the desired creamy consistency.

2. To make the gravy, heat the olive oil over medium heat in a skillet. Add the mushrooms and the salt and sauté until soft and moist. Add the water and bring to a boil. Season with the shoyu, mirin, and brown rice vinegar. Simmer for 5 minutes. Add the tahini, mix, and simmer for 1 more minute.

3. Add the dissolved kuzu to the simmering mixture and stir constantly as the kuzu thickens and comes to a boil. After the kuzu has boiled, the gravy is ready.

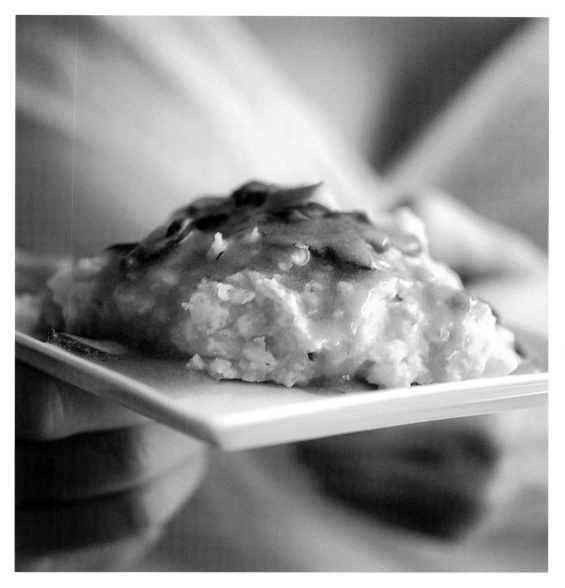

4. Heat the olive oil over medium heat in a small sauté pan. Add the garlic and a pinch of salt. Sauté for a few seconds. Add the rosemary and sauté all together, stirring constantly to avoid burning. Mix thoroughly and then fold into the millet mixture.

5. To serve, spoon the gravy over the millet mash on individual plates. Garnish with scallions, parsley, or chives.

Rice with Chestnuts

Serves 6 to 8

Mmmm . . . chestnuts. If you've never had them, you're going to love the soft, sweet taste of chestnuts cooked in rice. Due to a chestnut blight in the early 1900s, there are very few chestnut trees in North America, but the "nuts" themselves can be imported from Europe these days. You'll find them at better health food stores. This is an especially great dish in the fall and winter. Very warming and comforting.

---

1 cup dried peeled chestnuts, soaked in
   2 cups spring water (overnight if possible)
3 cups brown rice, soaking water reserved

4½ cups spring water (including rice- and
   chestnut-soaking water)
½ teaspoon sea salt

---

1. Before cooking, remove any brown or red skin from the chestnuts if necessary. Place the rice, chestnuts, and water in a pressure cooker. Bring to a boil over medium-high heat. Add the salt, cover the pot, and bring to full pressure.

2. Place a flame deflector under the pressure cooker, reduce the heat to low, and cook for 50 minutes (the pressure cooker should hiss very quietly). Remove from the heat and let the pressure come down naturally. Uncover and serve.

Lemony Quinoa Salad

Serves 4 to 6

This recipe is adapted from one by Chauvon Collins, a very talented MILF in the kitchen. It is the perfect summer dish.

---

1 cup quinoa
2 cups spring water
Sea salt
1 cup fresh corn kernels
2 tablespoons umeboshi vinegar
2 tablespoons mirin
¼ cup extra virgin olive oil

2 teaspoons ground cumin
1 to 2 teaspoons garlic powder
Juice of 1 lemon
½ medium red onion, finely chopped
1 cup chopped fresh cilantro
1 cup chopped fresh parsley

---

1. Rinse the quinoa well and place in a saucepan with the water and a pinch of sea salt. Bring to a boil, reduce the heat, and simmer with the lid on for 20 minutes.

2. Meanwhile, bring a small saucepan of water to a boil and toss the corn in for 2 to 5 minutes, until the color is bright yellow. Drain and let cool.

3. Whisk together the umeboshi vinegar, mirin, olive oil, cumin, garlic powder, and lemon juice.

4. When the quinoa is done cooking, fluff and let cool for a few minutes. Toss with the corn, onion, cilantro, and parsley and the vinaigrette.

Grain Products

Fried Noodles

Serves 4 generously

I live for fried noodles. They are a satisfying, delicious comfort food that can be enjoyed every week. Start with this recipe but then go crazy with your own ideas. You may add any other vegetable you like, as long as it sautés well. The only way you can screw up fried noodles is by adding too much water, which will make the noodles soggy. But barring that, it's game on.

One 8-ounce package whole wheat udon or soba noodles
2 tablespoons toasted sesame oil
1 medium onion, diced
Sea salt
½ carrot, cut into matchsticks

8 mushrooms, sliced
3 teaspoons shoyu
Kernels from 1 ear fresh corn
1 stalk bok choy, thinly sliced
¼ cup spring water
1 scallion, chopped

1. Cook the noodles according to the instructions on the package; drain, rinse with cold water, and set them aside.

2. Heat the oil in a skillet and when hot (but not smoking), add the onion. Add a small pinch of sea salt to bring out the onion's moisture and sweetness. Stir continually as the onion becomes soft and translucent. Add the carrots and another small pinch of salt and continue to stir until the matchsticks are slightly softened. Add the mushrooms and one more small pinch of salt and sauté until their moisture is released and they are soft. Season the vegetables with 1 teaspoon of the shoyu. Continue to stir as they cook for another 2 minutes.

3. Place the noodles on top of the vegetables. Do not stir them. Add the corn, bok choy, and the remaining 2 teaspoons shoyu. Dribble in the spring water, just to ensure that the vegetables on the bottom do not stick. Reduce the heat to low, cover, and cook for about 5 more minutes. The small amount of water should produce enough steam to cook the dish, but not enough to make the noodles soggy. Add the scallion and toss. Serve hot.

Soft Polenta with Braised Wild Mushrooms

Serves 5 to 8

With this recipe, MILFy Meredith McCarty hits the nail on the head. You will see her recipes throughout this book. She's a talented lady. This soft and delicious dish will keep you feeling taken care of.

SOFT POLENTA
1 cup polenta
4 cups spring water
1 teaspoon sea salt
1 teaspoon extra virgin olive oil
Kernels from 1 ear fresh corn

BRAISED WILD MUSHROOMS
2 teaspoons olive oil
8 large cloves garlic, sliced
1 pound wild mushrooms, stems trimmed, caps left whole if small, or halved or quartered if large

½ teaspoon sea salt
Freshly ground black pepper
1½ teaspoons chopped fresh rosemary and/or oregano
Generous splash of light white wine or spring water (if needed)
1½ teaspoons kuzu root starch or arrowroot powder, dissolved in cool water to cover (if needed)

Fresh Italian parsley, for garnish

1. To prepare the polenta, soak it in the water for 1 hour to overnight, or all day. Drain the water from the polenta into a measuring cup and take note of the amount. Discard. In a 3-quart saucepan, bring that same amount of fresh spring water to a boil with the salt and oil. Stir in the polenta and the corn. When the boiling resumes, turn the heat to low. Cook, covered, until thick and creamy, about 20 minutes. Stir or whisk occasionally.

2. To cook the mushrooms, heat the oil in a large skillet. Add the garlic, mushrooms, salt, pepper, and herb(s). Cover and stir occasionally until the mushrooms release their juices, about 5 minutes. Add the liquid (wine or water) if needed, cover, and cook until quite tender and flavorful, about 5 more minutes. Stir occasionally. If needed to thicken, stir in the kuzu or arrowroot.

3. Transfer the polenta to a casserole dish or polenta board. Spoon the mushroom mixture over the top and garnish with Italian parsley. Serve hot.

NOTE: Enjoy this dish year-round with whatever mushrooms are in season, such as porcini, chanterelle, morel, oyster, shiitake, or royal trumpet. To reheat leftovers, whisk the polenta with boiling water in a small saucepan, or slice the polenta and fry in a little hot olive oil.

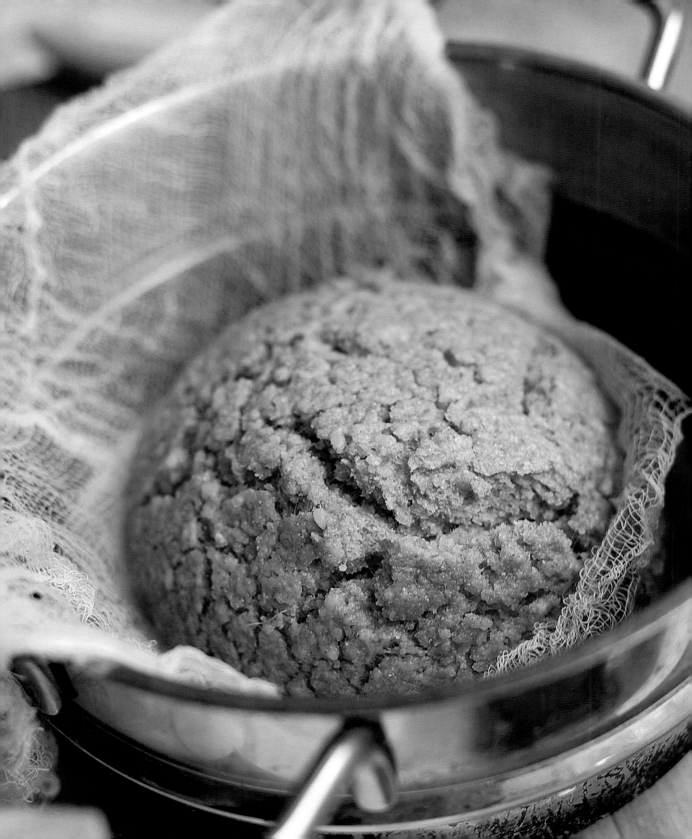

Steamed Sourdough Bread

Makes 2 small loaves (12 thin slices)

I know, steamed . . . what? This way of making bread is really fun and easy, and the results are very nice. Baked flour products can cause the body to feel tight and contracted, but by steaming the dough, it is softer and easier to digest. If you suffer from upper-back, shoulder, or neck pain, try skipping baked flour products and just eating noodles and steamed bread. You'll notice a difference.

2 tablespoons miso
3 cups leftover rice or other cooked grain
2½ cups whole wheat bread flour
½ cup whole wheat pastry flour

Spring water
Raisins, seeds, sautéed onion, grated carrot,
  or other ingredients to add variety (optional)
Olive oil

1. Add the miso to the leftover rice, using your hands to mix them together. Put aside for at least 2 days (I do 3 sometimes) in a warmish place. Massage the mixture once a day to get the fermentation to occur. This will become a little smelly and wet. It is your sourdough "starter."

2. The night before you plan to cook the bread, add the bread and pastry flours and water, a little at a time, until you are kneading a dense, but not inflexible, dough. Knead in any optional ingredients, if using. Knead for a few minutes, until the dough has a little springiness to it. (Note that this dough will always be denser and less springy than white flour dough made with conventional ingredients.) Divide into 2 small loaves. Coat them lightly with olive oil. Cover with cheesecloth and then a warm, damp dish towel. Let sit overnight.

3. In the morning, place the dough (wrapped in the cheesecloth) in a stainless steel or bamboo steamer above a pot of boiling water. If you don't have a steamer, you might try putting the loaves in a colander in a pot of boiling water, as long as the water doesn't come up to the level of the dough. Since the dough needs to steam for 1 hour, you must keep adding water to the pot. Check every 15 minutes or so to make sure you don't ruin your pot or your bread! Let cool on a rack and serve.

Crostini Hearts with Black Olive Tapenade

Serves 6

This lovely and elegant appetizer is also by Meredith McCarty. You can see her doing yoga on page 351. She's sixty-five. Can you believe it?

BLACK OLIVE TAPENADE
1 cup (about 4 ounces) pitted black olives
   (kalamata preferred, or regular canned
   black olives, drained)
1 small to medium tomato, chopped
1 clove garlic, chopped
2 tablespoons drained capers

1½ teaspoons fresh thyme leaves,
   or ½ teaspoon dried
1 teaspoon fresh lemon juice

CROSTINI HEARTS
14 slices whole grain-sourdough bread
Fresh thyme leaves, for garnish

1. To make the spread, first press each olive to be sure it is pitted. Puree all of the tapenade ingredients to the desired consistency, chunky or smooth. The tapenade may be stored in the refrigerator for up to 1 week. Makes 1 cup.

2. Preheat the oven to 400°F. To make the crostini, cut the bread slices with a 3-inch-wide heart-shaped cookie cutter. Spread the tapenade on the bread slices and transfer to a parchment paper–lined baking sheet. Bake for 15 minutes. Garnish with thyme leaves and serve.

Vegetables

We are all familiar with vegetables, but the MILF diet will introduce you to a couple of new ones. They are:

Burdock: This root vegetable is very hearty and earthy. In fact, it smells like dirt . . . but in a really good way. You may be familiar with the plant attached to this root—it's the one that leaves burrs on your coat in the fall and winter. Burdock has a ton of medicinal properties and is especially good for strengthening and purifying the blood. It is also very supportive of DILFy energy, especially the kind a DILF needs in bed—if you catch my drift. Burdock, with its earthy, gutsy, grounding taste, is great sautéed, in stews, and in soups, but is too bitter when eaten raw unless it's pickled. Burdock needs to be cleaned before use, but don't scrub all the brown stuff off—that's its skin. This new vegetable will seem expensive, but because the taste of burdock is strong, a little goes a long way. Use a little and then store the rest, wrapped in a damp tea towel, in a veggie drawer of the fridge.

Daikon: Pronounced "die-con," this long, white radish is very popular in Asia but grows easily in most climates. Daikon is cooling, is relaxing, and has a natural diuretic effect. You'll see it later in a recipe to help you lose weight fast. However, you can enjoy its properties on a daily basis by including daikon in recipes here and there; it's great in soups, stews, sautés, and salads; simply blanched; and especially as a pickle. Like a red radish, daikon is pungent when raw and pleasantly bland or even sweet when cooked. Raw daikon is often served with tempura and sashimi at Japanese restaurants because it helps to break down protein and fat.

Both burdock and daikon are regularly available at Whole Foods Markets and better health food stores. If they don't carry them, ask them to order some.

Brad Pitt Vegetables

Makes as much as you want

This recipe used to be called "Blanched Vegetables" or "Boiled Salad," but those names just didn't cut it. I mean, hey, it's pretty hard to get people excited about blanched veggies, but I'm a bit of a nerd on the topic. You see, quickly blanched vegetables offer a fresh, uplifting, and very important energy to your cooking; done right, they are very good-quality yin. Overcooked, they are just *bleccch*.

So look this recipe over carefully. Blanching vegetables correctly is not about dunking them in boiling water and walking away to check your e-mail. You must be present and pay attention and then you will get the most amazing results. Brad Pitt isn't easy, ladies!

Assorted vegetables, with at least one representative from the upward-growing category, one from the round or ground vegetable category, and one from the downward-growing category. That makes a more balanced Brad Pitt vegetable dish.
Upward-growing or leafy green: kale, collard greens, napa cabbage, bok choy, leeks, celery, mustard greens, watercress

Round or ground: yellow onions, red onions, winter squash, summer squash, broccoli, cauliflower, cabbage, snow peas, string beans
Downward-growing or root: carrots, red radishes, daikon, parsnips, burdock
Sea salt

---

1. Rinse the vegetables of your choice and cut them into medium-thin slices. Bring a pot of water to a boil. Add the sea salt—no more than 1 grain (I know that's impossible, but try). Even 1 grain of sea salt draws the minerals and taste to the periphery of each vegetable.

2. Take one type of vegetable and place it in the boiling water. Immediately *turn off the heat.* Just let the vegetable sit in the water for anywhere from 15 seconds (for delicate veggies like bok choy, napa cabbage, and thinly sliced onions) to 30 seconds (corn kernels, carrots, thinly sliced daikon) to a few minutes (tougher greens like collards, kale, and cabbage, and tougher root vegetables like parsnip and burdock). Because the water is no longer actively boiling, the minerals and flavor stay in the vegetable instead of being released into the water. This is what makes Brad Pitt Vegetables so delicious.

3. Remove the slices with a slotted spoon and set aside. You can, if you wish, run cold water over the vegetable to stop the cooking process and maintain a bright color.

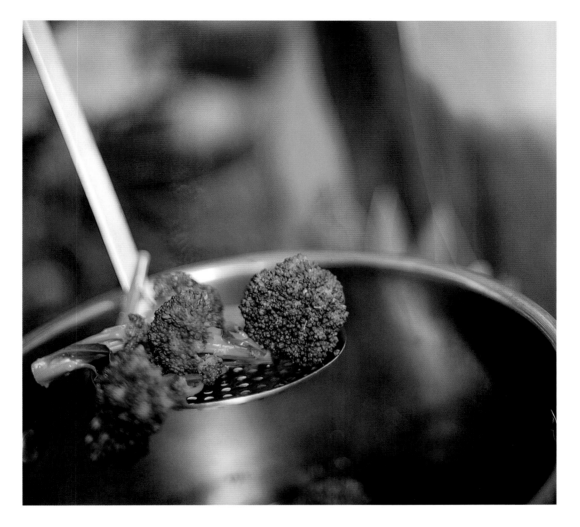

4. Bring the water to a boil again (no need to add more salt) and cook the next vegetable. Turn off the heat and repeat as above.

5. When all the vegetables are done, arrange them in an attractive way on a platter. Serve as is or with a dressing (page 239).

TIP: Cook any vegetables with a strong taste, like mustard greens, watercress, and radishes, at the end, since they make the cooking water kind of bitter.

Leafy Green Vegetable Roll

If you have large bunches and heads of greens, you should be able to make at least 4 rolls; each makes 8 pieces.

This recipe was donated by Gabriele Kushi, a lovely MILFy lady from Minneapolis who has been cooking this way for her whole adult life. These rolls are easy and refreshing, and she swears that kids love them. They go really well with her Green-Life Veggie Dip (page 241).

---

1 bunch collard greens (whole leaves)
1 head napa or Chinese cabbage (whole leaves)
Umeboshi paste

1 package bean sprouts, raw or slightly steamed
Toasted sesame seeds, for garnish

---

1. Boil the whole leaves of the vegetables in water for a few minutes. Let them cool.

2. Place 2 or 3 collard leaves on a bamboo sushi mat; cover the mat completely. Place 3 napa cabbage leaves horizontally along the mat, over the collard leaves, alternating their tops and bottoms. Then spread about ½ teaspoon umeboshi paste evenly in a line along the greens and add some sprouts.

3. Roll the vegetables into a cylinder with the sushi mat and squeeze out any excess liquid.

4. Cut the roll into 8 even pieces. Arrange them on a serving platter, adding a few sprinkles of sesame seeds, and serve.

VARIATION: You can roll basically anything in these vegetables. Try carrots, scallions, panfried tofu, or even cooked beans or grains. Enjoy and be creative.

Shanghai Bean Sprout Salad

Serves 4

This crunchy, refreshing, and exotic salad came from MILFy Suzanne Landry, the queen of vegetables. She really has a knack!

½ cup snow peas
1 stalk celery
2 Roma tomatoes, sliced into wedges
  (optional)
1 cup mung bean sprouts
2 scallions, finely chopped
¼ cup chopped unsalted roasted peanuts

DRESSING

2 tablespoons fresh lemon juice (juice
  of 1 lemon)
2 tablespoons brown rice vinegar
½ teaspoon shoyu
1 tablespoon mirin
¼ teaspoon prepared yellow mustard
2 tablespoons toasted sesame oil
½ teaspoon grated fresh ginger
¼ cup chopped fresh cilantro (optional)

1. Remove the strings from the snow peas by pinching the top of each snow pea and pulling down the string. Slice the snow peas in half. Blanch in boiling water for 30 seconds. Immediately remove to a colander and rinse with cold water, or transfer to a bowl of ice water, to stop the cooking process. Drain and place in a large bowl.

2. Slice the celery stalk down the middle lengthwise and then crosscut diagonally into ¼-inch pieces. Combine with the snow peas. Add the tomato wedges (if using), bean sprouts, and scallions to the snow peas along with the peanuts.

3. In a separate bowl, mix together the dressing ingredients. Toss with the salad and let it stand for 1 hour before serving, to marinate the vegetables. Without the dressing, the salad will last for 3 days, refrigerated.

Lemony Vegetable Salad

Serves 4 or 5

Pressed salads are lightly fermented foods; when you press raw vegetables with salt or another salty agent, the vegetables begin to release their liquid, their fiber softens, and they become easier to digest. This pressed salad was invented by Gabriele Kushi, Minneapolis MILF.

---

4 cups thinly sliced assorted green vegetables (Chinese cabbage, celery, cilantro, chicory, parsley, kale)
$\frac{1}{3}$ cup carrot matchsticks
3 scallions, white and green parts, thinly sliced

$\frac{1}{4}$ teaspoon sea salt
Juice and grated zest of 1 lemon
1 teaspoon dulse flakes
1 teaspoon walnut oil

---

1. Combine the vegetables in a glass bowl. Add the sea salt, lemon juice, zest, and dulse flakes. Mix, then squeeze the vegetables between your hands until they begin to release some moisture. Massage the vegetables for a minute or so. Let the vegetables marinate for a few hours before serving. You can also press in a salad press or with a heavy weight to aid the marinating process.

2. Drain off excess liquid. Serve as a side dish, drizzled with the walnut oil. This salad keeps in a cool place for 2 to 3 days.

Baked Parsnips

Serves 6

This recipe comes to us from MILFy Eliza Eller of Alaska. The mother of thirteen, she knows how to make food taste good. In her words, "Everybody, especially kids, hates parsnips—or that's what they think, because the ones that are sold are generally bitter, bland, and mealy. However, in Alaska, we have year-round access to the sweetest parsnips in the world, grown organically in ten feet of rich dark Matunuska Valley topsoil." But, hey, since we're not all going to move to Alaska, Eliza recommends that you and I just ask for the sweetest parsnips at our farmers' market, and this recipe will make them even better. She serves them with rice salad and simple black beans.

Sea salt

6 to 8 parsnips, cut diagonally, twirling the parsnip as you go so as to create large chunky triangles

Olive oil

Shoyu

1. Preheat the oven to 400°F. Bring a large pot of water to a boil with 2 pinches of salt.

2. Drop the parsnips into the water and boil for 7 minutes, or until just barely tender. Scoop out with a slotted spoon into a large mixing bowl.

3. Mix the hot parsnips well with plenty of olive oil and a dash of shoyu. Spread them out in a baking dish and bake in the oven for 30 to 40 minutes. During baking, stir the parsnips several times in their dish so they will cook evenly. They are done when they are soft all the way through and getting crispy and golden brown. Serve hot!

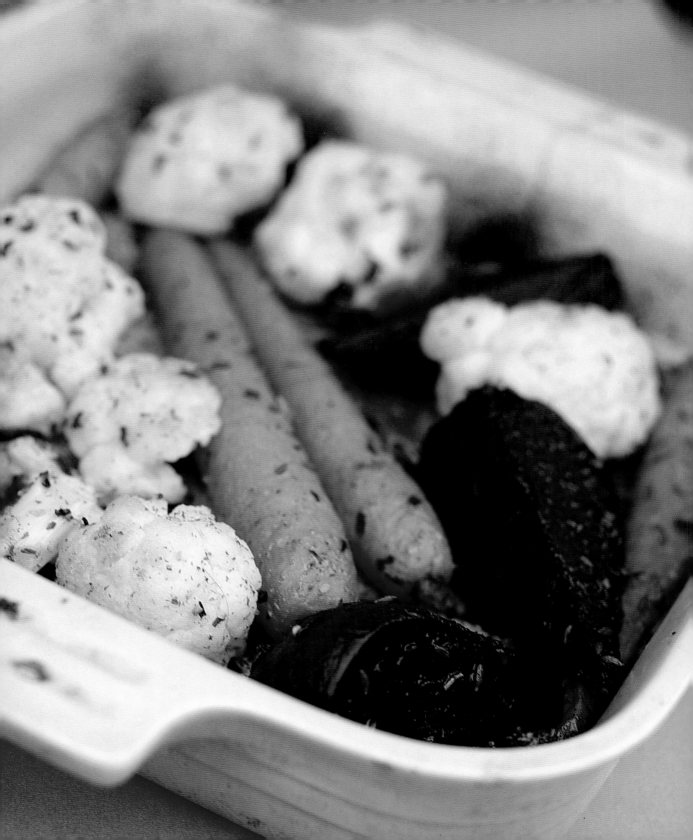

Oven-Roasted Root Vegetables with Garlic, Cumin, and Herbs

Serves 6 to 8

I *love* roasted vegetables. They are easy, delicious, and incredibly satisfying. I make them a lot. This recipe is from Meredith McCarty, and the cumin seeds make all the difference.

2 pounds mixed root vegetables (carrots, turnips, parsnips, rutabagas, red or gold potatoes, sweet potatoes, yams, beets), peeled where needed and cut into medium or large chunks (about 7 cups)

4 large cloves garlic, sliced
2 teaspoons extra virgin olive oil
1 teaspoon *each* cumin seeds and Italian seasoning
¾ teaspoon sea salt

Preheat the oven to 450°F. In a bowl, mix the cut-up vegetables with the remaining ingredients. Transfer to a 2-quart baking dish. Cover with the lid or with a sheet of parchment paper topped with aluminum foil (the parchment paper will protect the food from contact with the aluminum). Roast until completely tender, about 1 hour. Remove the cover to brown the top, 5 to 15 more minutes.

Daikon Rounds with Sesame Sauce

Serves 4 to 6 (depending on the size of the daikon)

Another Eliza Eller recipe from Alaska, this is a great way to eat daikon. She says this recipe is a favorite of all her kids, even the babies and the teens.

---

1 cup tahini
3 tablespoons shoyu, or to taste

2 large daikon, cut into 1-inch-thick rounds
Sea salt

---

1. Mix the tahini with about 1 cup water and the shoyu.

2. Boil the daikon rounds in water salted with 1 tablespoon sea salt until tender all the way through, 5 to 7 minutes, then drain. Mix the hot daikon with the tahini sauce and serve immediately.

Arugula Salad with Fennel, Bosc Pear, and White Balsamic Vinaigrette

Serves 8

This recipe by Meredith McCarty is an explosion of tastes: the bitterness and pungency of the arugula, mixed with the sweetness of the pear; the licorice taste of the fennel; and the tanginess of the dressing. . . . Very nice.

WHITE BALSAMIC VINAIGRETTE
3 tablespoons white balsamic vinegar
2 tablespoons spring water
1 teaspoon extra virgin olive oil
¼ teaspoon sea salt
Freshly ground black pepper to taste

ARUGULA SALAD
8 ounces mixed lettuces, predominantly arugula
½ small fennel bulb, very thinly sliced
1 medium tomato, thinly sliced into wedges (optional)
1 small Bosc pear, thinly sliced into wedges

1. Mix the dressing ingredients and allow to sit for a few minutes to meld the flavors. Makes ⅓ cup.

2. Toss the greens and fennel with the dressing to taste. Serve topped with the tomato, if using, and pear.

VARIATION: Meredith recommends using this balsamic vinaigrette on other veggies, like blanched broccoli and kale.

Carrot-Burdock Sauté

Serves 4

You may have had this at a Japanese restaurant. Also known as kinpira, it is sweet, earthy, and satisfying and gives really strong energy. It's a great side dish a couple of times a week, and although it's good for the whole family, it's very supportive of DILF energy.

1 to 2 tablespoons toasted sesame oil or olive oil
1 medium burdock root, cut into fine matchsticks
Sea salt

2 medium carrots, cut into fine matchsticks
1 tablespoon spring water
About 1 teaspoon shoyu
1 teaspoon grated fresh ginger

1. Heat the oil in a heavy skillet that has a lid. Sauté the burdock first with a tiny pinch of salt, stirring constantly for about 3 minutes. Add the carrots and another small pinch of salt, stirring constantly for another 3 minutes. Sprinkle the water over the vegetables, cover, and reduce the heat to low, allowing the vegetables to steam.

2. After 10 to 15 minutes, uncover and check to see that the dish is relatively dry. Sprinkle in the shoyu. Cover and cook for 5 more minutes. Squeeze the grated ginger to add a few drops of ginger juice to the dish, and discard the ginger pulp. Serve while hot.

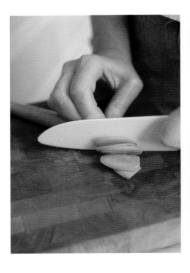 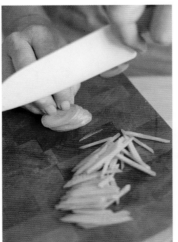 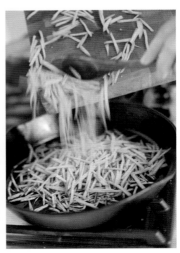

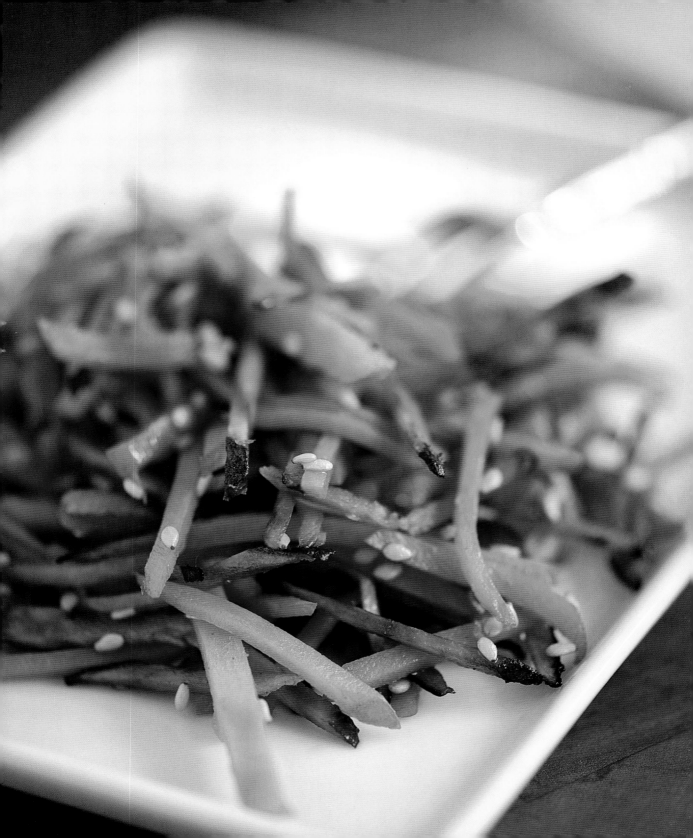

Sweet Stewed Carrots with Corn Sauce

Serves 4 to 6

Another Howard Wallen hit.

One 2-inch piece kombu sea vegetable

---

1 medium onion, cut into thick half-moons
4 large carrots, cut diagonally into ½-inch
    slices and then cut in half again, lengthwise
Sea salt

Kernels from 4 ears fresh corn
¼ teaspoon shoyu

---

1. In a heavy saucepan (with a heavy lid), soak the kombu in 1 inch of water. After 10 to 15 minutes, or when it is soft, remove the kombu from the water and slice into thin strips. Discard the soaking water and place the strips of kombu on the bottom of the pan. Layer in the onion and then the carrots on top. Pour water down the side of the pan to come just halfway up the onions. Add a pinch of salt. Cover, bring to a boil, and then reduce the heat to low. Let simmer for about 10 minutes, or until the carrots are tender.

2. Meanwhile, blend the corn kernels in a blender until they have a relatively creamy consistency. Pour off the excess cooking liquid from the carrots (keeping about ½ cup of it aside). Add the corn cream to the carrots and season with the shoyu. Cover and let simmer for 3 more minutes. Remove from the heat and shake the covered pan carefully to thoroughly mix the corn and the carrots together. If you need more liquid, use a bit of the reserved cooking water. Serve hot.

VARIATION: Add diagonally sliced green beans when the carrots are almost done.

Stir-fry

Serves 4

Stir-fries are great. First of all, they're easy; second, they're fast; third, they're delicious; and finally, there are endless permutations of the standard stir-fry, so they are a great opportunity for your kitchen creativity to roll.

1 red bell pepper
Toasted sesame oil
2 cloves garlic, minced
Sea salt
Splash of umeboshi vinegar
8 ounces button or cremini mushrooms, thinly sliced
8 stalks bok choy, sliced diagonally into 1-inch pieces

1 cup spring water
2 tablespoons shoyu
1 heaping tablespoon kuzu root starch, dissolved in about ¼ cup cold water
1 teaspoon grated fresh ginger, squeezed for juice
Toasted sesame seeds, for garnish

1. Roast the red pepper either by placing it on the flame of your gas stove and turning it with tongs as it chars or by coating the pepper with a little oil, slicing it in half, and placing it, cut side down, on a baking sheet in a 450°F oven for 30 to 40 minutes. Turn it with tongs every 5 minutes or so as well.

2. Place the charred pepper in a paper bag and let it sweat for 15 minutes. Remove the pepper and gently massage the skin so that it comes off. Do not put the pepper under running water, as that will dilute its taste. If some black skin is left on, that's okay.

3. Cut the pepper into thin slices and set aside.

4. Heat 1 tablespoon sesame oil over medium-high heat in a wok or a large stainless-steel skillet that has a lid. Throw in the garlic and a tiny pinch of salt and sauté for 10 seconds. Add the red pepper and sauté for 30 seconds with a splash of umeboshi vinegar to help the pepper hold its red color. Add the mushrooms and another pinch of salt. Sauté vigorously until the mushrooms wilt and sweat, about 3 minutes. Place the bok choy on top and pour the water down the side of the wok. Sprinkle 1 tablespoon of the shoyu over everything, cover the wok, and let the water you've added steam for 2 to 3 minutes. Don't let it cook for too long or the bok choy will become mushy. Uncover the wok and pour the kuzu mixture, ginger juice, and the remaining tablespoon of shoyu into the bottom and stir vigorously as the liquid sets into a gravy-like consistency. Toss, garnish with a sprinkle of sesame seeds, and serve hot.

VARIATIONS: These are endless. Start with the heartier vegetables and finish with the lighter ones being steamed at the end. Try matchstick carrots, mushrooms, napa cabbage, and corn kernels. Green beans, red bell peppers, carrots, lacinato kale, and tofu. Throw in seeds, pine nuts, roasted almonds. . . . You are limited only by your imagination.

Yams with Roasted Garlic

Serves 4 to 6

This is a very sexy recipe, donated by Sarah Loring, a Connecticut MILF and mother of four. There is something about the sweetness of the yams and the zing of the garlic that makes this dish a winner.

About 3 pounds garnet yams (or other yams or sweet potatoes)
Sea salt

1 head garlic
Olive oil (optional)
Freshly ground black pepper (optional)

---

1. Scrub the yams with a vegetable brush and remove any blemishes. Place in a medium-size saucepan and cover with water. Add a pinch of sea salt and cover. Bring to a boil and reduce the heat to medium-low. Simmer for 30 minutes, or until the yams are tender to the middle. You can test them by piercing with a fork. When the yams are done, remove them to a plate to cool.

2. Meanwhile, wrap the garlic in aluminum foil and roast in the oven (or a toaster oven) at 400°F for 30 minutes. Let the garlic cool. Cut off the base of the head and squeeze out the garlic pulp. Set aside.

3. The yams can be peeled or left with the skins on. Place the yams in a food processor and add a pinch of sea salt and one-half of the roasted garlic pulp. Process until smooth. (Do not overprocess.) Taste and adjust the seasoning and the amount of garlic. If you want to add a little olive oil and black pepper, this is the time. Sometimes the yam flavor is so vibrant that you want to capture that, not hide it. It will be a little different every time.

NOTE: Instead of using a food processor, you can also mash the yams with a potato masher or in a suribachi. Follow the same process: adding just a little seasoning, then tasting.

Leeks au Gratin

Serves 6 to 8

This recipe is an adaptation of one sent to me by Suzanne Landry, California MILF. She is particularly adept at cooking vegetables, and her soon-to-be-published book is called *The Passionate Vegetable*.

CASSEROLE
4 leeks
⅔ cup vegetable stock or spring water
¼ teaspoon sea salt
1 teaspoon dried rosemary
3 tablespoons dry white wine
2 tablespoons soy margarine or olive oil
¼ cup unbleached white flour

1¼ cups almond milk

TOPPING
½ cup whole wheat bread crumbs
½ cup soy margarine (Earth Balance is best)
2 tablespoons chopped fresh parsley
1 cup Daiya Cheddar "cheese" shreds

---

1. Preheat the oven to 350°F. Separate the white and green parts of each leek. Cut a vertical slit along the length of the bottom; wash thoroughly by pulling back the leaves. Slice the leeks into ½-inch pieces on the diagonal. Do the same for the green tops, using only the tender inner leaves and removing any tough outer leaves. Place the leeks in a large bowl and fill with water to wash them thoroughly. Place in a colander to drain.

2. Mix the stock or water, salt, rosemary, and wine in a large skillet and bring to a boil. Add the leeks, cover, and simmer over medium-low heat for 5 minutes, or until the leeks begin to soften.

3. With a slotted spoon, transfer the leeks to an oven-safe dish. Simmer the liquid in the pan without a lid until it reduces to half its volume.

4. Heat the soy margarine or oil in a small saucepan, stir in the flour, and cook for 1 to 2 minutes, making sure it doesn't burn. Slowly add the almond milk, stirring well, until it becomes a smooth sauce. Now pour in the remaining stock from the cooked leeks. Simmer for 2 to 3 minutes and pour over the leeks.

5. Mix all the topping ingredients together and sprinkle over the leeks. Bake in the oven, uncovered, for 20 to 25 minutes, until golden and the cheese is melted. Place the casserole under the broiler for 5 minutes, or until the cheese becomes a deep gold and crispy. Let cool a little before serving.

VARIATION: This recipe is great with a number of vegetables: cauliflower, carrots, squash, Brussels sprouts. . . . Go crazy.

Hurry-Curry Vegetables

Serves 6

This is another hit from Suzanne Landry, who says, "Creamy, hot, and sweet . . . all at the same time! Great served over brown rice, couscous, or quinoa."

---

1 small onion, chopped
1 tablespoon expeller-pressed vegetable oil
3 red potatoes, cut into ½-inch chunks (optional)
2 medium carrots, chopped into ½-inch rounds
½ green or red bell pepper, chopped
3½ tablespoons curry powder

¼ teaspoon sea salt
1 cup spring water
1 cup bite-size cauliflower pieces
1 cup fresh or frozen peas
¼ cup chopped fresh cilantro
1 tablespoon kuzu root starch, arrowroot, or organic cornstarch
One 13.5- to 14-ounce can light coconut milk

---

1. Sauté the onion in the oil over low heat for 2 to 3 minutes. Add the potatoes, if using, the carrots, green or red pepper, curry powder, salt, and ¾ cup of the water. Cover and cook until the vegetables are tender, about 10 minutes.

2. Increase the heat to medium and add the cauliflower; cover and cook for 5 minutes, or until tender. Add the peas and cilantro and warm through for another 1 to 2 minutes.

3. Add the kuzu to the remaining ¼ cup water and stir to dissolve until the liquid appears milky. Add the coconut milk and stir again. Stir into the vegetables and simmer for an additional 2 to 3 minutes, until the liquid has thickened.

Squochi

Serves 4 to 6 (depending on the size of the squash)

This is a favorite of mine and was a big hit with my mother. It combines the lovely sweetness of onions and winter squash with the gooeyness of melted mochi. A great dish for fall and winter.

1 tablespoon olive oil or sesame oil
1 large or two small onions, cut into thin half-moon slices (from top to bottom of the onion, not across)
Pinch of sea salt
½ winter squash, also cut into half-moon slices, up to ½ inch thick

1 tablespoon shoyu
1½ teaspoons mirin
½ cup spring water
Half a 12-ounce package plain mochi, grated

1. In a heavy saucepan (enameled cast iron is best), heat the oil and begin to sauté the onions with a pinch of salt. After they have started to sweat, cover them, reduce the heat, and let them cook down until caramelized. This may take 15 minutes or so. Check them regularly to make sure the heat isn't too high, but if they are covered with a heavy lid, they should be fine—onions release a lot of liquid that will just get recycled in the pan.

2. Layer the squash on top of the onions. Mix together the shoyu, mirin, and water and pour carefully down the side of the pan. This liquid will steam the squash. Cover and let the squash cook until it's soft, about 10 minutes.

3. Sprinkle the mochi evenly on top of the squash and cover once more. The mochi should melt in 3 to 5 minutes. Remove from the heat and serve hot.

VARIATIONS: It doesn't hurt to add more onions; they cook down and they are totally delicious, so play with the ratio of onions to squash.

For a meltier mochi "cheese" on top, melt the mochi in a little water in a saucepan on the side. As the mochi melts, slowly add more water until you get a cheesy consistency. Add a few sprinkles of shoyu and mirin, or to taste. When it's all melted, pour on top of the squash, let the dish simmer for 1 or 2 minutes, and then serve.

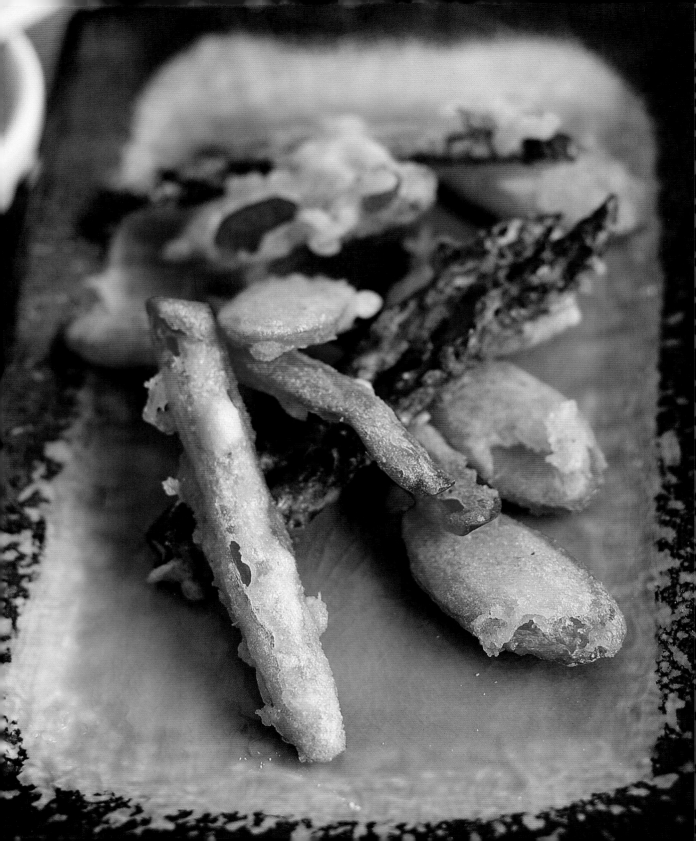

The Art of Making Tempura

Each batter recipe is enough for 12 to 20 pieces of tempura, depending on the size of the vegetable or the cut-up ingredient

This information is from Simone Parris, a MILF currently living in India. Her sweet and soothing voice comes through in her recipes. Tempura is best when made with high-quality vegetable oil and very fresh vegetables.

The best type of vessel for deep-frying is a thick, old-fashioned copper pot, a heavy cast-iron Dutch oven, or a deep skillet. You can also use a heavy stainless-steel pan; but remember, the thinner the pan, the less well it will hold the heat, and your tempura will come out less crispy, or even soggy.

The temperature of the oil needs to remain fairly constant at all times, between 350° and 375°F or 180° and 190°C. If you do not have a thermometer, heat the oil and drop a little batter into it. If the batter stays on the bottom, the oil is not hot enough. If the batter hits the bottom and comes up fairly quickly, it is hot enough. If the oil smokes, it is too hot and should be discarded. Start again with fresh oil.

Hundreds of different vegetables and fruits can be cooked tempura-style. Some of my favorites are carrots, cauliflower, broccoli, Brussels sprouts, mushrooms, string beans, parsley, onions, pumpkin (winter squash), sweet potatoes, zucchini flowers, kombu sea vegetable, seitan, tofu, apples, bananas, and many more!

Also, seafood such as shrimp, haddock, sole, squid, clams, oysters, smelt, and others can be deep-fried in basically the same manner.

TEMPURA BATTER NUMBER 1
$2/3$ cup unbleached white or whole wheat flour
$1/3$ cup cornstarch
$1/4$ teaspoon fine sea salt
$1/2$ cup cold beer
$1/2$ to 1 cup spring or filtered water
Sunflower oil or safflower oil (see Note)

TEMPURA BATTER NUMBER 2
$1/2$ cup unbleached white or whole wheat flour
$1/2$ cup sweet rice or rice flour
1 tablespoon cornstarch
$1/2$ teaspoon baking powder
$1/4$ teaspoon sea salt
1 to $1 1/4$ cups spring or filtered water
Sunflower oil or safflower oil (see Note)

---

1. Mix together the dry ingredients. Add the liquids and stir briefly. (It doesn't matter whether or not the batter is smooth; a few lumps mean crunchier tempura.) Refrigerate for at least 20 minutes before using.

2. Once you have rinsed the vegetables and cut them into large pieces (you might keep some whole, like mushrooms and green beans), place one type of vegetable at a time in an airtight plastic container. Add a few tablespoons of unbleached white flour, and once you have fastened the lid, shake well. Remove each piece, shaking well to get rid of the excess flour, and place on a platter.

3. Heat the oil in a deep, heavy pot over medium-high heat. When the temperature is between 350° and 375°F on a deep-fry thermometer, or when a dollop of batter rises to the surface quickly, you are ready to make tempura.

4. Dip the flour-coated vegetables into the batter quickly and drop gently into the hot oil. Some of the batter will separate from the vegetables when they are added to the hot oil. If too much separates, the batter is too thin. Simply add a little more flour. If none of the batter separates, the batter is probably too thick. Just add a little more water to thin it out.

5. Fry as many vegetables at once as you can without crowding the pot. When the batter appears golden and is crispy-looking, use a slotted spoon or tongs to remove the vegetables one at a time to a stack of paper towels or a paper bag to drain. Serve immediately, with one of the following dipping sauces, which not only are delicious but also aid in digestion. Serve your choice of sauce in small bowls. Each person should have his or her own dish of the sauce to dip the tempura in.

SHOYU-DAIKON DIPPING SAUCE
¼ teaspoon grated daikon
1 tablespoon shoyu
2 tablespoons spring water

SHOYU-GINGER DIPPING SAUCE
⅛ teaspoon grated fresh ginger
1 tablespoon shoyu

2 tablespoons spring water

SWEET GINGER–SHOYU DIPPING SAUCE
1 teaspoon fresh ginger juice
1 tablespoon shoyu
1 teaspoon rice syrup, or to taste
2 tablespoons spring water

Whisk together! Each recipe serves 1 as a personal dipping sauce.

NOTE: I have found that organic sunflower oil or organic safflower oil works best for tempura. If you live in a hot climate, try organic coconut oil.

VARIATION: Grated daikon (about 1 tablespoon with 1 drop of shoyu poured on it, for each person) can be served instead of the dipping sauce or in addition to the dipping sauce.

TIPS: To clean the oil, use an oil skimmer to remove chunks of batter debris. Also, you can drop an umeboshi plum pit into the hot oil and deep-fry it until it becomes charred. This will remove any odors from the oil. For instance, if fish has previously been deep-fried, it is desirable to remove the fish odor before frying vegetables.
   The oil can be stored in a glass jar. It should be tightly covered and kept in a cool, dark place. I find I can usually reuse the oil 4 or 5 times—depending on what I am frying. When the oil gets a dark hue or smells bad, discard and start fresh.

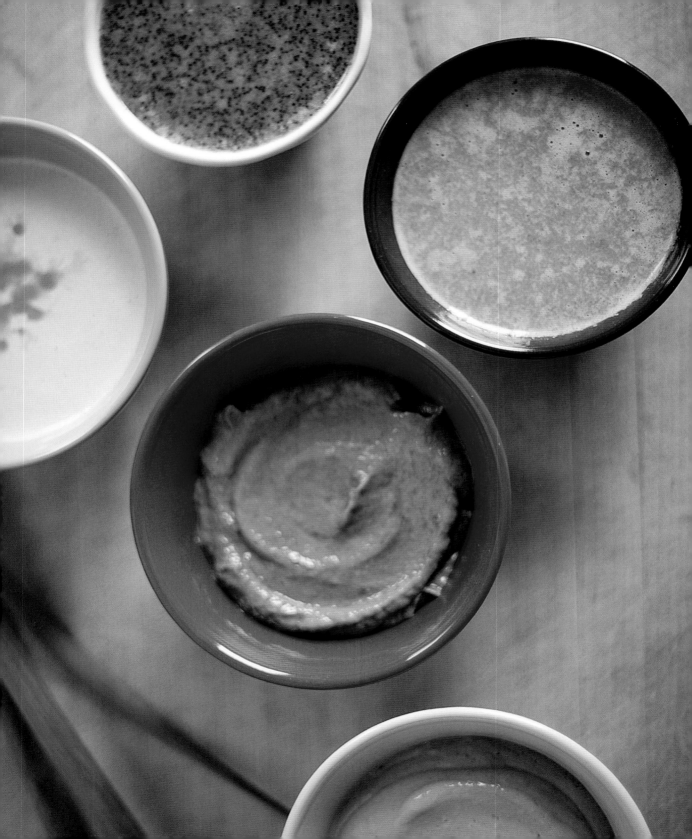

Umeboshi Pickles
Serves 6

6 red radishes, rinsed and thinly sliced   ¾ cup spring water
¼ cup umeboshi vinegar

1. Place the radish slices in a Pyrex cup or a mason jar. Cover with a piece of cheesecloth and secure with a rubber band. Pour the brine through the cheesecloth, being sure to cover all the slices. FYI: No matter the amount, the brine ratio is 1 part vinegar to 3 parts water.

2. Place the jar in an unhurried, room-temperature spot in the kitchen. Let it sit for 1 day. Using a clean utensil, remove some lightly pickled radishes, as needed, over the next 3 days. If they are really salty, give them a quick rinse.

3. After 3 days, pour off the brine and store the leftover pickles in a ziplock bag and refrigerate; they should last for a week or so. Or just start another batch; there's no reason not to have some light pickles going all the time.

VARIATIONS: This recipe can be used with carrots, onions, broccoli, cauliflower, daikon, turnips, or any other relatively hearty vegetable. And you can pickle a bunch of vegetables in one jar together.
Do this recipe the same way using shoyu instead of umeboshi vinegar.

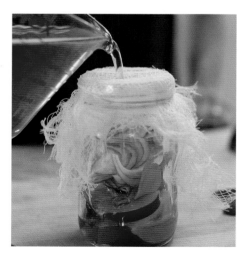

Miso Pickles

These are fun and very easy.

A variety of root vegetables   **A crock or jar full of miso**

---

1. Rinse the vegetables under running water, scrubbing with a vegetable brush. Let them sit, whole, in a cool, shaded place for about a day, until they soften a little. Ideally, you should be able to bend each vegetable into a curve.

2. If you are pickling whole vegetables, cut a number of slits in each root. Otherwise, cut the vegetables into medium-thick diagonal slices. Place the vegetables in the miso so that they are completely covered.

3. The sliced vegetables will be done in 3 to 7 days, and whole vegetables will take 1 to 2 weeks. Rinse before serving and take only small amounts, for these pickles are very strong.

Beans and Other Proteins

Bean Cooking Tips

Soaking: Most beans need to be soaked for 3 to 8 hours before cooking. The exceptions are lentils, split peas, and mung beans, which need no soaking.

Kombu: Beans taste better, soften faster, and don't become as gas-producing when cooked with kombu sea vegetable. Just an inch of dried kombu per pot of beans should suffice. You can soak it beforehand and slice it up, or just place it in the pot whole and pull it out at the end if it hasn't disintegrated.

Boiling: If you are boiling your beans, use 3 to 3½ cups of water per cup of soaked beans. Bring to a boil and let simmer until tender. Most beans take between 45 and 90 minutes. You can also just cover the beans with water and check them regularly. When they get dry, add cold water, as needed, by pouring it carefully down the side of the pot.

Pressure-Cooking: If you are pressure-cooking your beans, just cover the beans with about an inch of water, bring them to a boil, skim off any foam that rises, and place the lid on the pressure cooker. Let it come up to full pressure, then reduce the heat and let the pressure come down to a quiet, intermittent hiss. Let cook for 30 to 60 minutes, depending on the bean. Remove from the heat and let the pressure come down naturally. Open the pressure cooker and season the beans, letting them simmer 5 more minutes (if using shoyu or miso) or 10 more minutes (if using sea salt).

Seasoning: Whether you're boiling or pressure-cooking, you should never season beans before they are tender. Salt is yang, and if introduced too early—at the beginning of cooking—it will keep beans hard and contracted. Use seasonings only at the end of cooking.

Other Bean Products

In this section, you will be introduced to tofu, tempeh, and seitan. Technically, seitan (pronounced "say-tan") is not a bean product, as it's made from wheat gluten, but it belongs in this section because it's remarkably high in protein and is used as a meat substitute.

Tofu: Made from soybeans, tofu is incredibly versatile. It comes in different consistencies (silken, soft, firm, and extra-firm) and can be used in a million different ways. Because it's quick and convenient, tofu has become the go-to protein for many vegans and vegetarians, but I discourage MILFs from treating it that way. Enjoy its ease of use, but don't make it a substitute for other bean dishes. Whereas long-cooked bean dishes are warming, hearty, and give long-lasting energy, tofu is cooling to the body and should be used only a couple of times a week.

Tempeh: This wonderful food from Indonesia is made from soybeans as well, although these are fermented. Dense and satisfying, tempeh is great in many different forms: deep fried, as "bacon," in stews, or even as the principal food in the "tuna" salad on page 160. No matter how you season or finish it, tempeh needs to be steamed, boiled, or pressure-cooked for 20 minutes at some point in the process in order to be well digested.

Seitan: This spongy mass of wheat protein might sound weird, but it tastes great. Made from flour that has been kneaded and rinsed until only the gluten remains, it is then cooked in a salty broth. *Mmmm.* Seitan is a great meat substitute. It's delicious in stews, panfried, dipped in sauces, and in sandwiches. It's also really easy to make at home. But I'll save that for my next book . . . *Selling My Soul to Seitan*!

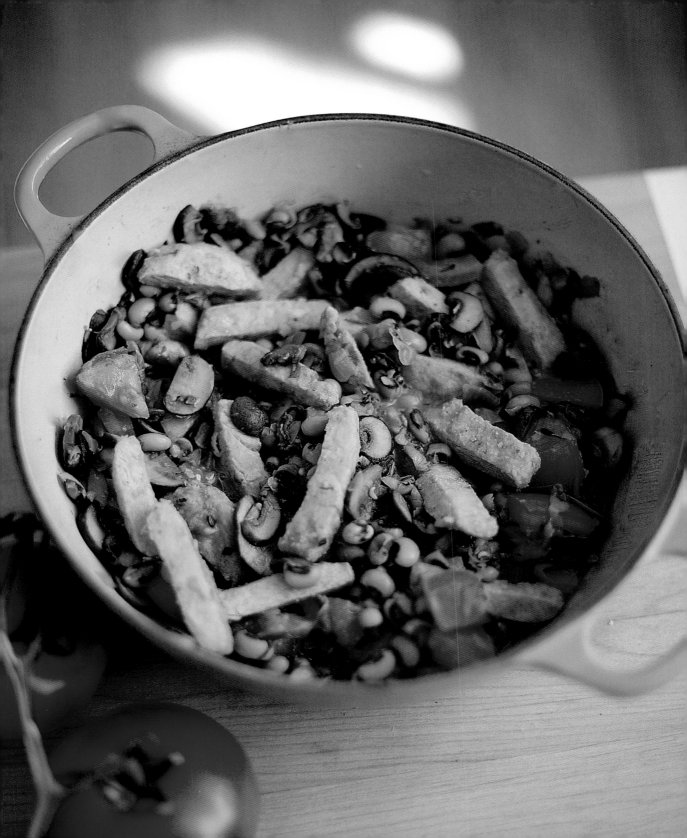

Black-Eyed Peas with "Chicken"

Serves 4

This recipe is oddly good. There's something about black-eyed peas; they have a mild but distinct taste. Add to them the chewy fried "chicken" and a hint of marjoram and thyme, and it's a really nice, unique dish.

1 cup black-eyed peas, soaked in spring water overnight
One 1-inch strip of kombu
2 teaspoons shoyu
1 package Gardein "chicken" strips, or ½ box WestSoy chicken-style seitan
½ cup whole wheat flour
1 teaspoon sea salt
¼ teaspoon ground black pepper

3 tablespoons safflower oil (or more if needed), for frying
1 small onion, chopped
1 pound fresh mushrooms, sliced
2 cloves garlic, finely chopped
1 teaspoon dried thyme
½ teaspoon dried marjoram
½ cup white wine or vegetable stock
1 medium tomato, chopped (optional)

1. Discard the bean soaking water. Bring the beans, kombu, and fresh water to cover to a boil in a medium saucepan. Skim off any foam on the surface. Cover and simmer for 45 minutes to 1 hour, checking the beans regularly and adding water when necessary. When the beans are soft, season with the shoyu and let simmer for 5 more minutes. Remove from the heat.

2. Cut up the "chicken" into serving-size pieces. Season the flour with ½ teaspoon of the salt and the pepper and coat the "chicken." Heat the oil, and brown the "chicken" pieces on all sides. Remove from heat and set aside. Add the onion, mushrooms, and garlic to the skillet and cook until tender, stirring occasionally. Stir in the herbs, the remaining ½ teaspoon salt, the wine, and the black-eyed peas (drained of most of their liquid if they are watery). Return the "chicken" pieces to the skillet, top with the tomato (if using), and cover the pan tightly. Simmer for 10 minutes. Serve from the pan.

Tempeh-Collard Wraps with Peanut Sauce

Serves 4 to 6

This recipe is from Melanie Brown Waxman, Philadelphia MILF and mother of seven. It is a great combination of tastes: sour, salty, sweet, and pungent, and the collard greens have a slight bitterness. Very satisfying.

4 to 6 collard green leaves
One 8-ounce package tempeh, cut into
  squares
One 1-inch strip of kombu
1 to 2 tablespoons shoyu
1 teaspoon minced fresh ginger
Dijon or whole-grain mustard
Safflower oil, for deep-frying
1 tablespoon sauerkraut

1 tablespoon grated carrot

PEANUT SAUCE
1 tablespoon creamy peanut butter
1 tablespoon mirin
1 to 2 tablespoons shoyu
1 tablespoon fresh orange juice
1 to 2 tablespoons spring water

1. Place water in a saucepan and bring to a boil. Lightly blanch the collard greens for 2 to 3 minutes, drain, and place on a plate.

2. Place the tempeh and kombu in a saucepan. Add enough water to cover. Bring to a boil, then add the shoyu and ginger. Simmer for about 20 minutes. Remove, drain, and spread 1 side of each tempeh square with mustard.

3. Meanwhile, pour oil into a deep, heavy pot and warm slowly over low heat. Before deep-frying the tempeh, increase the heat to medium. Test whether the oil is hot enough by dropping a small piece of tempeh into the hot oil. If the tempeh sizzles immediately on the surface, the oil is hot enough.

4. Deep-fry the tempeh until golden, about 3 minutes. Remove and drain on a paper bag or paper towels.

5. Place all of the ingredients for the peanut sauce in a bowl. Whisk to a smooth, creamy texture.

6. Place some of the tempeh, sauerkraut, and carrot in the middle of each collard leaf. Drizzle the peanut sauce on top. Fold up the sides of the leaf and roll to make a wrap. Cut in half and serve.

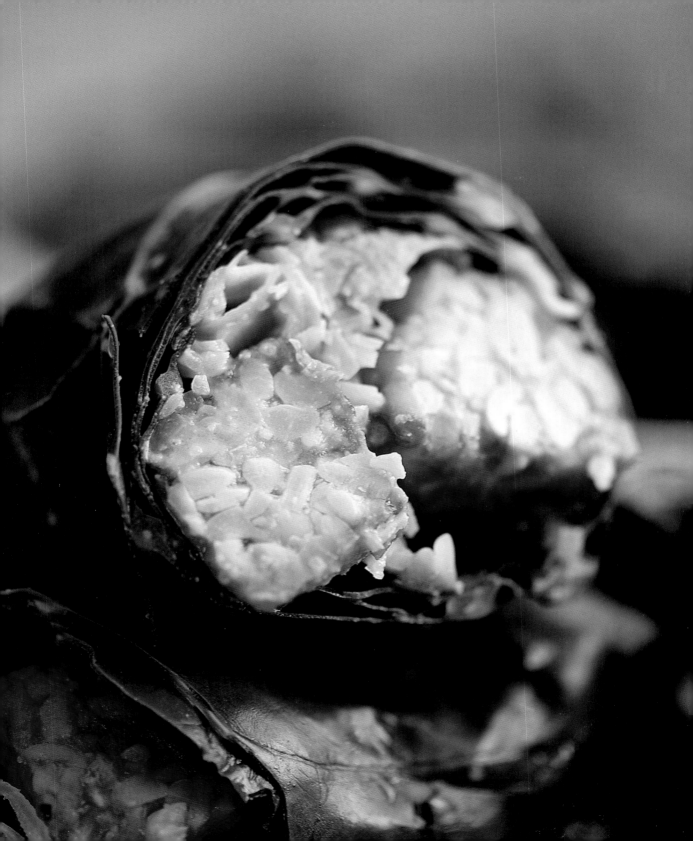

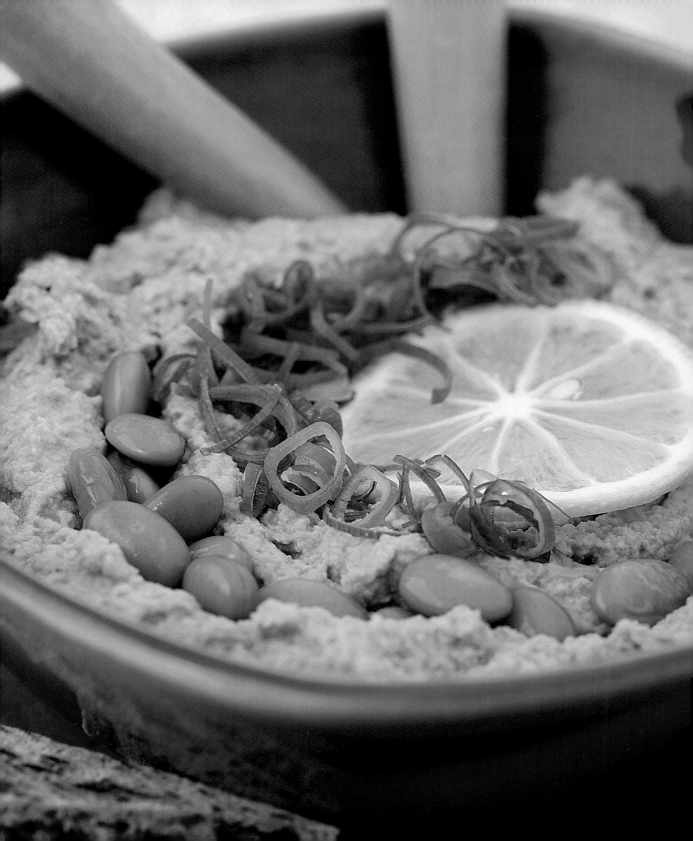

Edamame Dip

Serves 4

This recipe, donated by Sarah Loring, surprised me. I didn't expect such a strong, dynamic, and *yowza* taste from simple edamame. It's *really* good.

One 10-ounce package frozen organic shelled edamame

Sea salt

2 teaspoons shoyu

2 teaspoons brown rice vinegar

1 to 2 teaspoons toasted sesame oil

½ teaspoon minced fresh ginger

1 clove garlic, minced

⅛ teaspoon red pepper flakes

1 scallion, thinly sliced

1. Place the edamame in a steamer basket in a small pot. Add water to just under the basket. Sprinkle a pinch of salt over the beans. Cover. Bring to a boil and steam for 20 minutes. Remove from the heat and transfer to a dish to cool slightly.

2. Place the cooked edamame in a food processor. Add all of the remaining ingredients except the scallion. Process until smooth. If you need to add a little water to loosen it up, go for it. Taste and adjust the seasonings, if desired.

3. The scallion can be mixed into the dip or used as a garnish. This is great served with rice crackers.

You-Ain't-Kidding Kidney Beans

Serves 8

This dish combines the heartiness of kidney beans with the chewiness of seitan and the freshness of green beans, all topped with a lovely parsley sauce. Howard Wallen made it up, and his daughter, Hana, declares it a favorite.

---

2 cups dried kidney beans, soaked in spring water overnight
4 cups spring water
One 2-inch strip kombu
1 bay leaf
Sea salt
1½ cups 1-inch pieces green beans, sliced diagonally
1 tablespoon toasted sesame oil
1 small (or ½ medium) red onion, sliced into quarter moons
1 cup sliced shiitake mushrooms (optional)

1 package seitan, cut into bite-size dice
8 dandelion greens leaves, chopped into 1-inch pieces (avoid the tough bottoms of the stalks)
1 tablespoon shoyu

DRESSING
2 cups reserved bean cooking liquid
½ bunch fresh parsley
1 tablespoon umeboshi paste

Dash of umeboshi vinegar

---

1. Bring the drained kidney beans, the 4 cups water, the kombu, and bay leaf to a boil in an uncovered pressure cooker. Skim off any foam that might form. Cover the pressure cooker and bring to full pressure. Reduce the heat and simmer for 35 minutes. Remove from the heat and let the pressure come down fully. Uncover the pressure cooker and add 1 teaspoon salt; simmer for 10 more minutes over low heat. Remove bay leaf and discard. Drain the beans, but keep the cooking liquid.

2. In a small saucepan of boiling water, cook the green beans for 1 minute or so. Remove from the water and set aside.

3. In a skillet, heat the sesame oil and sauté the onion with a pinch of salt until the onion is soft and releases some of its moisture. Add the shiitakes, if using, and another pinch of salt. Add the seitan, dandelion leaves, and the shoyu. Stir well to integrate the ingredients. Cover and simmer for 3 minutes over low heat. This sauté should be a little salty.

4. Blend the dressing ingredients in a blender and adjust the seasoning to taste.

5. Toss the kidney beans, green beans, dressing, and sautéed vegetables together. Mix well and add a dash of umeboshi vinegar. This tastes even better if the ingredients are allowed to sit and blend their flavors for an hour or so. Great the next day.

Adzuki Beans with Winter Squash

Serves 6

This is a simple, delicious, and healing recipe. The adzuki beans are a tonic to your poor kidneys, which take quite a battering thanks to meat, sugar, alcohol, cold drinks, caffeine, and stress. Combined with the sweet squash, which helps to stabilize your blood sugar, this dish packs a medicinal punch. Kombu, the sea vegetable used to help soften the beans, is rich in nourishing minerals.

One 2- to 4-inch piece of kombu, soaked in spring water for 5 to 10 minutes
1 cup adzuki beans, soaked in spring water overnight

Spring water
2 cups winter squash chunks (unpeeled if organic)
1 teaspoon shoyu

1. After soaking the kombu and beans, discard both soaking liquids. Slice the reconstituted kombu into 1 by 1-inch squares and place it on the bottom of a heavy pot with a heavy lid, preferably enameled cast iron.

2. Add the beans on top of the kombu. Add fresh spring water to just cover the beans. Bring to a boil uncovered. When the water boils, skim off any foam that might be floating on top. Let the beans boil for about 5 minutes uncovered, as this allows the gases to release into the air, and not through you later on. Cover the pot, place a flame deflector beneath it, and reduce the heat to a simmer. Cook the beans for about 40 minutes, adding water when the liquid appears to dip down below the bean level. Check the beans every 10 minutes or so.

3. Add the squash on top of the beans and add more water (to cover the beans) if necessary. Cook for another 20 minutes. When the beans seem soft and tender, add the shoyu and cook for 10 more minutes. Gently stir the mixture to integrate the seasoning, but not so much that you break the larger chunks of squash. Serve.

VARIATIONS: Add the squash from the beginning of the simmering of the beans. This will make the squash melt more into the beans, creating a softer dish.

Use carrots instead of squash.

Add corn kernels at the end for an even sweeter dish.

Tempeh "Tuna"

Serves 3 or 4

Because tuna is high in mercury, it's important to let it go. But don't despair; this is a great substitute for tuna salad and is perfect in a sandwich, in a salad, or right off the spoon.

One 8-ounce package tempeh, cut into chunks
2½ tablespoons umeboshi vinegar
2½ cups spring water, or to cover tempeh
⅓ cup Vegenaise

Any spices you desire—cumin, curry, paprika, saffron (optional)
Freshly ground black pepper (optional)
1 stalk celery, diced
Small handful of chives, thinly sliced

1. Bring the tempeh, the umeboshi vinegar, and water to cover to a boil in a saucepan. Reduce the heat to low and simmer for 20 minutes. Remove from the heat, drain the excess liquid, and let the tempeh cool for a few minutes.

2. Mash with a potato masher or fork until there are no longer any big chunks, but the tempeh is not entirely smooth. Let it cool completely.

3. Add the Vegenaise, seasonings, celery, and chives. Mix well. Serve with pita bread or as a sandwich.

VARIATIONS: Add any herb or spice you like. Tempeh works well with everything.

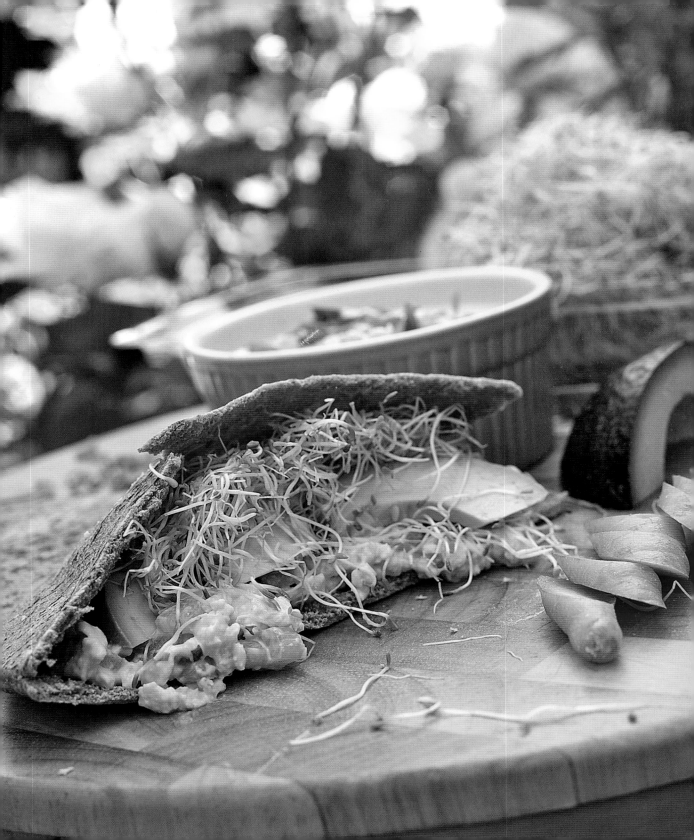

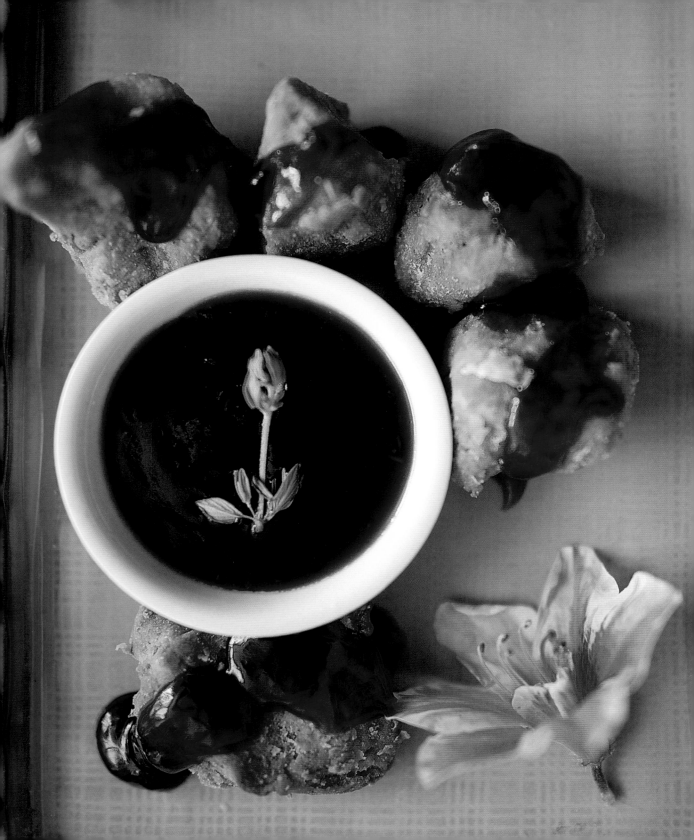

Deep-Fried Seitan with Sweet-and-Sour Hibiscus Dipping Sauce

Serves 2 or 3

Deep-fried seitan feels sinful. . . . Savory, chewy, and crispy, it is very satisfying. With this elegant dipping sauce as its perfect complement, this is an easy and fun dish to serve the whole family. Try it with some brown basmati rice and a fresh salad.

SWEET-AND-SOUR HIBISCUS DIPPING SAUCE
2 tablespoons olive oil
2 large shallots, minced
Pinch of sea salt
¼ cup dried hibiscus flowers
2 cups white wine (or water)
1 teaspoon umeboshi vinegar
2 tablespoons soy margarine

¼ cup brown rice syrup
2 teaspoons kuzu root starch
2 tablespoons cold spring water
Leaves from 2 or 3 sprigs of fresh thyme

1 package WestSoy seitan
Safflower oil
Unbleached white flour, for dredging

1. To prepare the sauce, heat the olive oil in a small saucepan. Add the shallots and salt, stirring until the shallots are soft. Add the hibiscus flowers and stir over low heat for a couple of minutes. Add the wine and umeboshi vinegar, bring to a boil, and simmer until reduced by about half. The liquid should be a nice burgundy color.

2. Strain the mixture to remove the flowers and shallots. Return to low heat. Add the margarine and rice syrup, stirring well to blend. Dissolve the kuzu in the cold water and add to the sauce, stirring constantly. Bring to a boil, allowing the kuzu to thicken the sauce, and then simmer for 1 minute. Add the thyme and simmer for 1 more minute.

3. To prepare the seitan, remove it from the package, draining off the excess liquid. Heat about ½ inch of safflower oil in a heavy or stainless-steel skillet over medium heat. Do not let it smoke. Dredge the pieces of seitan in the flour and place in the hot oil. Let the pieces of seitan fry for 2 to 3 minutes before flipping and cooking the other side. Let drain on parchment paper or paper towels.

4. Dip the fried seitan in the sweet-and-sour hibiscus sauce. Delicious!

Burrito Bar

MILFy Sarah Loring gives us a great lesson in burrito making: "This is a great quick lunch or light supper made from leftovers and whatever you have on hand. It is a familiar way to introduce your kids to the sustenance of eating grains and beans. After I make the filling, I put a variety of toppings out and let each child choose their own creation. If they don't have a good burrito-rolling technique, I take a minute and give them assistance and instruction so they can make their own.

"About 1 cup of rice and beans make a hearty burrito. You can use more beans or rice in the proportion you like.

"Make the filling with grains and beans, adding seasonings and veggies as desired. You can warm or toast the tortillas in the oven or over an open flame. Set up the toppings on the table or counter. Give each person a plate with a tortilla and a scoop of filling, and let him or her choose the rest.

"Any leftover filling can be rolled into a tortilla, wrapped in parchment and then foil, and frozen. For lunch, thaw in the fridge the night before and warm for 15 to 20 minutes in a toaster oven. Rewrap and go."

---

1 teaspoon olive oil per 2 cups rice and beans

OPTIONAL VEGGIE ADDITIONS
Diced onion
Diced bell pepper
Diced tomato
Fresh corn kernels
Chopped fresh cilantro

OPTIONAL SEASONING ADDITIONS
(FOR EVERY 2 CUPS OF RICE AND BEANS)
½ teaspoon ground cumin
¼ teaspoon ground coriander
1 teaspoon chopped garlic
1 teaspoon chili powder
2 teaspoons dried oregano or basil
⅛ teaspoon salt
Pinch of freshly ground black pepper

FILLINGS
Leftover rice or quinoa
Leftover black beans, or a can of black beans, drained

Large whole wheat tortillas (or sprouted corn, or spinach, or whatever you want)

SOME TOPPING IDEAS
Salsa (store-bought or homemade)
Chopped avocado
Chopped red onion
Chopped fresh cilantro or scallions
Grated nondairy cheese
Toasted pumpkin seeds

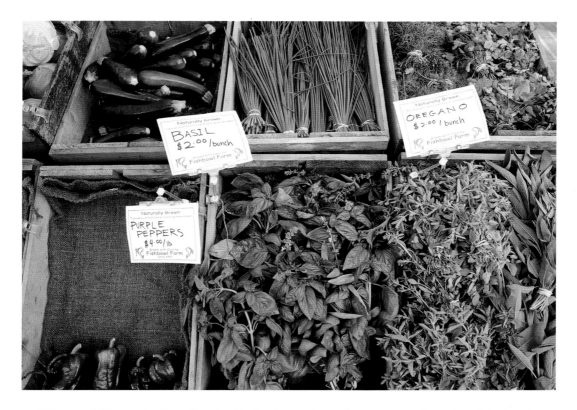

Warm a skillet with olive oil and add the chopped veggies and seasonings. Sauté for 5 minutes (stirring frequently), then add the rice and beans. Continue to cook for a few minutes, until the mixture is thoroughly heated. Taste and adjust the seasonings. Serve the filling on individual plates with the tortillas, with the toppings within reach.

Garbanzo Bean Burgers

Serves 6 to 8

Maine MILF Lisa Silverman contributed this total hit. I always find a way to get invited over when she serves these burgers.

1½ cups garbanzo beans, soaked for 6 to 8 hours
One 1-inch piece kombu
About 4½ cups spring water
½ cup old-fashioned rolled oats, ground into flour, or quick-cooking rolled oats
2 dill pickles, finely chopped
1 medium carrot, finely diced and blanched
1 medium red onion, minced and blanched

2 teaspoons umeboshi vinegar
1 tablespoon brown rice syrup
2 teaspoons Dijon or whole-grain mustard
2 teaspoons white miso
Cornmeal and ½ teaspoon sea salt, for dredging
3 tablespoons safflower oil, plus extra as needed

---

1. Cook the garbanzo beans and kombu together in the fresh water to cover for 45 minutes in a pressure cooker, or 1½ hours in a heavy pot. Once the beans are cooked, drain them and mash them with a potato masher. Mix in the oats, pickles, carrot, and onion. Blend together the vinegar, brown rice syrup, mustard, and miso, and add to the mixture.

2. Form into patties, and dredge in the cornmeal and salt. Heat the oil over medium heat. Fry the patties for 4 minutes per side. When the oil is gone, add more to the pan for the next round of patties.

NOTE: This mixture freezes well for later use.

Sea Vegetables

Baked Wakame

Serves 6 to 8

Because this wakame recipe contains more oil and seasoning, and is baked, it's a better choice for fall and winter, when we need to keep warm and toasty. It's easy and very delicious.

½ cup wakame pieces, well rinsed in cold
   water and drained
1 tablespoon sesame oil
2 cups sliced onions
Pinch of salt

⅔ cup tahini
2 tablespoons shoyu
2 cups spring water
¼ cup toasted sesame seeds

1. Preheat the oven to 350°F. Soak the wakame in cold water for 10 to 15 minutes.

2. Meanwhile, in a large skillet, heat the oil and sauté the onions with the salt until the onions are soft.

3. Drain the wakame. Set aside.

4. In a large bowl, stir together the tahini, shoyu, and 2 cups water. Mix in the drained wakame and the sautéed onion.

5. Turn the mixture into a 9 by 12-inch baking pan and sprinkle the seeds on top. Bake, covered, for 50 minutes. Serve immediately.

Refreshing Summer Wakame Salad

Serves 4

This recipe is from Eliza Eller of Alaska, where the summers are short but burn bright.

---

3 small Persian cucumbers, or 1 large cucumber
½ teaspoon sea salt
¼ cup wakame pieces, soaked in cold water for 10 minutes and drained

1 orange, peeled, sectioned, and cut into bite-size pieces
Dash of brown rice vinegar

Slice the cucumbers thinly and add the salt. Massage the cucumber slices until they become moist, releasing their water. Add the wakame and orange and let sit for 1 hour in the bowl, using a smaller, weighted bowl to press on the mixture. After an hour, drain the excess juice, toss the salad with the vinegar, and serve. Very refreshing!

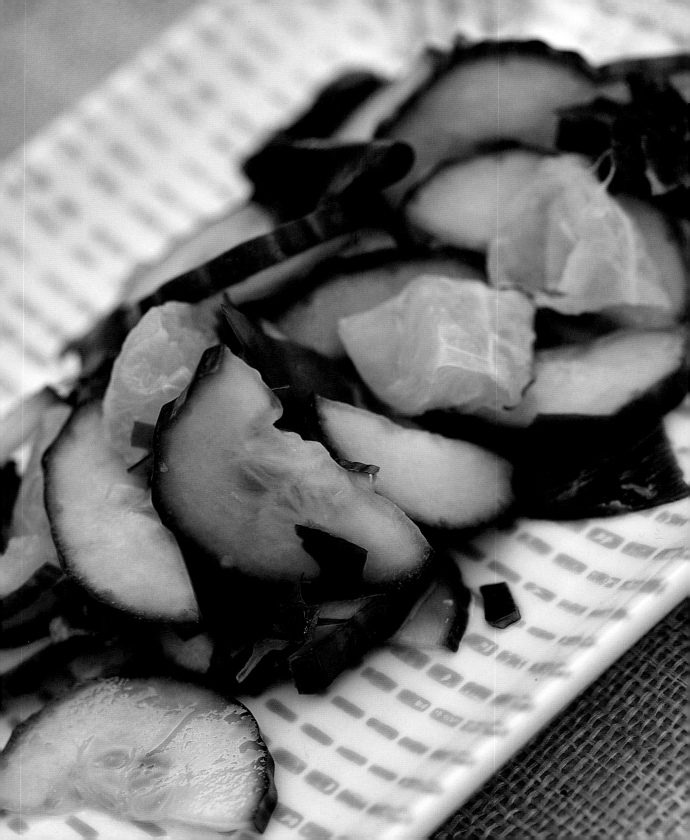

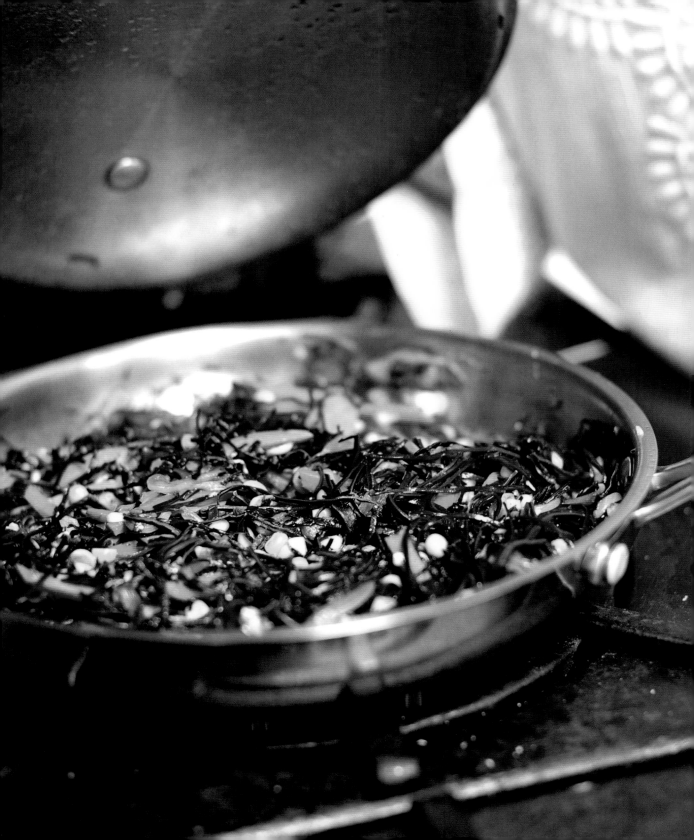

Arame with Onion, Carrot, and Corn

Serves 2 or 3

Arame is a delicate sea vegetable that goes really well with sweet vegetables. It's not too strong or fishy-tasting, so the whole family should enjoy this dish.

½ ounce arame (¼ of an average 2-ounce package)
1 tablespoon olive oil
1 medium onion, diced

Sea salt
1 medium carrot, cut into matchsticks
Kernels from 1 ear fresh corn
1 to 2 teaspoons shoyu

1. Rinse the arame and soak for 2 minutes. Drain and set aside.

2. In a skillet, heat the olive oil over medium heat and add the onion and a pinch of salt. Sauté the onion until it is translucent. Add the carrot and a tiny pinch of salt and continue to sauté until the matchsticks are slightly soft.

3. Lay the arame evenly over the onion and carrot and add water to come halfway up the vegetables. Bring to a boil, cover, and reduce the heat. Simmer for 10 minutes.

4. Add the corn kernels and shoyu, and if there is still lots of liquid, keep the lid off and cook for 5 more minutes, or until the liquid is almost gone. Mix and serve.

Hijiki, Fresh Corn, and Tofu Salad on Arugula with Toasted Sesame Dressing

Serves 4 to 6

Hijiki is so mineral-rich that it's really the granddaddy of sea vegetables. Make either a hijiki or an arame dish once a week, with enough to serve at lunch the next day. Two small servings of a sea vegetable will keep your bones strong and your hair nice and shiny. Meredith McCarty created this lovely dish.

¼ cup hijiki seaweed (about ½ ounce)
Kernels from 2 large ears fresh yellow or bicolored corn
6 ounces fresh firm tofu, cut into ½-inch cubes
3 scallions, thinly sliced

TOASTED SESAME VINAIGRETTE
2 tablespoons brown rice vinegar
1 tablespoon shoyu

1 tablespoon mirin (Japanese sweet rice cooking wine)
1 teaspoon toasted sesame oil
⅛ teaspoon shichimi, Japanese powdered chili pepper blend (optional)

2 ounces arugula, cut into 2-inch pieces (3 to 4 cups)
2 teaspoons sesame seeds, toasted

1. Soak the hijiki in 1 cup hot water for 30 minutes. Drain, reserving the mineral-rich liquid for your plants.

2. In a 2-quart saucepan, bring 2 cups water to a boil. Add the corn and tofu, and cook for 3 to 5 minutes. Drain, reserving the stock and returning it to the pan. Add the hijiki and cook for 2 to 3 minutes. Drain. Cut the hijiki into bite-size pieces if the strands are very long. Mix together the hijiki, corn, tofu, and scallions.

3. Mix together the dressing ingredients and toss with the salad.

4. Serve on a bed of arugula. Sprinkle the sesame seeds on top.

VARIATION: Substitute watercress or shredded lettuce for the arugula.

Nori Rolls

Makes 6 rolls, 48 pieces

Nori rolls aren't really a sea vegetable dish per se, because they also contain grains, vegetables, and often bean products, but they are a lovely way to get your nori. Rolling sushi takes some practice, so go easy on yourself. No matter how sloppy your experiments may be, they will still be delicious!

---

3 cups short-grain brown rice
5 cups spring water
¼ teaspoon sea salt
2 tablespoons plus 1 teaspoon mirin
1 teaspoon brown rice vinegar
2 tablespoons toasted sesame oil
One 8-ounce package tempeh,
  cut into 6 strips

2 tablespoons shoyu
2 medium or large carrots, cut into 6 long
  strips
3 scallions, cut in half lengthwise
¼ cup tahini
1 to 2 teaspoons umeboshi paste
6 sheets nori
1 ripe avocado, cut into 12 slices

---

1. Bring the rice and 4½ cups of the water to a boil in a pressure cooker. When boiling, add the salt, cover the pressure cooker, and bring to full pressure. When it's hissing strongly, reduce the heat and place a flame deflector under the pressure cooker. You should hear only a quiet hissing when the pressure is full but the heat is reduced. Cook for 50 minutes. Remove from the heat. Let the pressure come down completely. Remove the rice and set aside to cool. When cooled, mix together 1 teaspoon of the mirin and the brown rice vinegar and sprinkle into the rice as you mix it well.

2. Meanwhile, heat the oil in a skillet over medium heat and add the tempeh strips. Brown them on all sides, reducing the heat if necessary—don't let the oil smoke. Mix the shoyu and the remaining 2 tablespoons mirin with the remaining ½ cup water and pour the mixture over the browned tempeh. Reduce the heat to low and simmer for 20 minutes. Check the tempeh a couple of times to make sure the liquid hasn't completely cooked off before the 20 minutes have elapsed. If it has, add a tiny bit of water to keep it moist.

3. While the tempeh is cooking, bring a pot of water to a boil. Add first the carrots and then the scallions. The carrot strips need about 1 minute and the scallions only about 15 seconds. Remove from the water and set aside.

4. Mix the tahini and 1 teaspoon umeboshi paste and taste to see if it's seasoned to your liking. Add a second teaspoon of umboshi paste if you'd like it to taste stronger.

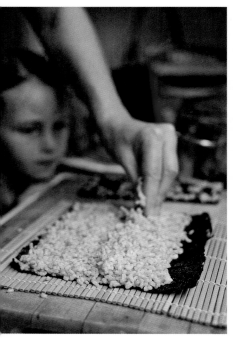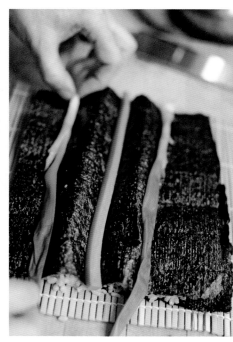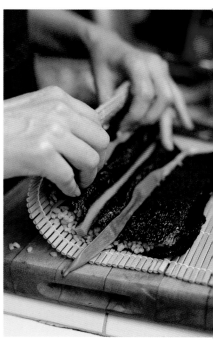

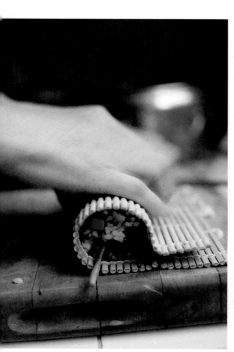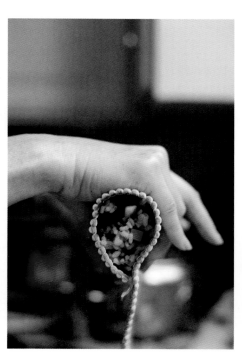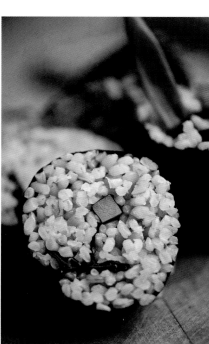

5. To assemble the rolls, have at the ready the nori sheets, a bowl of warm water, the cooled rice, the tahini-umeboshi mixture, the tempeh strips, the carrot strips, the scallions, and the avocado slices.

6. Lay your sushi mat in front of you. Place a sheet of nori, horizontally and shiny side down, on the mat. With wet fingers, take about ½ cup rice and press it onto the sheet of nori, spreading it about ½ inch thick, all the way to the sides, but leaving about a ½-inch margin along the edge nearest you and a 1- to 2-inch margin along the far edge. As you get better at rolling sushi, you may use less rice, and even half-sheets of nori, but for now, we're using training wheels. FYI: The sushi roll being made in the photos opposite is a decorative variation called flower sushi. For regular sushi, follow these written instructions and roll as shown in the photos.

7. With a spoon, spread a line of the tahini-umboshi mixture across the rice, about 1 inch from the margin nearest you. Place a strip of tempeh, a strip of carrot, and some scallion along the line as well. Add 2 slices of avocado.

8. Now it's time to roll: Using your thumbs on the outside of the sushi mat while your fingers steady the rice-vegetable filling and guide the nori, begin to roll the sushi mat away from you. This will bring the sheet of nori and its contents with it, so be sure to use your fingers to tuck the nori back into the rice when it starts to become a cylinder and to carefully release pressure on the sushi mat at the same time. You should be able to continue to roll the cylinder of sushi while simultaneously releasing the top side of the sushi mat so that it doesn't get caught up in the food. The mat serves as a stabilizer and a guide for the sheet of nori.

9. When you get to the far edge of the nori, wet your finger and drag it along the exposed edge of the nori. This will make the exposed nori stick to the rest of the roll. Continue rolling to seal the sushi. Hopefully, your mat has come with you and you can squeeze the whole roll in your mat to make it nice and tight.

10. Remove the sushi mat and slice the roll in half with a wet vegetable knife. Then slice each half again, and again, to make 8 pieces. Wet the knife before each cut so that the rice will not stick to the knife.

VARIATION: Flower Sushi: Cover a sheet of nori, using the aforementioned margins, with a layer of rice. Then make two little mountain ranges of rice on top of it, running horizontally, so that a valley is created between them. Place another half sheet of nori, running horizontally as well, over these mountains, and push it down into the valley. Place a carrot strip in the valley and half a scallion on the outside edges of the mountain ranges. Holding everything carefully in place, roll the sushi as above. Slice, and they should look like flowers as in the photo!

Soups

Miso Soup

Serves 4

If you've ever eaten at a Japanese restaurant, you've had miso soup—yummy, salty, MSG-laden miso soup made with fish stock! Well, now we're going to start eating the real stuff. Miso soup is incredibly medicinal when it's made with good ingredients. Because miso contains natural probiotics, alkalizes the blood, and even has a tumor-blocking element called genistein, miso soup should be regular fare for every MILF and her family. There are a million and one ways to make good miso soup. You can use different misos, different vegetables, start with a sauté . . . you name it. The only consistent elements of miso soup are water, wakame, and no more than 1 teaspoon of miso per cup of fluid (which may taste mild if you're used to the restaurant stuff, but it's the perfect amount for good health). Everything else changes. This is a very simple recipe that can act as a springboard for your future soupfests.

2 dried shiitake mushrooms
1 cup warm spring or filtered water
4 cups spring or filtered water (or homemade vegetable stock)
2 teaspoons wakame flakes

One 1-inch piece daikon, thinly sliced into half-moons
4 teaspoons barley miso, aged at least 2 years
1 scallion, thinly sliced

1. Soak the shiitake mushrooms in the warm water for 10 minutes. Drain and reserve the soaking liquid. Remove and discard the tough stems of the shiitakes and slice the caps into thin strips.

2. In a saucepan, bring the 4 cups water, the wakame, the shiitakes, and the soaking liquid to a boil. Reduce the heat and simmer for 10 minutes. Add the daikon and simmer for 3 more minutes. Remove about ¼ cup of the stock and add the miso to it. Using a suribachi and surikogi (Japanese mortar and pestle)[1] or a cup and spoon, puree the miso until it is smoothly integrated into the stock.

3. Pour the miso liquid back into the soup. Simmer over very low heat for 3 more minutes. Do not let the seasoned soup come to a boil—boiling will overcook the live enzymes. Serve in individual bowls and garnish with the sliced scallion.

1. This serrated mortar and pestle from Japan is the best tool for dissolving and smoothing out miso for miso soup, so I urge you to order one from my website or from Amazon.com—they're cheap!

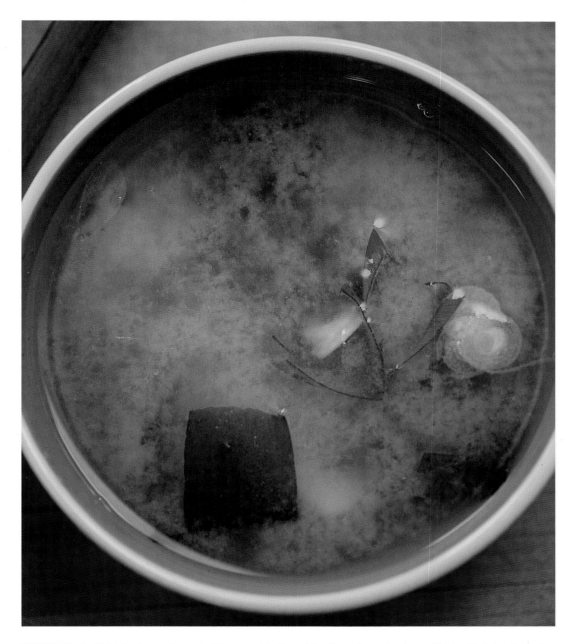

VARIATIONS: Sauté thinly sliced onion and winter squash before adding the water and wakame. Finish with light miso and fresh corn kernels. Garnish with parsley. Other options: cauliflower and fresh mushrooms, onion, summer squash, and tofu. Once in a while, add burdock to make your miso soup nice and strengthening. Squeeze some ginger juice into the soup at the end to make the soup more dynamic. Bake tiny cubes of mochi and float them in the soup as croutons.
Regularly add fresh greens like watercress and bok choy to the miso at the end of cooking.

Fake Chicken Soup for the Soul

Serves 10 to 12

I don't know what possessed me to create this soup, but I'm glad I did. It delivers a hearty, tasty warmth that just *begs* for a matzo ball. On a recent trip to Israel, my MILFy Jewish friends agreed it was a very good substitute for the real thing.

1 to 2 tablespoons extra virgin olive oil
2 medium onions, diced
1 red bell pepper, diced
2 cups red lentils, sorted and rinsed
10 cups spring or filtered water
2 medium carrots, diced
1 medium red-skinned potato, diced (optional)

1 package WestSoy chicken-style seitan, drained and liquid reserved, cut into bite-size pieces
1 small or ½ medium leek, cleaned and diagonally sliced
3 tablespoons shoyu
1 tablespoon mellow white miso
Fresh parsley, for garnish

1. In a large saucepan, heat the oil. Add the onions and sauté for 5 minutes, or until soft and translucent. *Do not add salt.* Add the red pepper and sauté with the onions until soft. Add the red lentils and stir in briefly. Then add the water.

2. Let it all come to a boil, then reduce to a simmer. Add the carrots, the potato, if using, and the seitan and seitan liquid. Simmer for about 30 minutes, or until the red lentils are dissolved.

3. Add the leek and shoyu. Dissolve the miso in a cup or suribachi with some of the soup stock. Make sure you smooth out any lumps. Add it to the soup. Stir and simmer for 5 more minutes.

4. Ladle into individual serving bowls and garnish with parsley. Eat. Send me an e-mail thanking me. It's that good. *Yum.*

Carrot-Coconut Bisque

Serves 6 to 8

This is a lovely, sweet, satisfying soup. It's great for those who live in warm climates, or as a sexy summer treat for the rest of us.

---

1 tablespoon safflower oil
1 large onion, diced
Sea salt
8 to 10 large carrots, cut into ½-inch rounds
Spring or filtered water

One 14-ounce can unsweetened organic
  coconut milk
Ground cinnamon
Ground nutmeg (optional)
Chopped fresh cilantro, for garnish

Heat the oil over medium heat in a large saucepan. Add the onion and a pinch of salt. Sauté for 5 minutes, or until the onion is translucent. Add the carrots and water just to cover the vegetables. Bring to a boil, add ½ teaspoon salt, and simmer for 20 minutes, or until the carrots are very soft. Whiz the soup either by transferring to a food processor or by using an immersion blender in the pan. Whiz until very smooth. Add the coconut milk and adjust the seasoning to taste. Add cinnamon and nutmeg, if using, to taste. Ladle into bowls, garnish with chopped cilantro, and serve.

VARIATION: Double the carrots and skip the coconut milk if you're not in the mood. Without the coconut, this is a very satisfying winter soup. You can also make it with butternut or kabocha squash. *Mmmm . . .*

Really Good Minestrone

Serves 8

I made this soup while cooking for a retreat called The Passage, developed by my good friend William Spear. In it, participants get down to core issues and work through difficult or stuck emotions. My job was to keep them nourished and satisfied in between all their hard work. Somehow, blessed by the soup gods, I came up with this. Because it includes a no-mato sauce, this recipe is a little complicated, but it's worth making a big batch and freezing half of it for soupy afternoons in the winter.

1 cup kidney beans, soaked overnight
1-inch strip of kombu, soaked 10 minutes
Sea salt
½ winter squash, preferably Hokkaido, pumpkin, or buttercup, cut into chunks
3 or 4 large carrots, cut into big chunks
1 medium beet, quartered or cut into chunks
Umeboshi vinegar
Shoyu
1 to 2 tablespoons olive oil
1 medium onion, diced

2 large stalks celery, diced
½ to 1 teaspoon dried oregano
½ to 1 teaspoon dried marjoram
6 cups vegetable stock (preferably homemade, but boxed is okay)
1 cup whole wheat or rice macaroni noodles (optional)
¼ head green cabbage, diced
1 cup diagonally sliced green beans
White miso, if needed, for extra flavor
Chopped fresh parsley, for garnish

1. Bring the kidney beans and kombu to a boil in fresh water to cover. As the water cooks away, add a cup of cold water, carefully poured down the side of the pan. This is the shocking method, and it works very well for cooking beans. Cook until the beans are soft. Salt to taste: remember, you want the beans to be tasty—inside and out—so don't skimp on the salt here.

2. While the beans are cooking, place the squash, carrots, and beet in a pressure cooker and add enough water to go about halfway up the vegetables. This will be your "no-mato" sauce that will make the soup taste tomatoey. Cover with the lid and bring to pressure. Reduce the heat and simmer for about 10 minutes. Let the pressure come down, and scoop the vegetables into a food processor, with the liquid.

3. Before whizzing the veggies, add umeboshi vinegar. This will give the "no-mato" sauce the tang and slight acidity of tomatoes. Keep adding until it tastes nice and tomatoey to you. It will permeate the whole soup, so don't be afraid of making it strong. Now whiz the veggies until smooth. Add a teaspoon or so of shoyu just to round out the taste and darken the sauce slightly. If needed, add more.

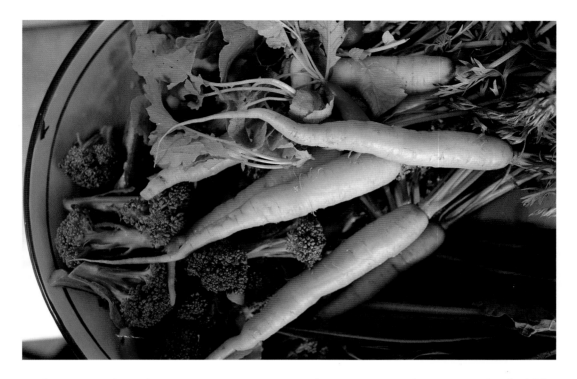

4. Heat the olive oil in a large, heavy pot over medium heat. Sauté the onion until soft. Add the celery and the herbs and continue to sauté for a few minutes. Pour in the vegetable stock and kidney beans and bring to a boil.

5. If you're using the noodles, now is a good time to cook them and rinse them with cold water; set aside until needed.

6. When the stock and beans are simmering, add the "no-mato" sauce. Let it all come together as a soup. Add the cabbage, the green beans, and miso, if you feel it needs more seasoning. Simmer for 10 minutes. Finally, if you're using the noodles, put them in last.

7. Serve garnished with chopped parsley.

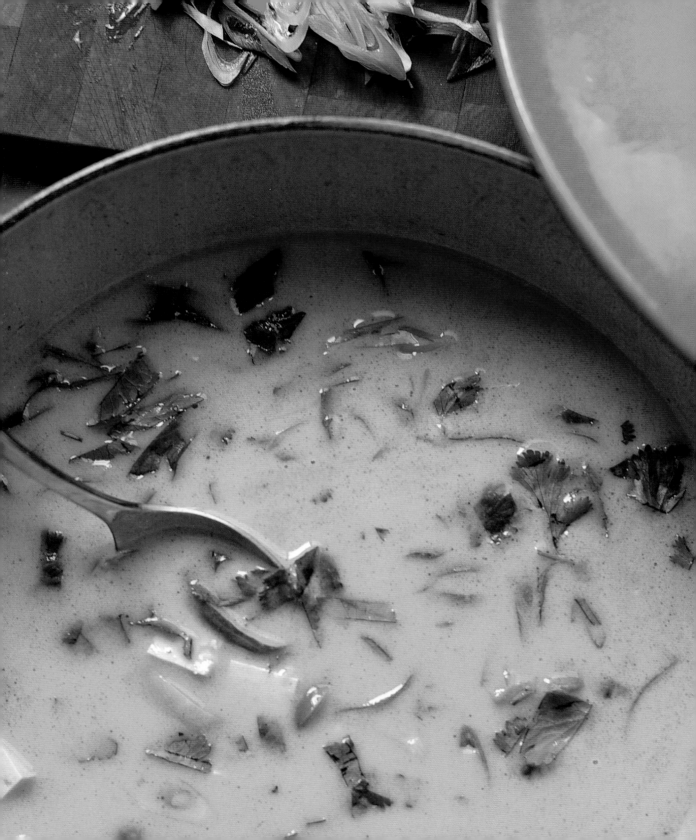

Tom Kha Ghai

Serves 6 to 8

Whenever I go out for Thai food, I check to see if the restaurant has vegetarian tom kha gai; but restaurants seldom do, so I put together this one.

1 tablespoon safflower oil
1 to 2 stalks lemongrass, outer sheath removed and bottom 3 inches trimmed, minced (3 tablespoons)
2 tablespoons minced fresh ginger
1 large clove garlic, minced
2 to 3 teaspoons Thai red curry paste
6 cups vegetable stock, homemade or low-sodium boxed
3 tablespoons shoyu, plus extra to taste
¼ cup agave or rice syrup
Two 14-ounce cans unsweetened organic coconut milk

One 14-ounce package firm tofu, cut into bite-size cubes
8 ounces button or cremini mushrooms, sliced
3 tablespoons fresh lime juice
1 tablespoon brown rice vinegar
1 tablespoon umeboshi vinegar
Grated zest of 1 lime
½ cup loosely packed fresh cilantro leaves, chopped, for garnish
3 scallions, green parts only, thinly sliced on the diagonal, for garnish

1. Heat the oil in a large saucepan over medium heat. Add the lemongrass, ginger, and garlic, and cook, stirring constantly, for about 1 minute. Add the curry paste and cook, stirring constantly, for 30 seconds.

2. Add ½ cup of the stock to the pan and stir to dissolve the curry paste. Add the remaining 5½ cups stock, the shoyu, and the sweetener, and bring to a boil over medium-high heat. Reduce the heat to low, partially cover, and simmer to blend the flavors, about 20 minutes.

3. Stir in the coconut milk, tofu, mushrooms, and lime juice. Taste for seasoning and add more shoyu if desired. Bring back to a simmer and cook for 5 more minutes. Add the vinegars and lime zest. Simmer for 1 more minute. Serve immediately, garnishing each bowl with the cilantro and scallions.

Corn Soup

Serves 4

This soup is very simple, so it really shows off the corn and lets it shine. A tonic to the energy of the heart, corn helps us to feel warm and expansive. . . . Don't be surprised if your cheeks flush a little after you eat a bowl of this soup.

8 ears fresh corn	Shoyu
Spring or filtered water	Chopped fresh cilantro or parsley, for garnish

On a plate or in a large bowl, grate the corncobs along a fine grater to get the pulp from the kernels. When all the cobs are grated, put the pulp into a saucepan, and if there's enough room, add a few of the cobs. Add water to equal the volume of the pulp. Let it come to a boil and then simmer for at least 10 minutes. Add shoyu to taste and simmer for 5 more minutes. Remove the cobs and discard. Ladle the soup into bowls and garnish with chopped cilantro or parsley.

Tuscan White Bean Soup

Serves 8

This is a recipe by Meredith McCarty, a stellar MILF and author of truly great cookbooks. I love her food.

---

2 cups dried white beans (lima, navy, cannellini, Great Northern)
8 cups spring or filtered water or mild-tasting vegetable stock (4 cups to soak, 4 cups to pressure-cook the beans)
2 tablespoons olive oil
2 medium onions, diced
2 large cloves garlic, pressed

One 6-inch piece kombu sea vegetable
2 bay leaves
1 teaspoon Italian seasoning
¼ cup white miso
½ teaspoon sea salt
¼ teaspoon freshly ground black pepper
½ cup minced fresh basil
Fresh Italian parsley leaves, for garnish

---

1. Sort through the beans for stones by spreading them on a white plate. Rinse the beans in water to cover. Drain, and soak in 4 cups of the spring water for 8 hours (all day or overnight), or until bubbles form, up to 24 hours.

2. In a pressure cooker, heat the oil and sauté the onions and garlic until barely tender, about 5 minutes.

3. Drain the beans, reserving the liquid for your plants or garden. Transfer the beans to the pressure cooker with the remaining 4 cups water. Bring to a boil and slowly boil, uncovered, for 5 minutes, to allow the initial gas to escape in the form of froth or steam. Add the kombu and bay leaves and cover to bring to pressure, then turn the heat to low to cook for 1 hour.

4. When the pressure subsides, set aside 1 cup of the stock. (Keep to add later, if needed. The exception is cannellini beans, for which you may need to add 1 cup water.) Remove the bay leaves. With a wire whisk or in a food processor or blender, puree the cooked beans, vegetables, and kombu with the Italian seasoning, miso, salt, and pepper until the mixture is almost smooth.

5. Return the soup to the pot. Add the fresh basil and heat through to blend the flavors, about 5 minutes. Adjust the seasonings, and adjust the amount of liquid to the consistency desired. Garnish with the parsley and serve.

Quinoa Soup with Corn

Serves 4

When I went on a trip to Peru in 1998, I got intimately acquainted with quinoa. It is a protein-rich, gluten-free superfood that grows high in the Andes, exposed to searing sunshine and freezing nights. It was quinoa that helped to make the Incan culture so rich and strong. The Peruvians eat it soft in the morning as a porridge, as a whole-grain dish at other meals, and often in a soup like this one.

½ cup quinoa, soaked overnight
4 cups spring or filtered water or vegetable stock
⅛ teaspoon cayenne pepper
Pinch of ground cumin
Pinch of ground turmeric
½ teaspoon celery seed
2 cloves garlic, finely minced

1 small onion, finely chopped
1 small carrot, diced
1 small stalk celery, finely chopped
1 teaspoon sea salt
1 cup fresh corn kernels
2 tablespoons chopped fresh parsley or cilantro
2 tablespoons fresh lime juice

1. Put the quinoa in a fine strainer and rinse well. It's important to rinse the quinoa to reduce the amount of saponin—the slightly bitter coating on the grain. As the quinoa soaks, you'll notice that the tails of the quinoa unwind a little. That's the beginning of the sprouting process.

2. In a medium saucepan, bring the quinoa and soaking liquid, cayenne pepper, cumin, turmeric, celery seed, garlic, onion, carrot, and celery to a boil. Add the salt. Reduce the heat to a simmer and cook for about 10 minutes. Add the corn and cook for another 3 minutes. Remove from the heat and add the parsley or cilantro. Stir in the lime juice and serve.

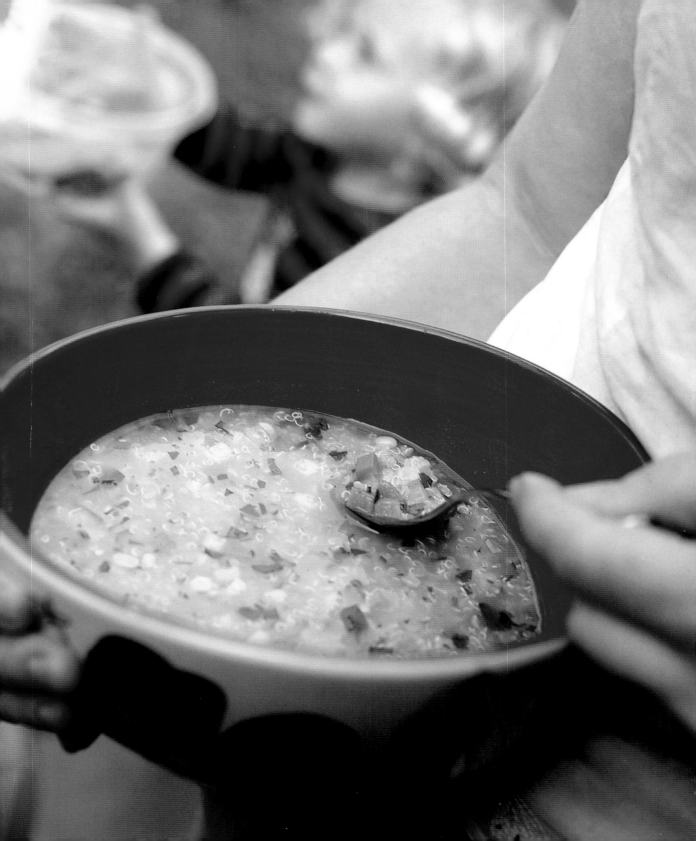

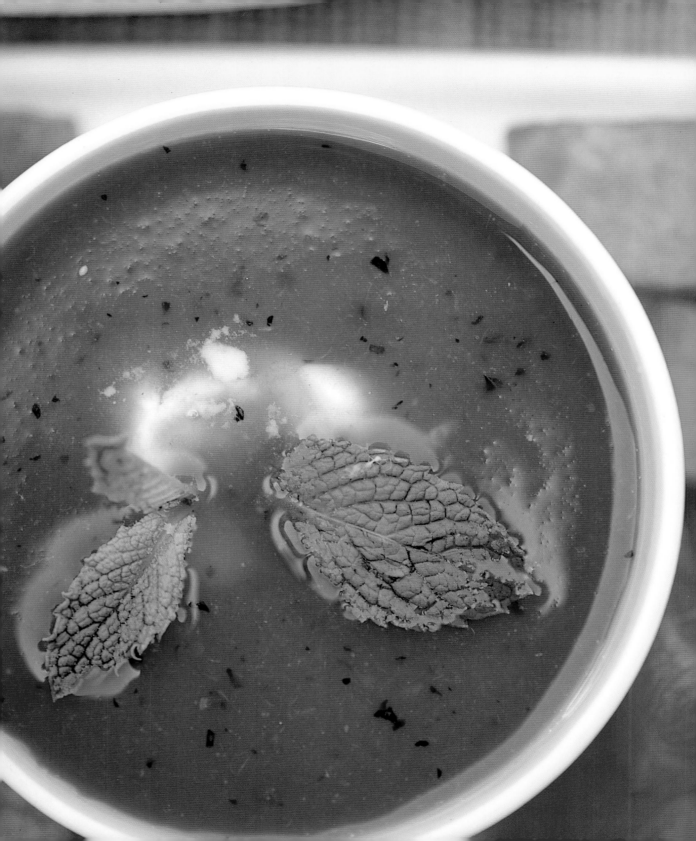

Watermelon Soup

Serves 6

This quick, easy recipe is perfect for a hot summer day. You won't realize how yang and cranky you've become until this soup cools you from the inside out and plants a big, stupid smile on your face. I mean it. It will make you smile and crack jokes.

---

4 cups cubed seeded watermelon
$\frac{1}{3}$ cup thawed apple juice concentrate
1 tablespoon chopped fresh mint leaves
1 knob ginger, grated and squeezed to make $\frac{1}{2}$ teaspoon ginger juice

$\frac{1}{3}$ cup plain unsweetened soy yogurt (see Note)
Freshly ground black pepper
6 mint sprigs

Dice enough of the watermelon to measure $\frac{1}{3}$ cup and reserve it for garnish. In a blender or food processor, process the remaining watermelon, the apple juice concentrate, mint leaves, and ginger juice until smooth. Place in the refrigerator, covered, for 1 hour, to let the flavors blend. Serve in small chilled bowls and garnish each with some diced watermelon, a dollop of the yogurt, a sprinkle of pepper, and a mint sprig.

Note: Unsweetened soy yogurt can be hard to find in small amounts. If you can't get your hands on it, skip it. The soup is still amazing.

Desserts

Birthday Cake for Chocolate Lovers

Serves 12

I got this cake from Lisa Silverman, my MILFy friend in Portland, Maine. She runs a cooking school there and hosts lots of potlucks. Lisa keeps Maine healthy!

FROSTING
2 cups grain-sweetened nondairy chocolate chips
1 cup maple syrup
7 ounces extra firm silken tofu (Mori-Nu is good)
Pinch of sea salt
1 tablespoon vanilla extract
1 cup soy milk powder

CAKE
1 cup whole wheat pastry flour
1 cup unbleached white flour
2 teaspoons aluminum-free baking powder
2 teaspoons baking soda
1 teaspoon sea salt
½ teaspoon ground cinnamon (optional)
½ cup plus 2 tablespoons organic cocoa powder
½ cup maple sugar
½ cup safflower oil
1 cup maple syrup
1 cup vanilla soy milk
1 cup spring water
1 teaspoon apple cider vinegar or balsamic vinegar
1 tablespoon vanilla extract

1. To prepare the frosting, in a double boiler, melt the chocolate chips and maple syrup, stirring occasionally to avoid burning the chocolate.

2. In a food processor, puree the tofu, salt, and vanilla. Pour the chocolate-maple mixture into the tofu and blend together well. Add the soy milk powder, a little bit at a time. Blend well.

3. Let the frosting cool in the refrigerator while you make the cake.

4. Preheat the oven to 350°F. Oil and flour two 9-inch cake pans.

5. Sift the whole wheat flour, white flour, baking powder, baking soda, sea salt, cinnamon (if using), cocoa powder, and maple sugar into a large bowl. Stir with a wire whisk to mix.

6. In another bowl, combine the safflower oil, maple syrup, soy milk, water, vinegar, and vanilla. Mix with a wire whisk until the mixture foams a little.

7. Pour the wet ingredients into the dry ingredients and mix until the batter is smooth. Pour the batter into the cake pans, dividing evenly.

8. Bake on the center rack of the oven for 25 to 30 minutes, until the center of the cake springs back when lightly touched and a toothpick inserted in the center of the cake comes out clean.

9. Let the cake layers cool in the pans on wire racks for 10 minutes. Run a knife along the sides of the pans to release the cakes. Turn the layers out of the pans directly onto racks and let cool completely.

10. Frost one layer of the cake. Place the second layer on top and frost. Using the remaining frosting, cover the sides of the cake. Enjoy!

White Almond Mousse with Stewed Apricots and Orange Sauce

Serves 8

This is a subtle, elegant, and silky dessert that is great to serve at a party. The flavors of the stewed apricots and fresh orange juice blend beautifully with the subtle sweetness of the white almond mousse. It's a wee bit labor intensive, so save it for when you want to impress. It was donated by Simone Parris.

16 dried apricots, cut into quarters
1 cup apple juice
1 cup spring water
Sea salt
4 cups rice milk, plus extra as needed
¼ cup agar-agar flakes
1 teaspoon vanilla extract

2 tablespoons kuzu root starch
Grated zest of 1 lemon
2 tablespoons almond butter
Rice syrup
1½ cups fresh orange juice
¼ cup toasted sliced almonds

1. To prepare the apricots, place the apricots, apple juice, water, and a pinch of sea salt in a heavy-bottomed saucepan and bring to a boil. Cover, reduce the heat, and simmer until the apricots are soft and puffy—about 25 minutes. Remove from the heat and set aside.

2. To prepare the mousse, in a heavy-bottomed saucepan, heat the rice milk with the agar-agar and vanilla. Bring to a gentle boil and then reduce the heat to a simmer. Simmer for about 15 minutes, or until the agar flakes are dissolved. Stir occasionally to prevent the agar-agar from sticking to the bottom of the pan.

3. Dissolve 1 tablespoon of the kuzu in a little cold rice milk or water and stir it into the rice milk mixture. Stir well to prevent lumping and continue to stir as you raise the heat back to a brief boil. (Kuzu needs to boil in order to thicken properly.) Reduce the heat and add the lemon zest and almond butter. Whisk briskly to blend.

4. Beginning with 1 tablespoon rice syrup and adding more if necessary to achieve a mild, balanced sweet flavor, sweeten the mousse mixture. Remember that the apricots will add a lot of sweetness, so there's no need for the mousse to be too sweet.

5. Remove the rice milk mixture from the heat and pour into a glass or stainless-steel baking dish to cool. Chill in the refrigerator until firm. Once it has set, put the thickened gel in a blender and blend until smooth and creamy; or you can use an immersion blender in the original saucepan.

6. To prepare the orange sauce, carefully bring the orange juice with a tiny pinch of sea salt to a simmer. Dissolve the remaining 1 tablespoon kuzu in a little cold water and stir into the simmering juice, adding enough of the kuzu mixture to achieve a saucy consistency.

7. Add a little rice syrup to cut the sourness of the orange juice—how much depends on how sweet or sour your oranges are.

8. To assemble the dessert, in 8 dessert bowls or parfait glasses, distribute the stewed apricots, spoon the mousse over the apricots, top with the orange sauce, and finish with the toasted almond slivers.

Creamy Lemon Pudding

Serves 6 to 8

Simone Parris just keeps making great desserts, so I keep passing them along. This recipe is light, refreshing, and the ideal complement to a rich meal. It'll make you go, *"Mmmm."*

---

2 cups apple juice	Juice from 3 lemons
1 cup spring water	2 cups amazake
6 tablespoons agar-agar flakes	¼ cup toasted slivered almonds
¼ cup brown rice syrup	Fresh raspberries, for garnish
2 teaspoons vanilla extract	

---

1. Place the juice, water, and agar-agar flakes in a saucepan. Bring to a boil over medium heat and simmer for 5 minutes, or until the flakes are dissolved. Stir occasionally to prevent sticking. Add the rice syrup and vanilla and mix gently. Remove from the heat; add the lemon juice and place in a dish to cool and set. You can place the dessert in the refrigerator to speed up the setting time.

2. When the gel is firm, blend with the amazake until smooth and creamy. Place in individual glasses and serve chilled, garnished with the almonds and fresh raspberries.

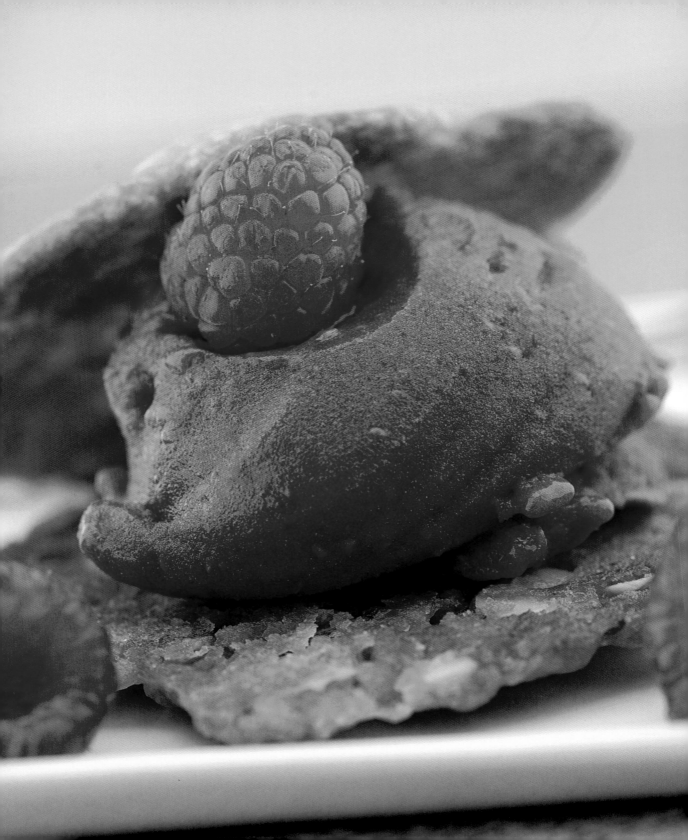

Raspberry Sorbet with Lace Cookies

Serves 6

I lifted this recipe from my good friend Eric LeChasseur, a world-class chef who has cooked for tons of celebs. He and his wife, Sanae, also own a cafe in Los Angeles called Seed Kitchen. These delicate, elegant cookies will wow your guests, but the sorbet alone should be on summertime standby in the freezer. It's easy enough for a kid to make. This comes from his book *Love, Eric*.

RASPBERRY SORBET
1 pound frozen organic raspberries
Pinch of sea salt
1 teaspoon fresh lemon juice
¼ cup maple syrup

LACE COOKIES
⅓ cup maple sugar
⅓ cup maple syrup
6 tablespoons nonhydrogenated soy margarine
⅔ cup unbleached white flour
Pinch of sea salt
⅔ cup sliced almonds

1. To make the sorbet, leave the frozen raspberries out at room temperature for 20 minutes. In a food processor, puree the raspberries until smooth. Add the sea salt, lemon juice, and maple syrup. Process for a few more seconds. Transfer to a freezer container and freeze for up to 2 weeks.

2. To make the cookies: preheat the oven to 350°F. In a large bowl, combine the maple sugar, maple syrup, margarine, flour, salt, and almonds to make a dough. Divide the dough into 12 pieces and roll them into 12 balls, about the size of apricots. On a baking sheet, evenly place 6 dough balls. Press on each dough ball to flatten it into a 4-inch-diameter circle. Bake for about 8 minutes, or until golden brown. Allow the cookies to cool on the pan. Using a stainless steel spatula, remove the cookies from the baking sheet and set aside. Do not stack them. Repeat with the second batch.

3. To serve, using an ice cream scoop or 2 soup spoons, make a small ball of the sorbet and set it in the middle of a crispy cookie. Add a second cookie over the ball of sorbet. Add one final scoop of sorbet to crown the dessert.

Super-Delicious Mystery "Cheese" Cake

Serves 8

Laura Taylor and Karen Bryson teach whole foods cooking classes in Los Angeles. They are totally MILFy and have come up with some amazing recipes. Here is their "cheese" cake, which has pleased every single palate it has crossed. Gluten-free, soy-free, it is remarkably satisfying, delicious, and easy. *You must try it.*

FILLING
¾ cup millet, soaked overnight in 2½ cups spring water
Pinch of sea salt
¾ cup cashews, pine nuts, or macadamia nuts, soaked overnight
½ cup fresh lemon juice
2 teaspoons lemon extract
2 teaspoons vanilla extract
¼ cup maple syrup or brown rice syrup, plus extra as needed

CRUST
2 cups toasted nuts (almonds, walnuts, or any combination), or 1 cup toasted nuts and 1 cup toasted gluten-free low-fat oatmeal

Pinch of sea salt
¾ cup pitted dates (soaked for 30 minutes and drained if dried)

FRUIT TOPPING
1 cup fruit-sweetened jam (strawberry and blueberry are both delicious choices)
Or, if you'd like to make a topping from scratch:
2 cups fresh berries
1 cup apple juice
½ cup maple syrup or brown rice syrup
Pinch of sea salt
2 tablespoons kuzu root starch

1. To prepare the filling, in the morning, cook the millet in the soaking liquid with the salt for 50 minutes. While the millet is cooking, drain the nuts and place in a blender with the lemon juice, lemon extract, vanilla, and sweetener. Process until very creamy.

2. To prepare the crust, grind the nuts and salt into a coarse meal in a food processor. Do not overprocess. Add the dates to the nut meal while the food processor is running, one date at a time. When the mixture holds together, it is done. Press onto the bottom of a 9-inch springform pan.

3. Let the cooked millet cool only slightly and add to the other filling ingredients in the blender. (If you let the millet cool completely, it won't blend well.) Process until very, very smooth. Check the sweetness and adjust if necessary. Pour into the crust and allow to set for at least 4 hours.

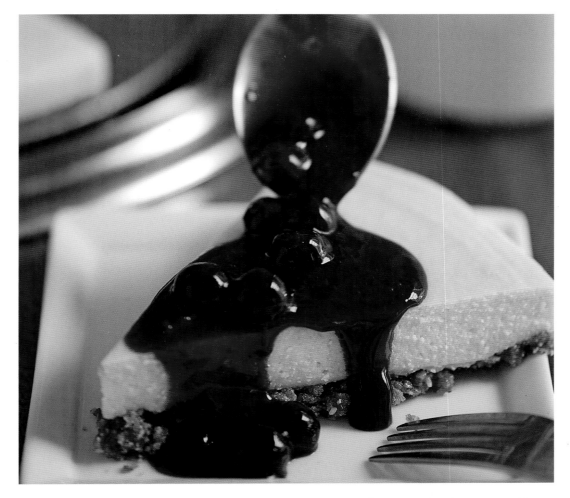

4. If you are not using the jam and are making the topping from scratch, place 1 cup of the berries, the juice, and the sweetener in a saucepan with the salt. Bring to a boil. Reduce the heat and simmer for 5 to 10 minutes, letting the fruit break down a little. Dilute the kuzu in cold water and whisk into the berries, bringing the mixture back to a boil for 1 minute. Reduce the heat. Add the remaining 1 cup berries and stir in, so you have a combination of well-cooked berries and almost fresh ones.

5. After 4 hours or when ready to serve, spoon the fruit jam or your homemade fruit topping over the cooled "cheese" cake or onto individual servings.

VARIATION: Substitute lime juice for lemon and the "cheese" cake tastes like Key lime pie.

Poached Pears with Raspberry Sauce

Serves 6 to 12, depending upon serving size

This is a lovely recipe contributed by Sarah Loring. She was one of my cooking teachers back in the day and I love her gentle spirit, subtle cooking, and fantastic results.

---

1 package frozen organic raspberries,
   or 1½ cups fresh raspberries
½ cup maple syrup
Sea salt
1 tablespoon kuzu root starch

6 pears
6 cups apple juice
½ teaspoon grated lemon zest (optional)
⅓ vanilla bean (optional)
Pinch of ground cardamom (optional)

---

1. Place the berries, maple syrup, and a pinch of sea salt in a small saucepan. Bring to a boil, reduce the heat to low, and simmer for 15 minutes (5 to 10 minutes if you're using fresh berries). Dissolve the kuzu in a little cold water, whisk into the raspberry mixture until it resumes boiling, let simmer for 1 minute, and remove from the heat.

2. Rinse and peel the pears. Halve them and remove the seeds with a melon baller to make a nice round indent in each half to hold the sauce. Turn the pear halves over and cut a little slice off their round backs so the halves will sit level when turned cut side up. Place the pears in a skillet and cover with the apple juice. Add a pinch of salt and the lemon zest, vanilla bean, and/or cardamom, if using.

3. Bring to a boil and reduce the heat to low. Cover and simmer until the pears are tender—15 to 45 minutes, depending on the ripeness of the pears. Remove the pears to a serving dish or individual plates.

4. Pour the raspberry sauce over the pears, filling their little indents and adding an artful drizzle.

VARIATIONS: If the pears are ripe, fresh, and in season, the optional ingredients may not be necessary; you can just enjoy the beauty and flavor of the pears.

This dish can be served hot or cold. The pears can be dressed up with chocolate sauce and soy or rice ice cream or dressed down, as leftovers, with hot oatmeal.

Cashew-Apricot Cookies

Makes about 12 cookies

This is another lovely dessert by Simone Parris. These chunky, nutty cookies were a huge hit at a recent dinner party.

1 cup unsalted raw cashew nuts
1 cup spelt or whole wheat pastry flour
1 cup fine rolled oats
½ cup organic soy margarine or coconut oil
⅓ cup maple syrup
¼ cup brown rice syrup
¼ cup unsweetened coconut flakes

¼ cup sesame seeds
½ teaspoon ground cinnamon
½ teaspoon vanilla extract
¼ teaspoon fine sea salt
1 teaspoon baking powder
1 cup dried apricots, cut into quarters

1. Preheat the oven to 300°F. Rinse the cashews and dry-roast for about 10 minutes. Remove the cashews. Turn the oven up to 350°F.

2. Combine all the ingredients and mix well. Roll into 1½-inch balls, place on a baking sheet, and press lightly with a fork. Bake for 15 minutes, or until golden brown. Remove from the oven and let cool before removing from the baking sheet.

VARIATIONS: Try replacing the apricots and cashews with other combinations of dried fruits and nuts. For a really sweet cookie, go for dates and pecans.

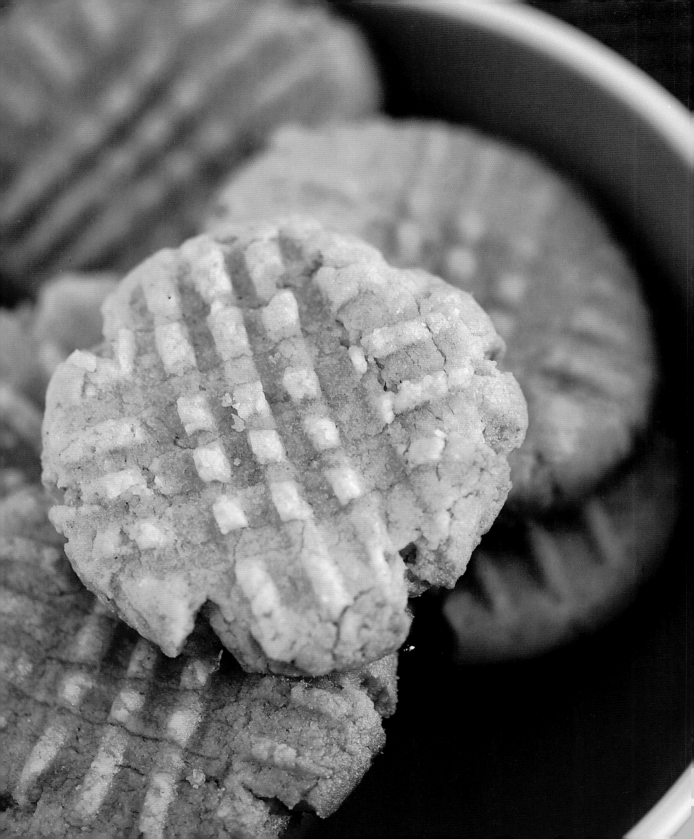

Peanut Butter Cookies

Makes about 12 cookies

Who doesn't—with the exception of those allergic—*love* peanut butter cookies? These are great. . . . I adapted a recipe from Meredith McCarty's dessert cookbook *Sweet and Natural* by adding Vegenaise. I know. Sounds weird. But it's *gooood*.

---

1 cup whole wheat pastry flour
1 cup unbleached white flour
2 teaspoons aluminum-free baking powder
¼ teaspoon sea salt
½ cup light vegetable oil

½ cup peanut butter (crunchy or smooth)
¼ cup Vegenaise
½ cup maple syrup
1 teaspoon vanilla extract

---

1. Preheat the oven to 350°F. Line 2 baking sheets with parchment paper, or brush with oil.

2. Mix together the pastry flour, white flour, baking powder, and salt.

3. Whisk together the oil, peanut butter, Vegenaise, maple syrup, and vanilla and add to the dry ingredients to form a dough.

4. Shape into small balls. Divide the dough balls between the prepared baking sheets. Press the tops with a fork in a classic crisscross design. Bake until the bottoms are golden, 12 to 15 minutes.

5. Let cool briefly on the baking sheets, then remove to a wire rack to cool completely.

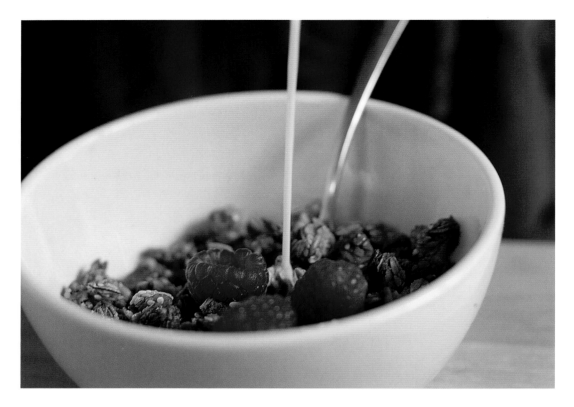

Breakfast Food

Breakfast can be either simple or sexy.

Simple: This generally consists of a grain porridge and some steamed or blanched leafy greens. You heard me: greens at breakfast. With strong upward energy, leafy greens are the perfect way to align yourself with the rising energy of the day. Many MILFs also take their miso soup in the morning. It may sound crazy, but miso soup tastes fantastic first thing in the morning. The simple breakfast may be rounded out with some roasted nuts, seeds, a nut butter, or maybe a little fruit.

Sexy: Scrambled tofu, breads, muffins, fruity spreads, granola, plant-based "milks," etc.—you name it. There are a bunch of breakfast foods in this section, and I recommend you explore them—especially when you have more time on the weekends—at your leisure.

Scrambled Tofu

Serves 4

I love this dish—and any variation on it—because it is quick, simple, and yet totally pleasing. This version is by Howard Wallen, DILF-at-large.

2 tablespoons extra virgin olive oil
½ medium onion, thinly sliced into
   quarter-moons
Sea salt
¼ cup fine burdock matchsticks
1 cup quartered mushrooms
2 tablespoons mirin
½ cup carrot matchsticks

½ cup fresh corn kernels
One 14-ounce package extra firm tofu,
   drained and crumbled
Pinch of freshly ground black pepper
¼ teaspoon ground turmeric
¾ cup broccoli florets
2 tablespoons shoyu
Splash of umeboshi vinegar

Heat the oil in a medium skillet or saucepan over medium heat. Add the onion and a pinch of salt and sauté until the onion becomes soft. Add the burdock and mushrooms, another small pinch of salt, and 1 tablespoon of the mirin. Sauté for 3 minutes. Add the carrot, corn, and another small pinch of salt, and sauté until the carrot softens a little. Lay the crumbled tofu over the sautéed vegetables and season with the black pepper and turmeric. Add the broccoli and about ½ cup water—enough to cover the bottom of the pan, but not to drown the broccoli. Cover and let the water steam the tofu and vegetables for 5 minutes. Season with the shoyu and the remaining 1 tablespoon mirin, remove the lid, and let any excess liquid cook off. Finish with a splash of umeboshi vinegar and serve.

VARIATION: Try this with any vegetable you like that sautés well. *Mmmm.* I also love adding nutritional yeast to scrambled tofu dishes for a cheesy flavor.

Pantastic Pancakes

Makes 4 small pancakes

---

1 cup whole wheat pastry flour
2 tablespoons aluminum-free baking powder
1/8 teaspoon sea salt
1 cup soy milk

2 tablespoons brown rice syrup
2 tablespoons safflower oil, plus extra for the pan
Maple syrup, for topping

---

1. Combine the flour, baking powder, and salt in a large bowl until well mixed.

2. Mix the soy milk, rice syrup, and oil together, then mix into the dry ingredients until the batter is smooth.

3. Drop 1/4 cup of the batter at a time onto a hot oiled griddle or into a well-greased skillet over medium-high heat. When bubbles appear on the surface of the pancake, after about 3 minutes, flip, and cook the other side for another 2 minutes. Re-oil the pan with each new pancake. Serve with maple syrup.

VARIATIONS: For an even sweeter version, add fresh or frozen strawberries to the batter. For a savory version, add sautéed onions to the batter after it's been poured onto the griddle.

Mochi Flips

Serves 2

I got this recipe from a lovely Irish MILF named Aine McAteer. She has cooked for all sorts of celebs and wrote a beautiful cookbook called *Recipes to Nurture.* Imagine her Irish lilt as she says, "The hardest part of making this dish is grating the mochi, so if there's a man around the house, put him to work."

---

2 sweet apples, peeled if not organic
½ cup apple juice, plus extra as needed
1 heaping teaspoon kuzu root starch or
   arrowroot

⅔ of a 12-ounce package mochi, grated like
   cheese (yields about 2 cups)
Safflower oil

---

1. Cut the apples into quarters, remove the cores, and dice the fruit. Place in a saucepan with the ½ cup apple juice. Bring to a boil, cover, and simmer on low heat for 10 to 12 minutes. When the apples are soft, remove from the pan with a slotted spoon and set aside. Dissolve the kuzu or arrowroot in a little cold apple juice or water and add to the fruit juice in the pan, stirring until thickened. Set aside.

2. To make each flip, place ½ cup of the grated mochi in a lightly oiled skillet. Spread about ½ cup of the cooked apple mixture on the mochi and top with another ½ cup mochi. Place the pan over medium heat until the pan is heated and then turn the heat to low. Cover the pan and allow the mochi to cook for 2 to 3 minutes, then carefully turn, using a stainless steel spatula. Continue to cook for a couple of minutes.

3. Cut the filled mochi into quarters while still in the pan and arrange on a serving plate. Drizzle with the apple juice–kuzu mixture or with maple or agave syrup.

VARIATIONS: Other fruits such as pears, peaches, mangoes, and berries can be used as a filling. The berries don't need to be cooked. If using strawberries, cut them into small pieces.

Sautéed mixed veggies can be used to make a delicious savory dish. Onions or leeks; carrots; zucchini; red, yellow, or green peppers; and cabbage would all work well. Simply heat a little olive oil in a pan and sauté the veggies until wilted. Season with sea salt and freshly ground black pepper or a drizzle of tamari, and use in the same way as the fruit.

For a sweeter dish, drizzle with maple or brown rice syrup.

Morning Porridges

Just about any leftover grain can be made into a morning porridge by adding water and cooking it for a while. Some quickly cooked cereals, like bulgur and polenta, can be made into fresh porridges. Here are a couple of recipes from the MILFs.

Bulgur Breakfast Bowl

Serves 3 to 4

From Eliza Eller in Alaska: "Bulgur wheat, I am discovering, makes a great breakfast—it's filling, delicious, and fast, and it satisfies some deep American need I have for wheat toast."

1 cup bulgur wheat
4 cups spring water
Sea salt

1 medium onion, sliced into half-moons
Olive or sesame oil

Bring the bulgur and water to a boil. Add a pinch of salt, reduce the heat to low, and cover. Simmer for 15 or 20 minutes, until soft and porridgy. Meanwhile, sauté the onion in some oil with another pinch of salt until it's golden. When the bulgur is ready, combine the porridge with the onion and serve.

Polenta Porridge

Serves 2

From Aine McAteer: "There are so many variations on this soft polenta porridge that once you get the basic method down, you can throw it together in a matter of minutes, giving it your own unique touches."

---

1 cup quick-cooking corn grits (polenta)   Big pinch of sea salt
3 cups water   1 cup fresh corn kernels

Bring the grits, water, and salt to a boil. Reduce the heat to low and simmer for 5 minutes. Stir in the corn kernels and cook for 2 more minutes.

VARIATIONS: Instead of adding fresh corn, you can add some chopped dried apricots, dates, figs, or raisins. You could also add fresh fruit such as diced apple, pear, peach, or apricot for a delicious fruity porridge.

You can cook the polenta in some orange juice or other fruit juice to make a sweeter dish. Alternatively, you could use half rice or nut milk and half water or juice. Sprinkle with toasted slivered almonds, hazelnuts, sunflower seeds, or some ground flaxseed.

You can make the polenta up the night before and spread it about 1 inch thick on a baking sheet or plate to cool. In the morning, slice it up and panfry it in a little organic oil and serve drizzled with syrup or with a dollop of stewed fruit, or to accompany scrambled tofu.

Morning Rice

Serves 4

Leftover rice makes a really creamy, nourishing, and warming breakfast porridge.

---

2 cups leftover cooked brown rice   **4 cups spring water**

---

1. Place the rice and water in a heavy-bottomed pot and break up the rice as best you can. Bring it to a boil, reduce the heat, and simmer, covered, for 45 minutes, until creamy. Stir occasionally to prevent sticking or burning.

2. Serve with toasted seeds or nuts, nut butters, dried fruit, and/or rice syrup. *Yum.*

Bagels and "Cream Cheese"

Serves 1 happy MILF

This isn't really a recipe per se. It's a reminder that life doesn't stop when you give up extreme foods. There are lots and lots of fake foods out there that are pretty darn good substitutes for the old stuff. As you transition, feel free to indulge. . . .

---

1 hemp-seed or whole wheat bagel   **Follow Your Heart cream cheese alternative**
Earth Balance soy margarine   **Fruit-sweetened jam**

Toast the bagel and slather with soy margarine and then cream cheese alternative. I know that may not be normal, but that's the way I like it. Top it off with jam. Oh, God.

Power Crunch Granola

Makes enough granola for about 24 servings (you can store the extra for later use)

I don't think of granola as an Irish dish, but Aine McAteer makes it really well. She suggests you make up a big batch of this; it's delicious served with soy, almond, or rice milk as a breakfast cereal or sprinkled on stewed fruit to make a great dessert.

6 cups rolled oats	1 teaspoon ground cinnamon
1 cup chopped or slivered almonds	Pinch of sea salt
1 cup chopped pecans	1 teaspoon grated orange zest
½ cup sunflower seeds	⅔ cup coconut oil
½ cup pumpkin seeds	⅔ cup agave syrup
½ cup sesame seeds	2 tablespoons fresh orange juice

1. Preheat the oven to 325°F and place a rack in the middle of the oven.

2. In a large mixing bowl, combine the oats, almonds, pecans, seeds, cinnamon, salt, and orange zest. Warm the coconut oil, mix together with the agave syrup and orange juice, and drizzle over the dry ingredients, mixing well, until all the ingredients are completely coated.

3. Spread the mixture on a baking sheet and put into the oven. Bake for about 35 minutes, stirring occasionally to make sure it bakes evenly. Let cool and store in an airtight container in a cool place.

4. Serve with some chopped fresh fruit and a dollop of soy yogurt or some rice, oat, or almond milk.

NOTE: For a gluten-free version, make sure to use certified "gluten-free" oats.

VARIATIONS: Other nuts can be added, such as chopped walnuts, hazelnuts, and cashews.

Instead of agave syrup, you can sweeten the granola with rice syrup, maple syrup, or honey. Honey is sweeter, so use a little less.

Other flavorings can be used in place of cinnamon and orange zest. Lemon zest and lemon juice can be added, or almond or vanilla extract.

Hopi Blue and Yellow Indian Corn Muffins

Makes 12 muffins

This is another killer recipe from Meredith McCarty. Great for breakfast or for serving with chili or any other dish that strikes your fancy. Here are her notes: "The intriguing swirl of marbled color in this corn bread comes from a combination of blue and yellow cornmeal batters. Soy milk acts as a mild leavening agent in addition to the baking powder. You can also make this into a corn bread loaf and cook it in a cast-iron pan for the best crust."

BLUE CORNMEAL BATTER
¾ cup blue cornmeal
¾ cup whole wheat pastry flour
2 teaspoons aluminum-free baking powder
¼ teaspoon sea salt
3 tablespoons light vegetable oil, such as walnut or canola
3 tablespoons brown rice malt syrup, barley malt syrup, or pure maple syrup
1 cup soy milk

YELLOW CORNMEAL BATTER
¾ cup yellow corn flour or cornmeal
¾ cup unbleached white pastry flour
2 teaspoons aluminum-free baking powder
¼ teaspoon sea salt
3 tablespoons light vegetable oil, such as walnut or canola
3 tablespoons brown rice malt syrup or pure maple syrup
1 cup soy milk
Kernels from 1 small ear fresh corn (optional; in season)

1. Preheat the oven to 350°F. Brush a 12-cup muffin tin with oil. Heat the muffin tin in the oven while you make the batter (this is an optional step).

2. To make both of the batters, in 2 bowls, mix the dry ingredients. Mix the wet ingredients in 2 separate bowls, and gently whisk with the corresponding dry ingredients. The batters should be thin and pourable.

3. Pour the blue cornmeal batter into the muffin tin. Pour the yellow batter on top. With a thin-bladed knife, draw a spiral through to the bottom of the batter in each cup. Bake until the muffins test done, approximately 12 minutes.

VARIATION: For a corn bread loaf, brush a 10-inch cast-iron skillet with oil and place in the oven while it preheats. Prepare the batters and pour into the hot skillet. Bake for 30 to 35 minutes.

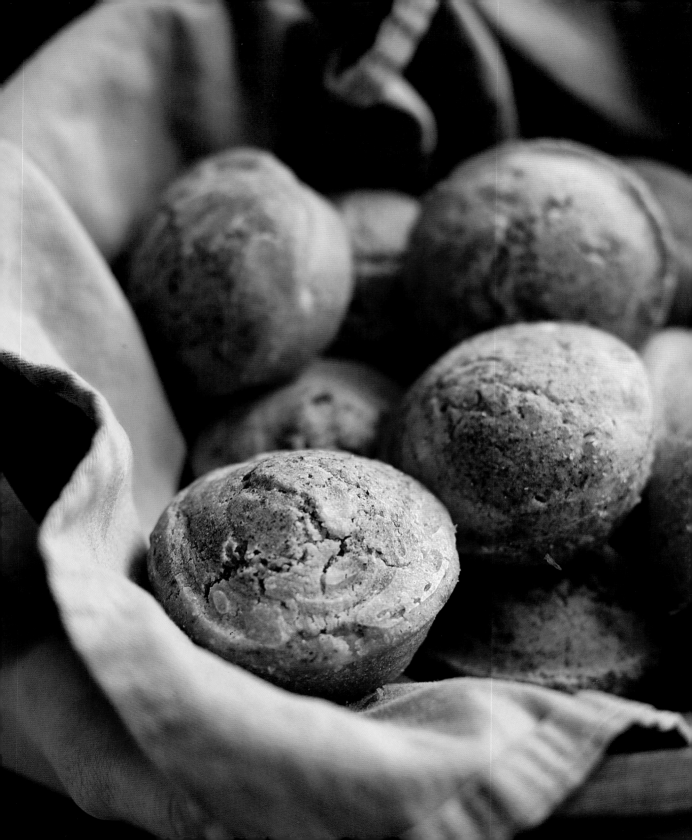

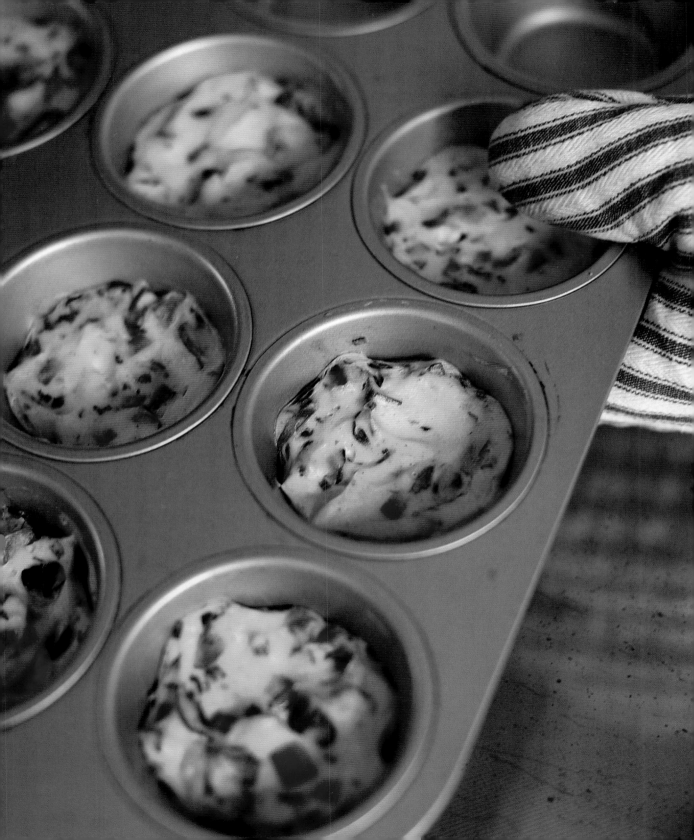

Mini Crust-Free Tofu Quiches

Makes 12 mini quiches, which serve 3 or 4

This is an adaptation of a recipe by Susan Voisin, creator of the healthy website fatfreevegan.com. They are really, really good. Try them for brunch with a big ol' mess of greens, a grain, and some tempeh bacon!

Extra virgin olive oil
1 teaspoon minced garlic
½ cup diced red bell pepper
1 cup sliced mushrooms
1 tablespoon minced fresh chives, or
　1 scallion, minced
1 teaspoon minced fresh rosemary,
　or ½ teaspoon dried, crushed
Freshly ground black pepper

One 12.3-ounce package firm silken tofu,
　drained
¼ cup soy milk
2 tablespoons nutritional yeast
1 tablespoon kuzu root starch
1 teaspoon tahini
¼ teaspoon onion powder
¼ teaspoon ground turmeric
½ to ¾ teaspoon sea salt

1. Preheat the oven to 375°F. Brush a 12-cup muffin tin with olive oil.

2. Heat about 1 tablespoon olive oil in a skillet over medium heat and sauté the garlic, red pepper, and mushrooms until the mushrooms begin to sweat. Stir in the chives, rosemary, and black pepper, and remove from the heat.

3. Place the tofu, soy milk, yeast, kuzu, tahini, onion powder, turmeric, and salt in a food processor or blender. Process until completely smooth. Add the tofu mixture to the vegetables and combine. Spoon into the muffin cups, filling each one about halfway.

4. Place the pan in the oven and reduce the heat to 350°F. Bake until the tops are golden and a knife inserted in the center of a quiche comes out clean, about 20 minutes. Remove from the oven and let cool for about 10 minutes.

For Kids

In this section, I've put together some recipes that kids love: chocolate chip rice treats, mac 'n' "cheese," alphabet soup, and more. It seems that any "normal" recipe—from soups to snacks to pizza and dessert—can be converted into a healthier version, so let this collection be a jumping-off place for more exploring. And although stuff like "seaweed nut crunch" may not—at first glance—seem like a winner, you and your kids will be amazed when you finally try it. As my photographer, Josh, said, "It's like sushi peanut brittle!"

Simply Delicious Alphabet Soup

Serves 4

This recipe is by teenager Eliana Finberg, daughter of Maine MILF Amy Rolnick. It is a quick, easy, and fun soup that kids will love.

1 to 2 tablespoons olive oil
1 large onion, diced
2 to 3 medium stalks celery, sliced
2 to 3 medium carrots, diced
2 cloves garlic, minced
¼ teaspoon paprika
¼ teaspoon dried oregano
¼ teaspoon celery salt
½ teaspoon dried basil

½ teaspoon mustard powder
½ teaspoon dried parsley
6 cups liquid (any combination of spring water or filtered water and your favorite vegetable stock)
½ cup uncooked alphabet noodles
½ to 1 teaspoon sea salt
Freshly ground black pepper (optional)
Fresh parsley, for garnish

Heat the oil over medium heat in a medium saucepan. Sauté the onion, celery, and carrots until the onion is translucent. Add the garlic and mix well. Add the paprika, oregano, celery salt, basil, mustard powder, and dried parsley, stirring well. Add the liquid, bring to a boil, then reduce the heat and simmer for 20 minutes. Add the alphabets, salt, and black pepper to taste. Simmer for 5 more minutes. Garnish with fresh parsley.

Killer No-Bake Drop Cookies

Makes 8 to 12 cookies, depending on the size of your spoonfuls

These are fun and easy and keep in the freezer . . . if they're not all gobbled up immediately!

⅔ cup maple syrup
¼ cup safflower or sunflower oil
5 tablespoons unsweetened cocoa powder
1 teaspoon ground cinnamon

½ cup peanut butter
1 cup rolled oats
1 teaspoon vanilla extract

---

1. In a saucepan over medium heat, combine the maple syrup, oil, cocoa, and cinnamon. Boil for 3 full minutes, stirring constantly.

2. Remove from the heat and stir in the peanut butter, rolled oats, and vanilla until well blended.

3. Drop by heaping spoonfuls onto waxed paper and chill in the freezer to set, about 30 minutes.

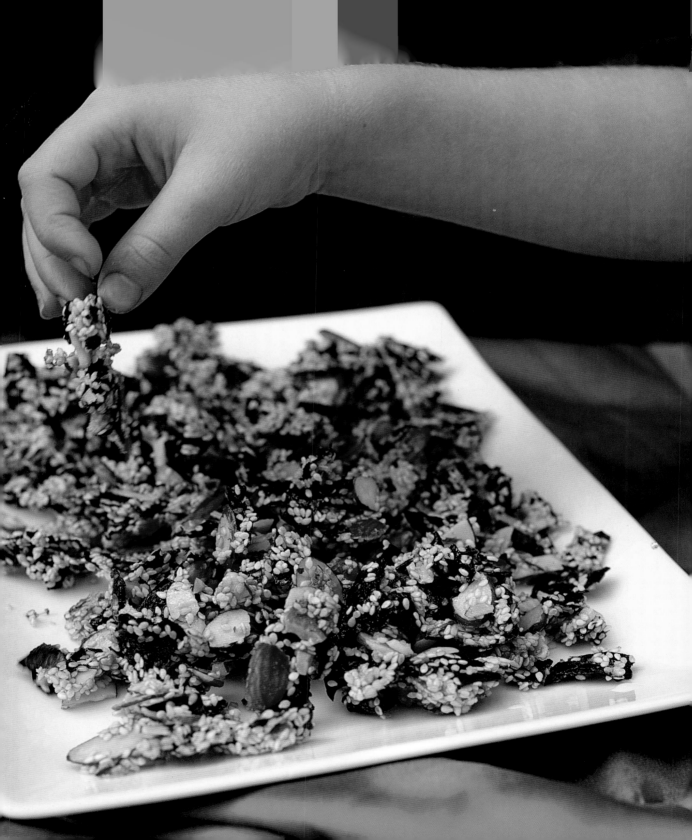

Seaweed-Nut Crunch

Serves 6

This recipe hails from the Rolnick household; as weird as it sounds, it is an *amazing* dessert or snack that woos kids and grown-ups alike. It's also easy.

---

2 tablespoons safflower or sunflower oil
½ cup maple syrup
1 cup sliced almonds

1 cup sesame seeds
6 sheets nori seaweed, torn into little pieces
1 teaspoon shoyu, or to taste

Preheat the oven to 350°F. Pour the oil and maple syrup into a large skillet. Bring to a frothy boil, and add the sliced almonds; stir, and add the sesame seeds and nori pieces. Sprinkle in the shoyu. Continue stirring until everything is coated. Pour into one layer on a baking sheet, or onto parchment paper on a baking sheet. Bake for 10 minutes. Let cool and eat.

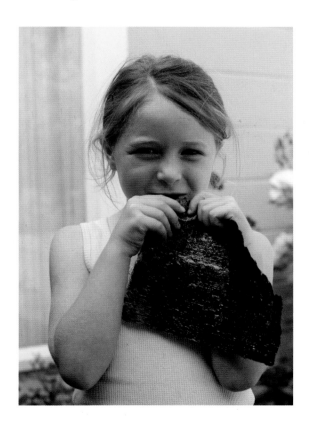

"Mac 'n' Cheese"

Serves 4

Chef Aaron Steinbach thought up this master "cheese" recipe and it works beautifully baked with noodles. You could also use it as a hollandaise sauce or another creamy "cheese" sauce.

---

2 cups dried macaroni or other noodles
1 cup raw cashews
1 cup spring water
1 tablespoon plus 1 teaspoon mellow white miso

1 teaspoon salt
¼ teaspoon ground turmeric
1 tablespoon kuzu root starch
½ cup plus 2 tablespoons safflower oil
½ cup whole wheat bread crumbs

---

1. Preheat the oven to 350°F. Boil the noodles in salted water according to the directions on the package. Drain, rinse, and set aside.

2. In a blender, grind the cashews into a fine meal. Add the water and blend into a creamy paste. Add the miso, salt, turmeric, and kuzu and blend together until smooth. Slowly add ½ cup oil while the mixture blends at high speed. This will emulsify the "cheese."

3. Place the noodles in a casserole dish and pour the "cheese" into it. Stir. Mix the remaining 2 tablespoons oil with the bread crumbs to form a paste, and spread over the noodles and "cheese." Bake for 40 minutes. Let cool for 20 minutes before serving.

"Mac 'n' Cheese" #2

For tofu lovers, this version is nice; it bakes into a slightly firmer dish and gets its cheesy taste from the nutritional yeast. Try them both!

2 cups whole wheat elbow macaroni
1 block soft tofu (usually 12 or 14 ounces)
½ cup olive oil
¼ cup nutritional yeast

¼ cup tahini
¼ cup spring water
2 tablespoons umeboshi vinegar

Preheat the oven to 350°F. Prepare the noodles according to the package directions and set aside in a large bowl. Blend the tofu, oil, nutritional yeast, tahini, water, and umeboshi vinegar until smooth. Pour the sauce onto the noodles and mix well. Put the mixture into a casserole dish and bake for 40 minutes. Let cool for 20 minutes before serving.

Crispy Kale

Serves about 4, depending on the size of the bunch of kale

This is a great way to get the kids to eat greens every once in a while. Not so bad for grown-ups either . . .

½ large bunch kale
1 teaspoon olive oil

½ teaspoon shoyu

Preheat the oven to 350°F. Tear the kale into large bite-size pieces. Combine the oil and shoyu and massage the kale with this mixture until well coated. Use more if necessary. Place on a baking sheet or in a Pyrex baking dish and put on the center rack of the oven. Bake for 15 to 20 minutes, until crispy. Serve.

Banana Wontons

Makes as many wontons as you like, depending on how many wonton skins you have

This recipe comes from Krista Berman, Florida MILF. When I first tasted these, I couldn't believe my mouth's good luck!

Bananas, sliced into ½-inch rounds
Square wonton skins (without egg, if you can find them—they exist)

Fruit-sweetened preserves
Sesame Salt (page 253)
Safflower oil

1. Place some banana slices in the middle of a wonton skin. Add a tiny bit of preserves and a sprinkle of sesame salt. Fold the wonton skin corners in, one corner at a time, over the banana slices, so that they all come together, as if you were wrapping a present or sealing an envelope. Seal closed with a touch of water on the last corner flap. Prepare the number of wontons you would like to serve.

2. Heat oil in a cast-iron skillet until very hot but not smoking and gently place as many wontons in the pan as you can without crowding them. Fry on each side until golden brown, paying close attention, as they cook quite quickly and can burn if the oil is too hot.

3. Drain briefly on paper towels and serve hot.

VARIATION: Try apple pie wontons with apple slices, cinnamon, and maple sugar; or raspberry-chocolate wontons made with a raspberry or two and some SunSpire nondairy chocolate chips.

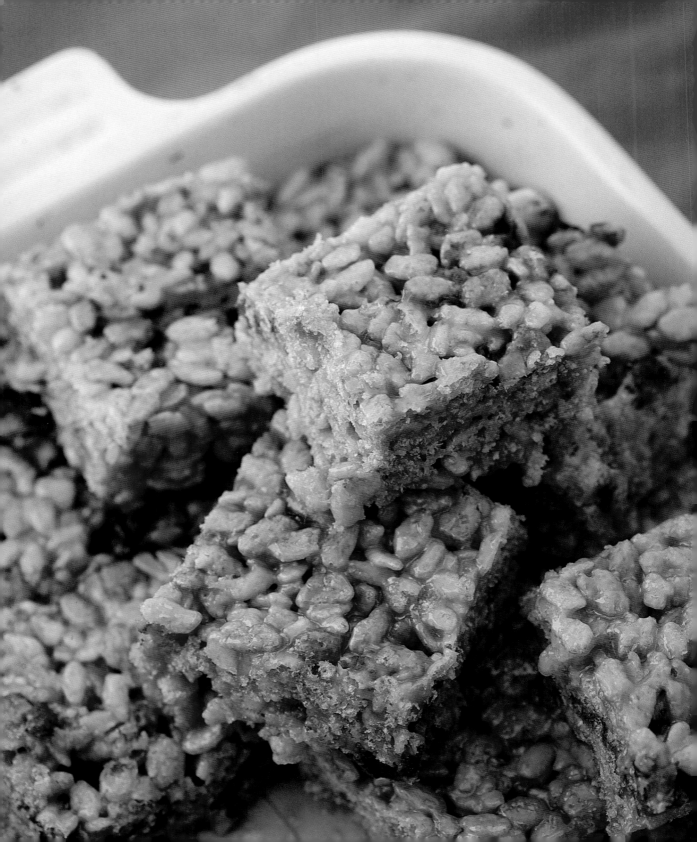

Chocolate Chip Rice Treats

Serves 8

I dare you not to like these.

---

4 cups crispy brown rice cereal
1 cup brown rice syrup
¾ cup peanut butter
Dash of umeboshi vinegar

Dash of vanilla extract
¼ to ½ cup grain-sweetened nondairy
    chocolate chips by SunSpire

Pour the cereal into a mixing bowl. In a saucepan over medium heat, heat the brown rice syrup, peanut butter, vinegar, and vanilla, stirring constantly until the mixture is smooth, thinned out, and bubbling a little. Reduce the heat to low and keep stirring while the mixture bubbles for at least 3 minutes. Pour the rice syrup mixture onto the cereal and blend with a wooden spoon. Mix well. Let cool until you can add the chocolate chips without melting them completely, 5 to 10 minutes. Fold in the chocolate chips. Pour into a Pyrex pan or baking pan and flatten with a wet spatula. Let cool. Slice and serve.

Divine Corn-Crust Pizza

Makes 2 pizzas

This is a slight adaptation of a recipe by lovely and talented Aine McAteer. She makes a delicious "no-mato" sauce for MILFs who want to avoid nightshade vegetables and the sore joints that can come with them. In the photograph, I've added Daiya "cheese" to the pizza, but this original recipe does without it. Try it both ways!

CRUST
1½ cups cornmeal
1½ cups white spelt flour, plus extra for the work surface
1 cup fresh corn kernels
2 teaspoons aluminum-free baking powder
½ teaspoon sea salt
About ½ cup spring water
2 tablespoons olive oil

"NO-MATO" SAUCE
½ medium onion, diced
3 medium carrots, diced
½ large beet (or 1 medium), diced
Sea salt
Olive oil
2 cloves garlic, minced
1 shallot, minced

½ teaspoon dried oregano
1 tablespoon umeboshi vinegar
Freshly ground black pepper

TOPPINGS
Vegan "cheese"
Shiitake or cremini mushrooms
Olives
Red, yellow, green bell peppers
Zucchini
Red onion
Broccoli (blanched)
Veggie or tofu sausage (thinly sliced)
Fresh basil
8 ounces crumbled firm tofu, mixed with 1 tablespoon olive oil and 1 tablespoon shoyu

1. To make the crust, combine the cornmeal, spelt flour, corn (I like to put the kernels in a food processor or blender first and break them up), baking powder, and salt in a bowl and add the water and olive oil. Mix well so that the mixture comes together and forms a dough, and transfer to a floured work surface. Knead for at least 5 minutes, until the dough is smooth and stretchy. Cover the dough and set aside as you prepare the rest of the ingredients.

2. To make the "no-mato" sauce, combine the onion, carrots, and beet in a saucepan and add enough water to just cover the vegetables; add a big pinch of sea salt. Bring to a boil, cover the pan, reduce the heat, and simmer for about 15 minutes.

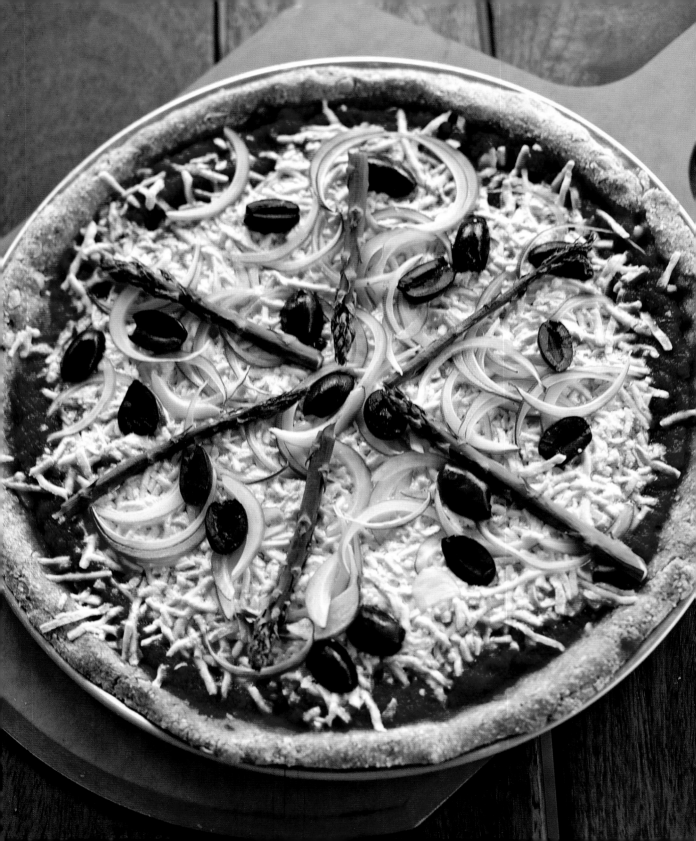

3. While the vegetables are cooking, heat 1 tablespoon olive oil in a sauté pan and add the garlic and shallot and a big pinch of sea salt. Sauté for a minute or so, then add the oregano and continue to sauté until the vegetables are soft and translucent.

4. When the onion, carrots, and beet are done, puree them in a blender, adding enough of the cooking water to get a thick-sauce consistency. Add the blended mixture to the shallot mixture and stir it in. Add the umeboshi vinegar for a tangier tomatoey taste Add black pepper to taste.

5. Preheat the oven to 375°F. Oil 2 pizza pans or baking sheets.

6. Divide the pizza dough in half. Roll out each half into a big circle and transfer it to a pizza pan. You can decoratively crimp the edges. I usually just roll the dough out a bit and then transfer it to the pan and continue to press it into the desired shape, circle or rectangle. Prick the dough all over with a fork and bake for about 5 minutes.

7. Remove from the oven and top with the sauce and your choice of toppings. I like to make 2 different pizzas, so there's a choice. Return to the oven for about 10 minutes, then slice and serve.

VARIATIONS: You can use another flour such as whole wheat pastry flour, or for a gluten-free version, rice or oat flour in place of the spelt.

Instead of "no-mato" sauce, you can top with pesto and veggies—this is one of my favorite variations. I make my own pesto with 2 cups fresh basil, 1 cup parsley, ⅓ cup pine nuts or almonds, 6 tablespoons olive oil, 1 clove garlic, and sea salt to taste, all whizzed in a blender or food processor.

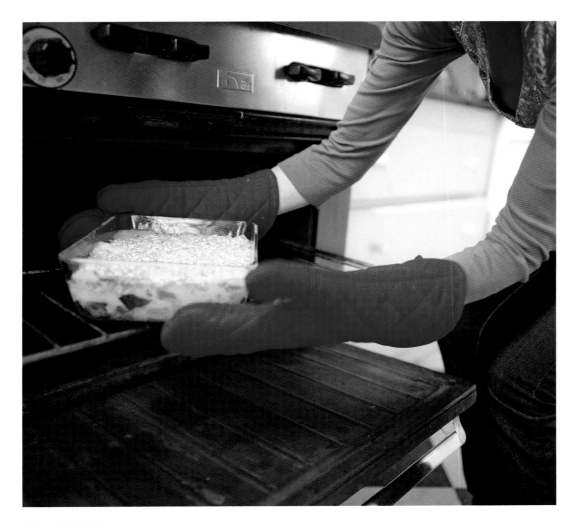

For DILFs

Most DILFs love to eat, and if you're lucky, you have one who enjoys just about everything put in front of him. In this section, I've put together a collection of recipes that are tried-and-true winners for the husband willing to try a plant-based diet. And if he's reluctant, sneak a little meat in here and there until his taste buds come around.

And of course, you, Ms. MILF, can enjoy these recipes, too!

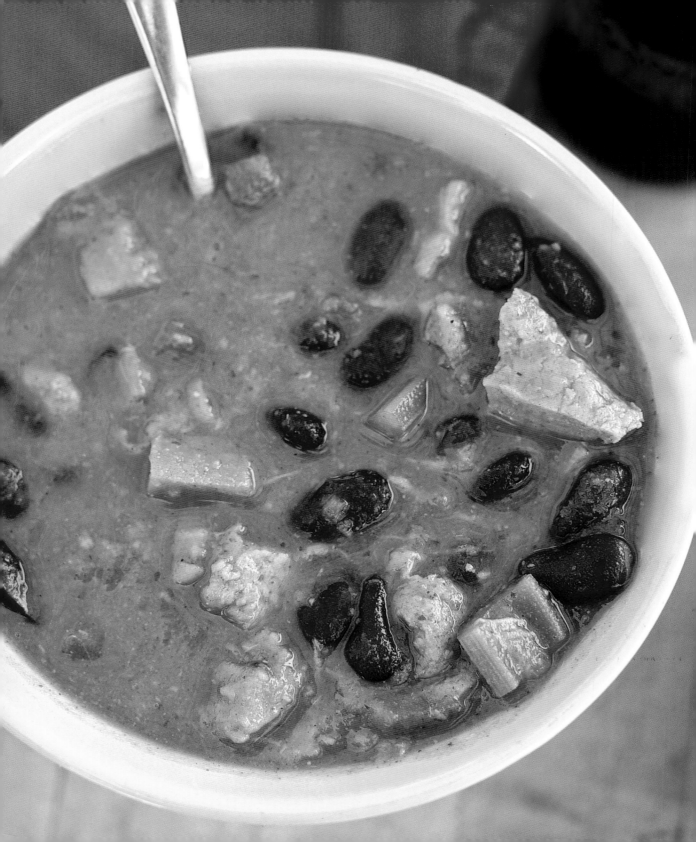

Vegetarian Chili

Serves 4

This is a recipe by Melanie Brown Waxman, and it is perfect for the DILF who loves his spicy food, a cold beer, and maybe a corn muffin for dipping. If he's eating meat, this is a great dish to hybridize.

---

2 tablespoons extra virgin olive oil
1 clove garlic, sliced
1 medium onion, cut into large cubes
One 1-inch piece kombu
2 medium tomatoes, diced
1 medium stalk celery, diced
1 small sweet potato, diced
1 medium carrot, diced
1 cup dried kidney beans, soaked overnight, or two 15-ounce cans cooked

Spring water
1 tablespoon sea salt
1 teaspoon chili powder
1 teaspoon ground cumin
$\frac{1}{4}$ to $\frac{1}{2}$ teaspoon cayenne pepper
1 cup diced seitan
1 tablespoon balsamic vinegar
2 tablespoons chopped fresh basil

---

1. Heat a pressure cooker and add the oil. Sauté the garlic and onion for about 2 minutes. Layer the following ingredients on top: the kombu, tomatoes, celery, sweet potato, carrot, and beans. Add enough water to just cover the beans. Use the bean soaking water and any additional water as needed.

2. Cover and bring up to pressure over medium heat. Reduce the heat to low and cook for 45 minutes (20 minutes if using canned beans). Remove from the heat and let the pressure drop.

3. Add the salt and return to medium heat. Add the chili powder, cumin, cayenne pepper, and seitan, and cook for about 10 minutes. Add the balsamic vinegar and cook for 1 more minute. Serve with the fresh basil.

Grilled "Cheese" Sandwiches with Portobello Mushrooms and Cashew-Garlic Aioli

Makes 4 sandwiches

This is a great recipe. It was inspired by a sandwich I would eat religiously every time I visited a sadly now-defunct restaurant in Toronto called Pulp Kitchen. Anyway, I've substituted my new favorite vegan "cheese" for the original's polenta, but feel free to try it any way you like. Great for DILFs, but it's not unreasonable for a MILF to enjoy this now and again . . .

GRILLED PORTOBELLOS
4 large portobello mushrooms
¼ cup olive oil
2 tablespoons shoyu
3 to 4 teaspoons balsamic vinegar
Pinch of sea salt
Couple of grinds of black pepper

CASHEW-GARLIC AIOLI
½ cup raw cashews

3 tablespoons fresh lemon juice
3 to 4 cloves garlic, chopped
¼ cup spring water
½ cup safflower or sunflower oil
Pinch of sea salt

Olive oil
8 slices sourdough bread (whole wheat is best)
Daiya cheddar "cheese" shreds

1. Preheat the oven to 450°F. Make sure the rack is in the middle of the oven. Brush the mushrooms to remove any obvious dirt. Remove the stems from the mushrooms.

2. Place the caps in a baking pan, gill side up. Mix the olive oil, shoyu, vinegar, salt, and pepper together well and pour over the mushroom caps. Marinate the caps for 10 minutes, and then turn them, making sure lots of surface area gets introduced to the marinade. Let them sit for at least 10 minutes and up to 1 hour.

3. Remove the mushrooms, but keep the leftover marinade. Oil a baking sheet and place the mushrooms on the sheet, gill side down. Brush with a little of the reserved marinade, and roast in the middle of the oven for about 5 minutes. Turn the mushrooms over, brush with marinade, and roast until they are tender, about 5 more minutes (see Note). No need to get neurotic about the timing—you can't really mess up portobello mushrooms unless you totally forget about them and they shrivel completely.

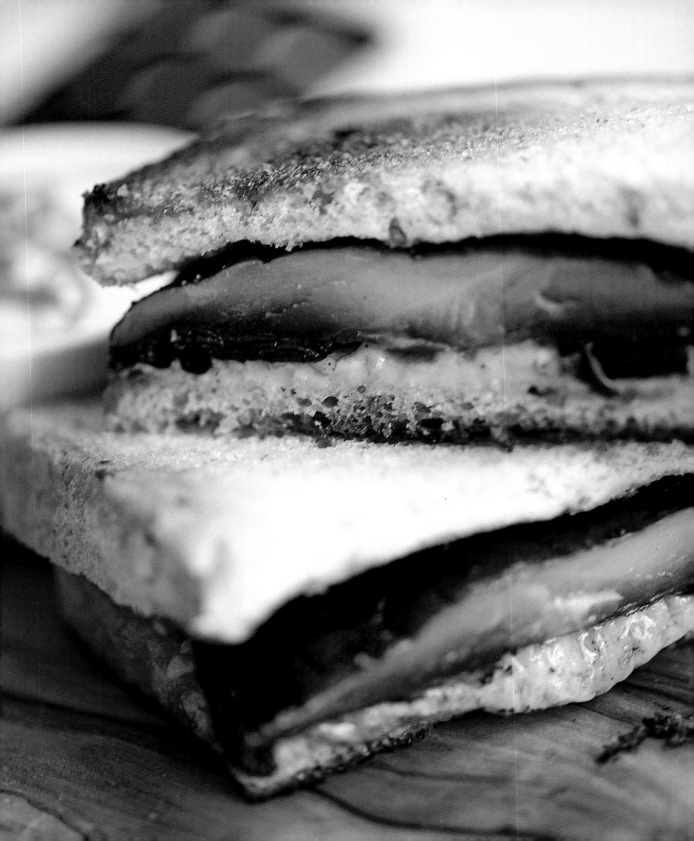

4. To prepare the aioli, in a food processor or blender, grind the cashews into a very fine meal. Add the lemon juice, garlic, and water and combine until you get a relatively smooth consistency. Begin to add the safflower or sunflower oil, slowly, until you get a creamy texture. Add the salt and process for another minute or so. Adjust the seasonings if necessary. Makes 1 cup.

5. To assemble the sandwiches, in a large, heavy skillet, heat 1 to 2 tablespoons olive oil over medium-low heat. Place the slices of bread in the skillet and sprinkle each slice with Daiya cheddar "cheese." Cover and let the "cheese" melt. This "cheese" won't appear (to your eye) to melt completely, but if you touch it, you'll see that it's soft. When it seems to have melted, remove the bread slices from the skillet, place on a platter, and place a grilled mushroom cap on 4 of the slices. Top with the remaining 4 slices, surrounding the mushrooms with cheese. Slice and serve with the aioli, for dipping. And you thought healthy food would be boring!

NOTE: If you're using an outdoor grill, cook the mushrooms about 6 inches from the flame (or coals) for about 5 minutes on each side, brushing with the marinade a couple of times.

Tempeh Reuben with Russian Dressing

Makes 2 sandwiches

This is lip-smackingly good.

RUSSIAN DRESSING
2 tablespoons fruit-sweetened ketchup or
    Sun-Dried Tomato Ketchup (page 110)
2 tablespoons organic relish
½ cup Vegenaise

SANDWICH
One 8-ounce package tempeh
½ cup spring water
2 tablespoons shoyu
2 tablespoons olive oil
4 slices whole-grain sourdough bread
1 tablespoon unsweetened sauerkraut or any
    unsweetened pickle

1. Mix the dressing ingredients together by hand and set aside.

2. Slice the block of tempeh in half. Simmer the tempeh in the water and shoyu until the liquid is absorbed, 15 to 20 minutes. Flip the tempeh at least once, so that each side gets seasoned.

3. Panfry the tempeh in the olive oil until crispy.

4. Steam the bread in a steamer for 1 minute (or grill it in a little olive oil until crispy). Slice the tempeh in half and place the tempeh, sauerkraut, and dressing on 2 pieces of the bread. Place the top slices on the sandwiches. Slice and serve.

VARIATIONS: Use different flavors of tempeh, like sea vegetable, three-grain, or quinoa. You can also quarter the tempeh lengthwise and use 8 slices of bread, so one package of tempeh will yield four sandwiches.
    Great additions are lettuce, sprouts, and raw red onion.

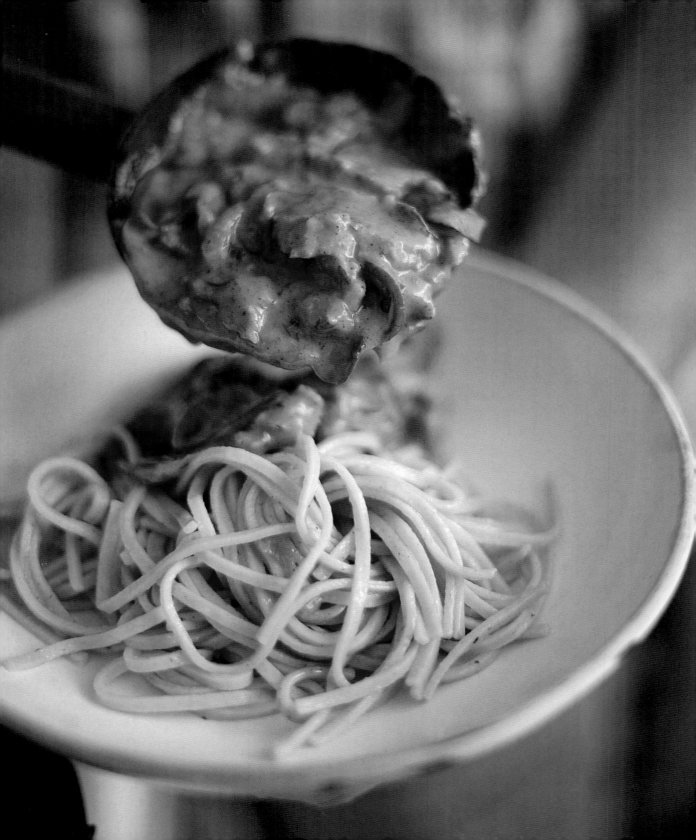

Seitan Stroganoff

Serves 2 or 3

My good friend Aaron Steinbach is a private chef who works for the rich and famous in Hollywood these days, but I met him when he was a young whipper-snapper eating brown rice and kale. I asked him to donate this recipe to the book because I couldn't forget it after eating it seventeen years ago. It's hearty, delicious, and, served over noodles or rice, perfect for a DILF. It's even quick!

1 tablespoon olive oil	2 cups spring water
1 medium onion, sliced into half-moons	1 tablespoon mirin
8 ounces cremini or button mushrooms, sliced	2 teaspoons kuzu root starch or arrowroot
1 teaspoon sea salt	2 to 4 tablespoons almond butter
One 8-ounce package WestSoy seitan, cut into bite-size slices	1 to 2 tablespoon shoyu
	Chopped fresh parsley, for garnish

In a skillet, heat the oil over medium heat. Add the onion and sauté until soft. Add the mushrooms and continue to sauté. Add the salt and allow the mushrooms to soften even more, releasing some of their liquid. Add the seitan, 2 cups water, and mirin. Bring to a boil. Dissolve the kuzu completely in a little bit of cold water and whisk into the mixture, continuing to stir to prevent lumps. Stir in the almond butter and shoyu, starting with the lower measurements and tasting as you go. Simmer for 3 to 4 minutes over low heat. Serve over noodles or rice and garnish with parsley.

Fried Rice for DILFs

Serves 2

Any dish can be made more yin or more yang, and fried rice is a great example of that. You've got the basics, which are the rice and vegetables, but all the other choices can tip the dish in one direction or the other. In this recipe, we are using short-grain rice (more yang than long-grain or basmati), a heartier oil, root vegetables, dense tempeh, and more salty seasoning. A MILFier version might have long-grain rice, more and lighter veggies (fresh corn, red bell pepper, snow peas, bok choy perhaps), tofu, olive oil, less shoyu, and a girlie splash of fresh lemon juice. The whole dish would have a fresher, lighter vibe. Of course, there are no hard-and-fast rules, but this fried rice should certainly satisfy a DILF on a cold day.

¼ cup cubed tempeh
3 tablespoons toasted sesame oil
1 tablespoon mirin
1 tablespoon plus 2 teaspoons shoyu
1 clove garlic, minced
Sea salt
1 medium onion, diced

1 medium carrot, diced
2 cups leftover short-grain rice
1 medium stalk celery, diced
2 tablespoons spring water
Knob of ginger, grated and squeezed to make
    1 teaspoon ginger juice
Chopped scallions, for garnish

---

1. Steam the tempeh for 20 minutes. In a skillet, heat 2 tablespoons of the oil and add the tempeh. After the cubes have browned a little, turn them and add the mirin and the 1 tablespoon shoyu. Let the liquid cook off. Remove from the heat and drain the tempeh on paper towels or a paper bag.

2. Heat the remaining 1 tablespoon oil in a skillet over medium heat. Add the garlic and a tiny pinch of salt, stirring quickly to avoid burning. After about 10 seconds, add the onion and another small pinch of salt, cooking until the onion is translucent. Add the carrot and another small pinch of salt. Sauté for a few minutes until the carrot is soft. Add the cooked rice, tempeh, celery, and the 2 teaspoons shoyu. Sprinkle the water carefully over the contents of the pan, cover, and reduce the heat. Let it steam for 4 minutes. Squeeze the ginger juice over the dish. Mix well. Garnish with chopped scallions.

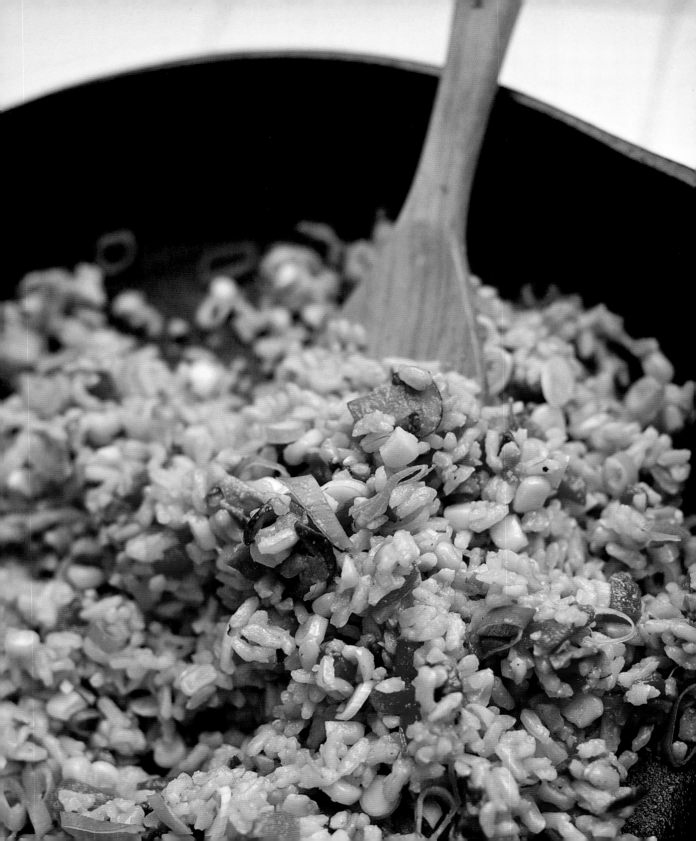

Palak Seitan Murg

Serves 4 to 6

This is a dish created by MILFy Simone Parris, who has spent the last few years living, and cooking, in India. *Palak murg* actually means "spinach chicken," but for the MILF diet, we've changed that to kale and seitan. Really tasty and great for DILFs who crave strong spices.

---

1 pound kale, finely chopped
Sea salt
1 tablespoon extra virgin olive oil
2 cups finely diced onions
1½ pounds seitan, cut into 1-inch cubes
1 tablespoon minced peeled fresh ginger
1 tablespoon minced garlic
½ teaspoon chili powder

2 teaspoons ground toasted coriander seeds, or ground coriander
2 tablespoons mirin or cooking wine
1 cup spring water
½ teaspoon garam masala
1 teaspoon shoyu
¼ cup finely chopped fresh cilantro

---

1. Cook the kale in a large pot of rapidly boiling salted water until just tender, 2 to 3 minutes. You will need to do this in 2 batches, at least. Drain and set aside.

2. In a skillet with a lid, heat the oil over medium heat and sauté the onions with a pinch of salt for 3 to 5 minutes, or until translucent. Stir in the seitan, ginger, garlic, chili powder, ½ teaspoon salt, and the coriander and sauté for another 2 minutes. Add the mirin and water, cover, reduce the heat to low, and simmer for 15 minutes.

3. Remove the lid, stir in the blanched kale, the garam masala, and the shoyu, and cook off any excess water. Garnish with the fresh cilantro and serve hot.

VARIATION: WestSoy now makes a "chicken" seitan, which is very nice for this dish, too.

Sauces and Dressings

Sexy, silky dressings can transform a ho-hum dish into a hit. I encourage you to try the following dressings and then begin to explore making them yourself; mix tastes, textures, and consistencies to keep your daily fare as MILFy as possible.

If you're short on kitchen time, you can now find a variety of delicious nondairy and sugar-free sauces and dressings at better health food stores. Vegenaise is a great mayonnaise substitute, and be sure to try Miso Mayo in its three zippy flavors. Wildwood also makes a lovely garlic aioli, and Amy's produces a number of great salad dressings. Explore and enjoy.

Miso-Tahini Sauce

Serves 4

This is a base for a number of different variations you could think up. Miso and tahini go beautifully together (salt and oil always do!), but you can add scallions, cilantro, parsley, citrus, garlic, ginger, grated onion, brown rice syrup, balsamic vinegar. . . . You name it. Miso-tahini sauce can go a million different ways.

⅔ cup tahini	½ teaspoon umeboshi paste, or ⅛ umeboshi
2 tablespoons miso	plum flesh
½ cup spring water	

Whiz all of the ingredients in a blender until smooth. Serve over Brad Pitt Vegetables (page 126) or a grain dish. *Mmmm* . . . makes everything better.

VARIATIONS: Use less water and it becomes a spread for the sourdough bread on page 123. Also, you can use light or dark miso; lighter misos are sweeter and darker misos are saltier.

Carrot-Ginger Dressing

Makes about 1 cup, which serves 4 to 6

I've always loved the dressing that comes on fresh salads at Japanese restaurants, and this is a great version of it.

1 tablespoon minced carrot
1 tablespoon minced peeled fresh ginger
⅓ medium onion, chopped
1 tablespoon finely chopped lemon (with some rind)
2½ tablespoons shoyu
¼ cup safflower or light olive oil
¼ cup brown rice vinegar

1 tablespoon brown rice syrup
¼ cup spring water
2 teaspoons sugar-sweetened ketchup or Sun-Dried Tomato Ketchup (page 110)
Pinch of sea salt (adjust depending on how salty your shoyu is; optional)
Pinch of freshly ground black pepper

Whiz all of the ingredients in a blender until creamy. Serve this dressing immediately or reblend before serving, as it tends to separate.

Lemon–Poppy Seed Dressing

Serves 4 to 6

Simone Parris donated this recipe. She says, "This is just an amazing salad dressing—people always rave about the delicious lemony taste and the crunchy texture." She's right. It's great.

¼ cup fresh lemon juice
Grated zest of 1 lemon (please use an organic lemon and only the yellow part; avoid the white part, as it is bitter)
1 teaspoon prepared Dijon or whole-grain mustard
1 teaspoon shoyu

4 drops lemon essential oil (optional)
2 tablespoons brown rice syrup
2 tablespoons diced onion
¼ cup sunflower oil
2 tablespoons untoasted sesame oil
1 tablespoon brown rice vinegar
¼ cup black poppy seeds

Combine all of the ingredients and blend in a blender.

Avocado Dressing

Serves 2

I made this dressing up to slather all over a salad of diced iceberg lettuce, red onion, and cucumbers one hot summer night. I LOVE ICEBERG LETTUCE!!!

½ **really ripe avocado**
½ **bunch fresh cilantro**
¼ **cup extra virgin olive oil, plus more as needed**

1 **teaspoon organic Dijon mustard**
1 **teaspoon umeboshi vinegar**
½ **teaspoon shoyu**
1 **teaspoon maple syrup**

Whiz all the ingredients in a food processor or blender. If the mixture is too thick, just add more olive oil until you have a nice, creamy consistency. Adjust the seasonings to taste. (You might need more umeboshi vinegar.)

Green-Life Veggie Dip

Serves 4 or 5

In this vegetable dip, Gabriele Kushi uses avocados, and she knows a thing or two about them: "Avocados contain oleic acid, a monounsaturated fat that may help lower cholesterol. Avocados are a good source of potassium, a mineral that helps regulate blood pressure." You can find more recipes like this in her book, *Embracing Menopause Naturally*.

4 **ounces soft tofu**
1 **tablespoon shoyu**
7 **fresh basil sprigs**
2 **avocados**

Juice and peel of 1 lemon
¼ **teaspoon sea salt**
Dash of spring water or extra virgin olive oil (optional)

Cube the tofu and simmer in 1 cup water and the shoyu for 5 minutes. Drain and set aside. Wash the basil sprigs and slice thinly. Peel the avocados and remove the pits. Combine the avocado flesh with the basil, lemon juice and peel, salt, and tofu in a blender or food processor. Purée until smooth while adding the water or oil, if using. Serve at room temperature.

VARIATIONS: Include a variety of finely chopped raw or steamed vegetables for different colors and tastes.

Beverages

These days, we are told to chug water—eight glasses a day, to be precise. In fact, the word on the street is that we should be drinking before we're even thirsty; that by the time we experience thirst, we are *dehydrated.* Cue scary music.

But if MILFs are looking to balance themselves and to harmonize with the natural environment, then having an external prescription for taking in fluids makes no sense. Think about it: You don't go to sleep early because "by the time you're tired, you're *exhausted*!" You don't have sex before you're aroused because "by the time you're horny, you're a *nymphomaniac*!" You don't argue with fatigue, arousal, hunger, or the many other signals your body gives you. To think that—given the incredible symphony of functions your body handles at any given moment—thirst is somehow inherently flawed is pretty weird. So let's not get all neurotic about thirst; it works just fine.

The eight-glasses-a-day prescription, by the way, is designed for a world consuming tons of meat, sugar, and salty, processed foods. And, yes, it may be a good idea to drink plenty of water to flush out the toxins and acids that tend to build up on that kind of diet. But by eating the whole grains, vegetables, and plant-based proteins of the MILF diet, you are choosing from a more balanced and fluid-rich menu, so you don't need to be overriding your own thirst mechanism.

Besides, you can get too much fluid. Just as overwatering a plant can kill it, filling ourselves with water is not benign. Your body's brilliant ability to maintain homeostasis means handling its temperature, electrolyte balance, and all sorts of fluid-based functions that only it can finesse to perfection. Excessive hydration can actually create imbalances in systems that depend on dryness or warmth or a certain ratio of this to that. So when it comes to water, enough is exactly enough.

MILFy Drinking Dos and Don'ts

DO: Invest in a good water filter or buy spring water. Because you are made of 70 percent water, it's important to replenish yourself with good-quality H_2O.

DO: Check the labels on bottled water carefully. Some are simply tap water or from city reservoirs. Look for real spring water with nothing added to it.

DO: Drink to satisfy thirst. But if you find that you're thirsty often, you may be getting too much salt, in the form of sea salt, shoyu, or miso. Your excessive thirst is a sign that your body is striking a wide balance. Dial down the salt and you should crave less fluid. Refined carbohydrates like white sugar and white flour also cause the body to crave fluid.

DON'T drink with meals, since water dilutes digestive enzymes. After a meal, however, have some tea (see below) or water if you feel like it.

DON'T drink cold or iced drinks, which can tax kidney energy and cool the body. Remember, your body is constantly seeking a temperature of 98°F. That's warm. By pouring ice-cold liquids into it day after day, you are throwing yourself out of balance and wasting a lot of your life force simply heating up fluid. Go for hot, warm, or room-temperature drinks. Even on hot days. FYI: Your attraction to icy drinks will lessen as you kick meat and sugar, which tend to overheat the body.

DO: Explore mild teas, especially the ones coming up. By *mild,* I mean "not too stimulating." The strong stuff can be used now and then, but for daily use, it's best to drink teas that are balanced and stabilizing.

Kukicha Tea

Serves 2

Kukicha is also known as "twig tea," because it comes from the young stems of the tea plant. This is a great daily beverage because it's alkalizing and it contains some calcium. Kukicha also has a nice, sort of woody taste. You can find it in tea bags, or you can buy and steep the twigs themselves.

2 to 3 cups spring water
1 level tablespoon kukicha twigs
(in a tea ball if desired)

Rice syrup (optional)

Bring the water to a boil. Add the twigs and reduce the heat. Simmer on very low heat for 5 minutes, then strain out the twigs. The tea should be light brown in color, not dark. Once in a while, serve it with a dollop of rice syrup.

Roasted Barley Tea

Serves 2

This is another tea that can be enjoyed on a daily basis, although, because barley has a naturally cooling effect on the body, it's best in the spring and summer. Barley is also great for the liver and gallbladder and will give you clear and glowing skin. Roasted barley tea is available mostly in a loose form and is often found at Asian supermarkets. Seriously old-school hard-core MILFs roast their own barley to make tea. This recipe is for pre-roasted barley.

2 to 3 cups spring water	**Barley malt (optional)**
1 level tablespoon roasted barley	

Boil the water. Pour it into a teapot with the barley. Let steep for 5 minutes. Strain and serve. If you want to sweeten it, try some barley malt in your cup.

Peppermint Tea

Serves 2

Peppermint is so great because you can either pluck it from your garden or find a MILFy friend who grows it; chances are she will be overrun by this hearty plant. Both peppermint and spearmint are cooling to the body, so they're great for spring and summer.

2 to 3 cups spring water	**12 to 15 fresh peppermint leaves**

Boil the water and pour over the peppermint leaves in a teapot. Let steep for 4 to 5 minutes. Strain and serve.

Healing Drinks

These are drinks used for specific reasons and conditions. Use them when you need them and not just for fun; they're powerful.

Umeboshi Tonic

Serves 1

This drink is a remedy for a number of ailments: diarrhea, hangovers from alcohol and sugar, weak digestion, and general listlessness. The umeboshi plum alkalizes your blood easily and quickly, while the kuzu has a binding effect in the intestines and is an intestinal tonifier. If you struggle with constipation but still want to use this drink, skip the kuzu.

1 cup spring water
½ umeboshi plum
1 heaping teaspoon kuzu root starch,
    dissolved in ¼ cup cold water

A few drops of shoyu

Bring the water and umeboshi plum to a boil. Simmer for about 3 minutes. Add the kuzu mixture, stirring constantly to avoid lumps. Bring back to a boil. Add the shoyu and simmer for about 4 more minutes. Drink/eat when it has come to a temperature you can handle, but the warmer, the better.

VARIATION: Umeboshi tea (½ umeboshi plum boiled in 1 cup spring water) is also good for hangovers and relieves heartburn and nausea.

Really Relaxing Tea

Serves 1

This tea is incredibly relaxing because shiitake mushrooms help to pull excess salt from the body. So if you're tense and salty after a restaurant meal, make this tea. Shiitake mushrooms also help to dissolve fat.

---

1 dried shiitake mushroom
1 cup spring water

1 or 2 drops shoyu

Soak the mushroom in the water for 20 minutes. Remove from the soaking liquid, discard the stem from the mushroom, and slice the cap into strips. Bring the soaking liquid and mushroom strips to a boil. Simmer for 10 minutes. Add the shoyu and simmer for 5 more minutes. Drink/eat.

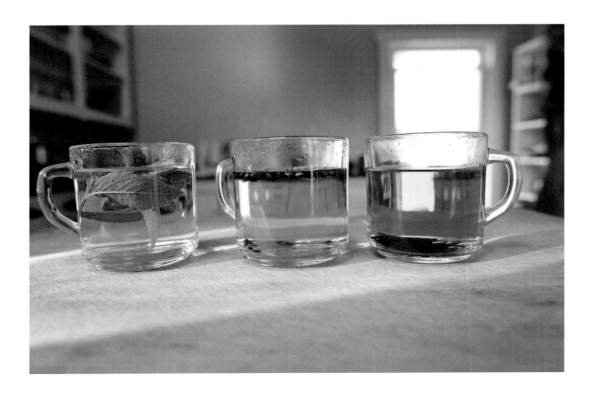

That-Time-of-the-Month Drink

Serves 1

This drink is great for menstrual cramps because it helps to relax the liver meridian, which runs through your uterus and ovaries. Sounds crazy? Try it. It won't be quite like taking a pill, but you'll find that it helps to relax that whole area of your body. The smell this drink makes when it's cooking is a little strong, but the taste is fine.

½ cup grated (into a pulp) daikon
½ cup spring water

1 to 2 drops shoyu

Bring the daikon and water to a boil. Add the shoyu. Simmer for a couple of minutes, so the daikon loses its pungency. Drink/eat when the temperature is right for you.

Carrot-Daikon Drink

Serves 1

This pulpy, slushy drink is great for weight loss, and you can drink/eat it for ten days straight, but then you need to dial it back to twice a week. Too much of it can start to demineralize your body. Do the ten-day regimen only once or twice a year.

½ cup grated (into a pulp) carrot
½ cup grated (into a pulp) daikon
¼ umeboshi plum
A few of drops of shoyu

1 cup spring water
¼ sheet nori seaweed, torn into little pieces (optional)

Bring the carrot, daikon, umeboshi plum, shoyu, and water to a boil. Simmer for about 3 minutes. Add the nori, if using. Remove from the heat and drink/eat.

Fun Drinks

Juices are a great-tasting and easy way to get lots of nutrients quickly. But juices shouldn't take the place of regular foods, or entire meals; juices lack fiber and wholeness and can be high in natural sugar. So treat them as fun drinks. Enjoy a veggie juice a couple of times a week and something fruitier a little less often.

Ari's "Tender Mix" Juice

Serves 1 or 2

My friend Ari Arom is a chef to the stars, an herbalist, and a master mixologist in Los Angeles. This juice recipe is packed full of nutrients, and the strawberries give it a relaxing, delicate MILFiness.

3 or 4 large carrots (to make about ¾ cup juice)
5 or 6 large strawberries or 8 medium, hulled
2 large stalks celery

1 large broccoli floret (about ¼ cup if chopped)
3 or 4 leaves romaine lettuce

Juice the carrots, strawberries, celery, broccoli, and lettuce. Drink immediately.

VARIATIONS: Add a touch of fresh apple, lemon juice, or ginger juice.

Enlightenment Smoothie

Serves 2

MILFy Lisa Silverman is into all things spiritual and she likes to drink this smoothie before doing all that woo-woo stuff. Wink.

1 ripe peach, pitted and chopped
1 cup strawberries
1 tablespoon chia seeds
1 teaspoon coconut oil
1 cup unsweetened soy milk, or almond, hemp, or oat milk

½ cup apple cider or juice
1 teaspoon ginger juice
½ teaspoon ground cinnamon
1 tablespoon almond butter

Place in a blender, whiz until smooth, and serve.

VARIATION: To make Lisa's favorite smoothie, substitute a pear for the peach and chopped mango for the strawberries. But, really, you can go crazy with any fruit you like.

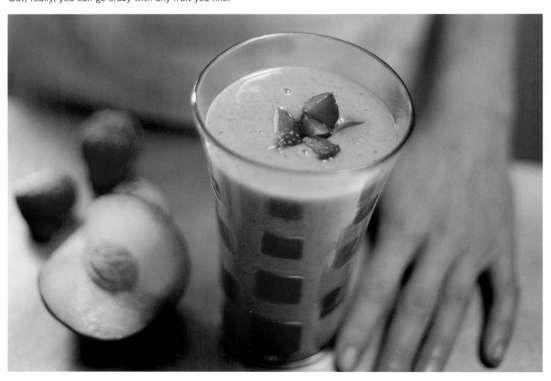

Seasonings and Condiments

Your New Basic MILF Seasonings

Unrefined sea salt: Unrefined sea salt, which is white and clumps a little, is the best salt for your body. Its mineral balance is very close to that of your blood, so it keeps you nice and balanced.

Refined sea salt, which may still be white but has been processed to pour freely, is not as balanced. Although you may want to play with gray, pink, or other exotic salts every once in a while, they often contain too many minerals, so it's best to keep the white, unrefined sea salt as your go-to in the kitchen.

Table salt, which is mostly sodium chloride, has been stripped of most of its original minerals and can cause real damage to the body; when people get all upset about the harmful effects of salt, they're generally talking about table salt. Chuck it out.

Sea salt should always be cooked into a dish and never set out on the table. It is too intense and contracted for the body to assimilate well.[2] Think about it: salt isn't found in crystals in the sea; it's integrated into the fluid, just as it should be in our bodies. When adding salt to soups and other dishes, make sure it is cooked for at least ten minutes.

Shoyu: This is what you think of as "soy sauce," but these days it's getting called by its Japanese name. It is a fermented food made from soybeans and salt. Used in rice, vegetable, and bean dishes and soups, shoyu imparts a lovely flavor. It is best if you buy it organic and even raw (unpasteurized), which is called "nama" shoyu. Like sea salt, shoyu should be cooked into dishes completely, needing at least four minutes of cooking. For gluten-free folk, it's best to use organic tamari, which is very similar to shoyu but is made without wheat.

Miso: This ancient food is made from a bean (usually soy) and often a grain, salt, and a mold starter called koji. Together they ferment and make miso, which continues to age, like a wine. The most medicinal miso is aged at least two years and is made from soybeans and barley.

---

2. Although sesame salt condiment appears to have undiluted salt in it, it is actually well integrated into the oil of the sesame seeds, making it easier for the body to assimilate.

However, there are many different types of miso and you should try them all for the sake of taste and variety. Lighter misos (white, chickpea), which are aged less than two years, need to be refrigerated, but older misos do not. If unrefrigerated miso develops a white mold, that's fine. It's just continued fermentation and you can mix it right into the miso. Miso needs to be simmered (but not boiled!) for two to three minutes before being served. Once in a while, you'll see a recipe where miso is not cooked, but go easy. It's salty.

Umeboshi plum or paste: The umeboshi plum imparts a very salty and sour taste to dishes. A fermented food as well, it is highly alkalizing and medicinal. You will see umeboshi or plum paste in dressings, sauces, and medicinal drinks. It can be cooked, but doesn't need to be.

Umeboshi vinegar: Umeboshi vinegar—like the plum—is both salty and sour and is best used sparingly, because it's strong. However, I have a little thing for umeboshi vinegar and tend to overdo it. It does not need to be cooked, but can be.

Brown rice vinegar: Made from fermented brown rice, brown rice vinegar is tasty. It shows up mostly in sauces and dressings for salads and other vegetable dishes. It does not need to be cooked.

Mirin: This is a cooking wine made from rice. It's sweet, delicate, and expensive. However, a little goes a long way, and it shows up in salad and dressing recipes every once in a while.

Herbs and spices: Herbs and spices make cooking interesting, varied, and delicious. However, it's best not to get into a deep rut with any herb or spice; each one has a strong energy and even sometimes a medicinal application, so change them up regularly. Most spices come from tropical climates and are great for cooling the body, so if your body needs to maintain balance throughout four distinct seasons, go easy on them, especially in fall and winter. No need to eat for Mumbai when you live in Minneapolis.

Sweeteners: Feel free to experiment with brown rice syrup, barley malt, and even maple syrup in your cooking. Sometimes the combination of sweet, salty, and sour in a rich bean or vegetable dish is a knockout.

Sesame Salt

This is the one condiment I recommend that you make. And the whole family will love it. If not, I'll come to your house and make dinner for you! The yin of the sesame oil and the yang of the salt make a very nice balance that is especially supportive of heart function. You'll need a suribachi (serrated bowl) and surikogi pestle for this, but they're cheap and you can order them at Amazon.com or through my website. Sesame salt gets stale after a couple of weeks, so be sure to make it fresh regularly.

1 teaspoon sea salt	½ cup black or tan sesame seeds

1. In a stainless steel or cast-iron skillet, toast the sea salt over medium heat. Keep it moving in the skillet and toast it until it becomes a sort of off-white color and emits an ammonia-like smell. This should take about 3 minutes. Place the toasted salt in a suribachi.

2. Rinse the sesame seeds in a strainer and place them in a skillet over medium heat. Move them constantly until they dry off. Reduce the heat to low and continue to stir regularly until most of the seeds have popped or have puffed up a little. Be careful not to let them burn.

3. In the suribachi, grind the salt with the surikogi until it no longer has any large granules. It should be a fine powder. Add the toasted sesame seeds and grind until about 75 percent of the seeds are cracked open. This may take 5 to 10 minutes of grinding, but the smell is amazing, and you can pass the task along to kids or others in the kitchen. Everyone likes making sesame salt.

8

· · · · · · · · · ·

Food
for
Thought

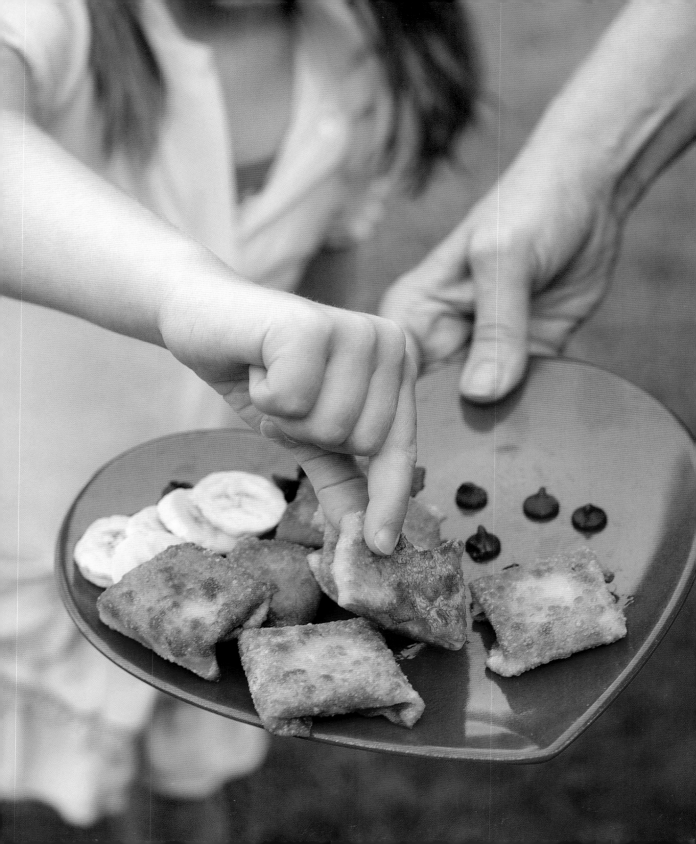

We eat every day. More than once. Chances are you've eaten within two hours of reading this book or will reach for something within the next two. Heck, I'm eating while I write.

Considering that we eat with such regularity—every single day of our lives—it makes sense to educate ourselves about what we ingest. Of course, people didn't always have to understand what they were eating, but that was before they had such a tremendous array of choices, both good and bad. Most MILFs throughout history didn't work at nine-to-five office jobs, so they spent lots of time interacting with their food—growing it, harvesting it, preparing it—which allowed them to "know" it on a deep, intuitive level. You can have that "knowing," too, in both your brain and your body.

So let's dive in. First, we'll look at meat and sugar, balancing the most popular—and extreme—seesaw on the playground these days. Then we'll look at dairy, caffeine, and what I call weird "foods," which only those of us lucky enough to have been plopped into the last couple of centuries have had to contend with.

From there, we'll start looking at nature's foods—the stuff that our bodies have known from time immemorial. Whole grains, vegetables, beans, sea vegetables, and natural sweets are not so weird, or extreme. They are designed for your body and, when eaten regularly, they allow it to function at its maximum MILFiness. You'll get all excited about them, I hope.

But first, the extremes.

Meat

Most of you holding this book grew up on meat. And I did, too. In our household, prosperity was written in beef. And bacon. And lamb. When I started my high school dieting years, I cooked skinless chicken breasts for myself, thinking that was the leaner way to go, but no matter the calorie count, flesh was being consumed.

I tend to tread a little lightly on the topic of meat. Not because I eat much (I have fish every once in a while—that's it), or because I was particularly fond of it growing up—I wasn't. It's just that the two sides of the meat debate can be so strident and righteous that it feels dangerous to even dip one's toe into the fray.

Truth be told, I feel for the strict vegans, because their cause is ethically sound; refraining from hurting animals is undeniably noble. It has a positive ripple effect for both humans and the planet as well. In fact, it turns out that eating a varied and balanced plant-based diet is one of the healthiest, smartest, and most ecological choices you can make in this lifetime. Not bad!

But let's be honest: Some ethical vegans can be pretty hard on their fellow humans in the name of loving animals. And harsh judgment is not always the best marketing tool. We need to love people for who they are, not for what they eat.

On the other hand, I feel for the carnivores, because they have history on their side and they're just doing what they grew up doing. And recently they're feeling judged and defensive about it. I honestly don't know anyone who raises a glass at dinner and proclaims: "Here's to supporting cruelty to animals today, James. . . . *Cheers!*"

The denial a meat-eater carries that her juicy burger was recently a creature's shoulder is more hardwired than a cruel, conscious choice. Humans have been eating flesh for hundreds of thousands of years, and a certain disconnect between the eater and the eaten may simply be part of the evolutionary picture, just as we're all in denial that an asteroid could come crashing down on us at any moment. Or that the carrot in our mouth had worms rubbing up against it last week. Or that we're all going to die one day. Denial is a natural thing. Of course, we now know that it's best for the meat-lover's health, the animal's well-being, and even the future of the planet if the meat-eater wakes up to what she's doing, but her denial doesn't make her an evil person. So let's just chill for a second, take a deep breath, and go hug a meat-eater with one arm while snuggling a vegan with the other.

Now that I've found a comfy space between extremes to present the issue of meat, here goes.

What is meat? Well, we all know what meat is: it is the muscle tissue of animals. Sometimes it's the organs, but in North America, we tend to eat the muscles.

Is meat more yin or more yang? Compared with plants, meat is very yang. It is dense, heavy, contracted, and full of minerals. Meat cells are more contracted than plant cells and their nuclei contain iron, a heavier element than the magnesium found in the nuclei of plant cells. Just as we humans are dense and heavy—compared with plants—animals are heavy.

In terms of yangness, animals are also warm-blooded (yang), active (compared with plants), and full of dense (yang) saturated fats. Plants are cool (yin) and inactive (yin) and contain mostly unsaturated (yin) fats.

Meat contains testosterone, which is a yang hormone: the cow itself is often male (I know "cow" is a term for a female, but it's basically gender neutral in the beef world), and that means there's lots of naturally occurring testosterone in its muscle. Add to that the injected hormones the cow is getting from the farmer in order to grow more muscle, and your rib-eye steak is designed to make you more muscular, active, and super yang, bordering on aggressive.

If we want to take it one step further, the stress hormones (adrenaline, cortisol) that the cow's glands release right before slaughter only serve to make the meat that much more stress inducing when it hits your bloodstream. Remember that women's natural default mode is to diffuse tension. We are the peacemakers. Estrogen literally calms things down. If you want to get a rush of testosterone, have more sex and get more exercise to raise your own levels of it. Because eating meat is not MILFy.

Meat is, as far as foods go, physically dense. Pick up a slab of beef and feel how heavy it is. Meat makes you feel grounded, concentrated, and sometimes stuck and rigid. All those things are expressions of yang force. Now, I'm not saying that women should never eat meat, but it certainly wouldn't be my first choice to support our natural femininity. If anything, too much meat pummels our beautiful magical essence into the barroom floor. Ouch.

What are the arguments for eating meat? The typical argument for eating meat is that it's a good source of protein, so let's sink our teeth into this topic.

Proteins are the building blocks of life. Your body, and just about everything in it, is made of proteins: hormones, enzymes, neurotransmitters, and your muscles, flesh, and blood. There are lots of different types of proteins, but they are all made up of some combination of what are called amino acids. There are only twenty known amino acids, but when you do the math to combine them all in different ways, they make up gazillions of different proteins.

Your body creates some amino acids itself, but not all of them. There are eight amino acids that the human body cannot make, so you must get them from food. They are called the eight essential amino acids.

Because meat contains all eight of the essential amino acids, it's been crowned a "complete protein." Roll out the red carpet! Flash! Pop! Hire a PR person! And the National Cattlemen's Beef Association has done just that. Meat's being a complete protein is the one hook the beef industry can hang its Stetson on.

Most plants, however, don't contain all eight amino acids, so we used to believe that vegetarians had to combine different foods together, like rice with beans, in order to get The Big 8 in one meal. God *forbid* you didn't combine correctly, or you'd be tossed to the curb—weak, skinny, and frail. Or so we thought. Turns out you don't have to combine carefully and that your super-duper body can do the mixing and brewing itself. Just as a cow stays healthy eating only grasses, your body uses what it can get from the foods you eat.[1]

How much do you need? Well, everyone's different, but the rule of thumb is that when you need protein, you will crave it; the body is very wise. Cavemen didn't have to pull out nutrition charts to figure out if they were getting enough protein, nor do massive, muscle-bound gorillas. Human breast milk contains 6 percent protein, so that tells us what nature has in mind for a rapidly growing baby. Vegetables contain an average of 22 percent protein. *Vegetables!* So you should be fine.

It's interesting that what no one seems to mention is the very real fact that you can get *too much* protein. That's right. You rarely hear it, but when it comes to protein, you need only so much, and too much is actually bad for you. I mean, if you build a house, you wouldn't build extra walls in the middle of the living room just because you had the plaster to do it. You wouldn't fill the bedrooms with bricks just for the hell of it. You need only what you need. Nothing more and nothing less.

---

1. In fact, most large animals get all the protein they need from plants. Gorillas, cows, pigs, horses, even *elephants,* get all the protein they need eating only vegetation and the occasional, unlucky bug.

In fact, my house analogy isn't exactly accurate, because, truth is, your body can't store protein for later use. Instead, excess protein is broken down into sugars, fatty acids, and amino acids. This causes your blood to become slightly acidic, which is a big biological no-no. This acidity overworks your liver and kidneys and can cause inflammation. But luckily, when your body becomes acidic, it does a neat trick to restore balance; it pulls minerals such as calcium from its secret storehouses and those minerals neutralize all the acid. Cool. The only problem is that your body's secret mineral storehouses are (drumroll, please . . .) your bones. Hello, osteoporosis. So all that extra building material actually causes your house to decay and fall down!

Iron

Premenopausal MILFs need their iron, especially pregnant ones. And the MILF diet can supply it. Here's the skinny on iron: there are two types of iron—heme and nonheme. Meat, poultry, and fish contain both heme and nonheme iron, but plant foods contain only nonheme iron. The heme iron found in meat is really easy for your body to absorb, so lots of people think they need to eat meat in order to get their iron. But that's not the case. Remember our vegetarian gorillas and elephants? They seem to be doing just fine.

Just because heme iron is easier to absorb, that doesn't mean that nonheme iron is *hard* to absorb; it's not. All you need is some vitamin C, and its absorbability increases sixfold. And, by the way, lots of plants, like broccoli and kale, contain both nonheme iron *and* vitamin C, so you don't need to think about it!

And that's good because, as with protein, it's possible to get too much iron. In fact, too much iron can create free radicals and, at its worst, is dangerously toxic. But your body can store iron, unlike protein, so it's actually good to eat mostly nonheme iron because it's better regulated by the body than heme iron.

Other foods that contain lots of nonheme iron include sea vegetables, beans, tofu, quinoa, tahini, tempeh, toasted pumpkin seeds, dried apricots, and many herbs. Foods rich in vitamin C include citrus fruits, papaya, Brussels sprouts, red bell pepper, peas, sweet potato, parsley, leafy greens, cauliflower, and strawberries.

By following the MILF diet, you will get these foods in combination all the time. Imagine a stir-fry with broccoli, bok choy, tofu, and toasted pumpkin seeds, smothered in a tahini sauce and ladled over a mound of quinoa. . . . *Mmmm.* Popeye would absolutely drool.

The Arguments Against Meat

Meat consumption is linked to heart disease. Heart disease is a big deal. It is the number one killer of women in this country and fells five times more women than breast cancer does. Contrary to common assumptions, more women than men die of heart disease each year.[2]

We all grew up hearing that meat-eating was a big factor in heart disease. For the last fifty years or so, it has been believed that ingesting saturated fat raises cholesterol, which then creates plaque in the arteries. When the arteries to the heart get all gummed up, oxygen is cut off to the heart and . . . some heart muscle dies and . . . ARGK! That's a heart attack. Until very recently, the conventional wisdom was that a diet of eggs, red meat, butter, cheese, and other foods high in saturated fats would put the eater at risk of a heart attack. This theory is known as the lipid hypothesis. "Lipid" is a fancy word for "fat" . . . as in "*lipo*suction."

However, as I write this, there is a growing debate about the issue of saturated fat and heart disease. In fact, a number of researchers are looking to *refined carbohydrates* as the bad guys gunning for our hearts. I will discuss this more in the section on sugar. For the sake of argument, let's go with the science of the last fifty years, which tells us that saturated fat leads to blocked arteries. Well, these arteries go not only to your heart, but to your brain, your limbs, and your sex organs. This dense and hard fat tends to create an overall sludginess in the body. Now, I know "sludginess" is not a medical term, but you know what I mean: circulation is restricted and sensitivity is reduced. Less blood flowing within your appendages means reduced blood flow to your hands, feet, and face. Fat builds up all over the body—and not just in the arteries. It's under the skin, around the belly, and even hugging your organs. An interesting study[3] conducted in 2009 showed a relationship between arterial blockage and stiffness of the trunk of the body, so if you're having a hard time doing that forward bend in yoga class, there may be something much deeper going on.

Whether it's by staying away from meat or refusing refined sugar, MILFs have less of this stiffness, sludginess, and insulation, and are less prone to heart disease. Yay!

---

2. http://www.womenheart.org/resources/cvdfactsheet.cfm.
3. http://ajpheart.physiology.org/content/297/4/H1314.short.

Meat is connected to cancer. The meat-cancer connection is tricky because no one is eating a burger and dropping dead of a newly minted tumor. Cancer can take years to develop, so it can be difficult to draw the perfectly straight line we like to see when proving something, but here are the curves . . .

Take, for instance, carcinogens and the creepy fact that an estimated 90 to 95 percent of all the environmental toxins you ingest get into your body via meat and dairy.[4] Not the air. Not products you use. Not even the pesticides on vegetables. Meat and dairy. The nasty toxins the animals take in (pesticides, herbicides, industrial chemicals) build up in the saturated fat of the animal—or her milk—and then she passes them on to you. And remember, cattle in the local feedlot aren't being fed organic broccoli. In fact, along with the heavily sprayed corn they eat, they're also chomping on the bits and pieces of diseased cows, manure, plastic, and lots of antibiotics.[5]

However, it may be that the toxins aren't the biggest factor when it comes to meat and cancer. In his book *The China Study,* Dr. T. Colin Campbell tells the story of stumbling upon the results of an Indian experiment in which rats that were fed a diet containing 20 percent animal protein and then heavily dosed with powerful carcinogens *all* developed liver cancer, while another group of rats eating only 5 percent animal protein and given just as much cancer-causing poison developed no cancers at all.

At the time, Dr. Campbell was a nutrition researcher committed to the idea that meat and dairy were superfoods poised to save the developing world, so he was skeptical and decided to repeat the experiments himself. Much to his surprise, the results were exactly the same: rats eating lots of animal protein got cancer, while the almost-veggie rats did not. He went on to conduct further studies that showed the growth of tumors moving in lock-step with the increase (or decrease) in animal protein in the rats' diets: the more animal protein they were given, the bigger their tumors grew; when the amount of animal protein was reduced, the tumors shrank. This study changed his career, his health, and his life. I strongly recommend

---

4. T. Colin Campbell and Thomas M. Campbell II, *The China Study: The Most Comprehensive Study of Nutrition Ever Conducted and the Startling Implications for Diet, Weight Loss, and Long-Term Health* (Dallas: BenBella Books, 2006), page 165.
5. http://www.ucsusa.org/food_and_agriculture/science_and_impacts/impacts_industrial_agriculture/they-eat-what-the-reality-of.html.

you read *The China Study* and share it with your DILF. It's great stuff for the science friendly and has convinced major-league athletes and major-league politicians to go plant based. If you don't feel like reading, see the movie *Forks over Knives*.

Dr. Campbell concludes that, although we ingest carcinogens, and although we may be genetically predisposed to certain conditions, animal protein seems to create the *environment* in which bad genes are activated and poisons take root. And it's not the saturated fat of the meat, but the protein itself. Huh. (By the way, Dr. Campbell is not the only brainiac out there who's anti-meat: Joel Fuhrman, Neal Barnard, Dean Ornish, Caldwell Esselstyn, and John McDougall are all physicians who have published books recommending a plant-based diet. Check them out.)

And red meat in particular may contain a special component that feeds cancer. Researchers have discovered a sialic acid sugar they've named Neu5Gc that is present in most mammals, but not humans. When we eat the meat of another mammal, we ingest Neu5Gc, which feeds any precancerous cells we might be brewing. Turns out cancer cells *love* Neu5Gc. Then, to top it all off, because Neu5Gc comes from the bodies of other species, it sets off our immune system alarms, keeping us in a chronic state of defensive inflammation as long as we're eating red meat.[6] This chronic immune response is also a perfect petri dish for cancer growth.

Meat contributes to osteoporosis. Guess what? Women who eat meat and dairy have weaker bones than their plant-eating counterparts. That's right. Countries that have the highest meat and dairy consumption rates (like the United States) have the highest osteoporosis rates. I can hear our bones snapping right now. But in countries that eat less meat and less dairy? Like China? When those woman fall down, they dust themselves off and get right up again. No snap, crackle, pop in the hip joints. Americans fracture their hips *five times more* than the Chinese do.[7]

As I said before (but it bears repeating, because you have been hypnotized about protein), excess protein breaks down into its original amino acids and these acids need to be neutralized by minerals. Minerals such as calcium. And where do you store lots of calcium in your body?

6. http://www.news-medical.net/news/20100726/Neu5Gc-in-drugs-provokes-strong-immune-response.aspx.
7. http://www.hindawi.com/journals/josteo/2010/757102/tab1/.

Your bones. So they offer up their calcium to buffer the acid building up in your blood. That's your blood maintaining homeostasis with a big, scary price tag.

The truth is that osteoporosis is not about getting enough calcium. It's about absorbing and properly utilizing the calcium you ingest. The MILF diet, rich in whole grains, leafy green vegetables, and especially sea vegetables, will give you tons of calcium, and if you're smart, you'll keep it. But if you chase the MILF diet down with meat, dairy, sugar, caffeine, carbonated drinks, and too much salt, you'll flush all that calcium right down the toilet.

Flesh-eating stinks. Meat and dairy are major contributors to bad breath[8] and unattractive body odors of all kinds.[9] Downright anti-MILFy.

As if you needed to hear any more. Meat is connected to rheumatoid arthritis,[10] ulcerative colitis,[11] and gout.[12]

Meat is getting freaky. Farmers give antibiotics to their livestock because factory-farmed animals are kept in overcrowded and unsanitary conditions—they basically stand around in their own feces—and prophylactic doses of antibiotics help to keep them disease free.

And strangely, antibiotics also serve as growth promoters in animals, so they make for bigger cows, or pigs, or chickens. Which makes for bigger paydays.

But the consequences of these choices are serious. You have microbes—friendly and unfriendly—throughout your body, but especially in your digestive tract. The friendly microbes are essential not only to your digestion but to your immune system and overall good health, so you want to keep those suckers. But when you eat meat that's dosed with antibiotics, these powerful medicines are being passed on to you, weakening or destroying the microbes—good and bad—in your intestinal tract. Over time, eating meat that's laden with antibiotics compromises your precious immune system.

---

8. http://www.animated-teeth.com/bad_breath/t3_causes_of_halitosis.htm.
9. http://chemse.oxfordjournals.org/content/31/8/747.abstract.
10. http://www.cbsnews.com/stories/2004/12/02/health/webmd/main658797.shtml.
11. http://www.ncbi.nlm.nih.gov/pmc/articles/PMC1774255/.
12. http://nydailynews.healthology.com/gout/article94.htm.

But this problem goes beyond your gut. Eventually dangerous microbes, like staphylococcus, get smart; having faced one antibiotic in a cow or pig, they mutate in order to become resistant to it. Then the pharmaceutical industry ups the ante by developing a newer, stronger antibiotic. After a while, the bug develops resistance to the second drug, and then the third. This is why there are over a hundred different antibiotics being used today. As the drugs get smarter, the bugs get smarter, and who do you think is going to win this battle—our brilliant scientific minds or Mother Nature?

The consequences have already arrived. Superbugs like MRSA (methicillin-resistant *Staphylococcus aureus*) are a very serious problem in the health care industry. We originally thought they were spawned in hospitals because open sores and surgical sutures were the perfect places for bacteria to travel and nest. But super staph seems to be creeping into the community as well . . . over the meat counter. As recently as 2011, researchers found *Staphylococcus aureus* bacteria in 47 percent of the chicken and beef samples they purchased at regular grocery stores. Of those, 52 percent were resistant to at least three classes of antibiotics. Dr. Lance B. Price, senior author of the study, said, "For the first time, we know how much of our meat and poultry is contaminated with antibiotic-resistant staph, and it is substantial."[13]

Staph infections can be very dangerous, resulting in amputations or life-threatening infections in the bones, joints, and even the heart. That's *sooo* not good. Even scarier, staph is becoming resistant to most of our antibiotics, so not only does medicating the animal fail to kill the bug, there's a decent chance that the drugs used on you or your kids might not work either, whether you eat meat or not. This problem is very real and growing rapidly, and the meat industry does *not* want you knowing about it.

It seems that the only way around this particular issue is to purchase all your meat from operations that do not use antibiotics, but that may be easier said than done: it is estimated that 99 percent of all the animals raised and slaughtered for food in the United States come from factory farms.[14] Another option is to forgo meat altogether. In a recent study, people who adopted a vegetarian diet for just five days saw the levels of antibiotics in their blood drop significantly.[15]

13. http://m.nypost.com/p/news/national/nearly_half_study_suggests_meat_q8zGMf5DW83MxBaOai6M7K.
14. http://www.farmforward.com/farming-forward/factory-farming.
15. http://www.environmentalhealthnews.org/ehs/newscience/phthalates-antibiotics-reduced-after-vegetarian-diet/.

Meat is a delivery system for excess sex hormones. Sounds like fun, but it's not. Adding growth and sex hormones to animals makes them grow bigger and heavier, and, because meat is sold by the pound, these extra hormones can increase a cow's value by a whopping eighty bucks.

The FDA claims that the hormones introduced into livestock don't cause the animals to exceed their normal levels of hormones, but confidential industry reports to the FDA cited in the *Los Angeles Times* seem to prove otherwise: "Following a single ear implant in steers of . . . a combination of estradiol and progesterone, estradiol levels in different meat products were up to twenty-fold higher than normal." [16] Estradiol, by the way, is a form of estrogen, which is directly linked to breast cancer.

Although the farmers are supposed to be introducing the hormones via a pellet implanted in the ear, pellets are often implanted in more muscular parts of the body, increasing the hormone levels of that particular part of the animal enormously. Unpublished results from a U.S. Department of Agriculture random check of thirty-two large feedlots noted that "as many as half the cattle had visible illegal 'misplaced implants' in muscle, rather than under ear skin." [17] Although the USDA swears up and down that hormone levels are not exceeding normal, according to the *Los Angeles Times,* "Of 130 million livestock commercially slaughtered in 1993, not one was tested for estradiol or any related hormone." So no one really knows.

What we do know is that exposure to estrogen is a critical factor in breast cancer. And while our beef is getting dosed with it, we're getting our panties all in a twist about the endocrine disruptors in plastics and cosmetics because they mimic estrogen in our bodies. Not to mention pummeling soy because of its plant-based (and very weak) estrogens. But we *don't* want to talk about the fact that we are bathing the blood of the vast majority of our beef in estrogen, progesterone, testosterone, and bovine growth hormone.

But, hey, who cares, right? Well, the Europeans do. In 1989, the European Union banned hormone-treated U.S. beef and they haven't gone back on their decision yet. Treating animals with hormones is not just frowned upon there, it's illegal.

---

16. http://www.preventcancer.com/press/editorials/march24_97.htm.
17. Ibid.

Meat contains no fiber. Fiber is a godsend. It is the indigestible stuff (the strings of celery, the pulp of a carrot, the sheath around a whole grain) that moves through your gut and gathers up all the bad stuff to be eliminated. It makes up the bulk of your stool. Think of fiber as a broom sweeping out your innards.

Because meat contains absolutely no fiber, it has a way of getting stuck in your gut and rotting you from the inside out. You see, your intestines are not designed like a true carnivore's, which provide a quick whoosh from mouth to anus.[18] Yours are longer and squiggly and take more time to digest your food. It's fine to let plant food stick around down there—it's alkaline and your body needs some time to extract the nutrients from it. But meat . . . well, it contains toxins and excess hormones, breaks down into an acid state in your gut, and just generally wreaks havoc down there.

Meat contains no carbohydrates. Although meat gives the eater a certain type of "energy," it isn't actually a fuel for the body. Meat, because it is so high in protein, is a building block. So unless you are working out like a madwoman and really trying to bulk up (and there are plant-based ways of doing that), meat delivers its protein, fat, and minerals and then it just sits around in your gut, decomposing. There is no real fuel for giving good-quality energy to your cells, or your mind, or your spirit. Notice how you feel after your next hamburger. Sluggish. Heavy. Not so MILFy.

We are going crazy with meat. In 1950, the average American consumed 144 pounds of meat—a combination of beef, pork, turkey, lamb, veal, and chicken. In 2007, that number had increased to 222 pounds, a more than 50 percent jump in less than sixty years. That's a lot of meat. And it seems we are setting the global pace: the worldwide meat supply grew from 71 million tons in 1961 to *284 million tons* in 2007, with global per capita consumption doubling in that time. Holy hamburger. The world's meat consumption is expected to double again by 2050.[19] Is it any accident that the world is getting faster, more pressurized, more competitive, and more yang?

---

18. You also have only four canine teeth for ripping flesh, while you have a mouthful of grain-grinding molars. And your stomach acids? Twenty times weaker than those of a true carnivore. Just sayin'.
19. http://www.nytimes.com/2008/01/27/weekinreview/27bittman.html.

Meat is big business. Remember when Oprah, during the scare over mad cow disease, said that she would never eat a hamburger again, and she was sued by cattle ranchers in Texas? You gotta have *deeeeep* Texan pockets to take on Oprah, but they went through with it because their industry has a lot to hide: unsanitary factory-farming conditions, sloppy slaughterhouse practices, high contamination rates (which I haven't even touched—just not enough room), the industry's devastating impact on the environment, and the bed it shares with Congress, not to mention that its products do real physical damage to its consumers. The ranchers were *not* willing to have a whistle-blower like Oprah spreading the truth to you and me. Hmm . . . You don't see the Artichoke Association taking Oprah to court. The Carrot Council hasn't sued anyone of late. The Barley Board isn't on the front page. Meat needs legal and financial muscle because it's a bad boy that has to stay out of jail.

Meat is taking its toll on the planet. This is a serious issue. The production of meat and other animal products is ridiculously resource heavy. It is estimated that it takes about *2,500 gallons* of water to produce a single pound of beef.[20] And get this: *70 percent* of the grains grown in this country are fed to livestock.[21] This requires huge amounts of fossil fuel and other resources. All so we can eat like gout-ridden kings.

And then there's the matter of cows grazing on land that is turning into desert, their manure leeching into the water table and contaminating local waterways, and their burps creating so much methane that it makes up 18 percent of the greenhouse gases emitted around the world. That's more than all the cars, trucks, and planes on the planet combined.[22]

The Amazon jungle is unparalleled in its biodiversity and produces 20 percent of the earth's oxygen supply and myriad species of exotic plants that are used for pharmaceutical drugs and medical research. Pretty neat. However, we are chopping down the precious Amazon rain forest to create . . . grazing land for cattle. Although deforestation rates have fallen since the global economic recession,[23] they peaked in 2002 with 10,000 square kilometers being destroyed that

---

20. http://www.earthsave.org/environment/water.htm.

21. http://www.tofurky.com/whyeatveg/meat_of_the_matter.html.

22. http://www.independent.co.uk/environment/climate-change/cow-emissions-more-damaging-to-planet-than-cosub2sub -from-cars-427843.html

23. http://www.guardian.co.uk/environment/2010/jul/23/amazon-deforestation-decline.

year alone.[24] And once the rain forest—with its oxygen production, rare species, and medicinal plants—is cut down . . . it ain't comin' back.

Clearly, modern meat production is unsustainable. Just think about it: There are between 6 billion and 7 billion humans on the planet right now. One billion of them don't have enough food or clean water. That's mothers, fathers, and children dying of preventable starvation and disease every day. And yet there are *20 billion* head of livestock on the planet—roughly triple the number of humans—and they are extremely well fed . . . fattened even . . . and are using up finite resources like clean water, fossil fuels, and topsoil that could be used to feed humans. That's just weird, if not downright immoral. We are neglecting human suffering and burning through our precious resources at an accelerated rate because we eat so much meat. Meat that is hurting us.

Yes, we evolved eating some meat. But it wasn't drugged, hormonally manipulated, and packaged, then delivered to our doorstep. You had to actually exert some energy and/or take some risks to get animal flesh. And the amount was negligible compared with the three-meal-a-day meatfests we are indulging in today. And, by the way, doesn't evolution imply, well . . . evolution? We are no longer cavemen. With the introduction of agriculture, we started building civilizations and coming together in relatively peaceful communities. Shouldn't we continue to evolve and maintain the planet as a livable space? Ask your gut: Does that picture include more or less animal food?

---

24. http://www.nytimes.com/2003/06/28/international/americas/28BRAZ.html?ex=1057377600&en=2b4d6f346c07c215&ei=5062&partner=GOOGLE.

What About Poultry, Eggs, and Fish?

Poultry: Just watch a chicken dart around pecking for a while. Chickens have intense, yang energy. Chicken also contains animal protein, and it is close to beef in terms of cholesterol content* and can contain significant amounts of saturated fat, depending on the part of the chicken consumed. And everything I said about heart disease, cancer, osteoporosis, and arthritis? And antibiotics? Chicken is in that club. Yuck.

Eggs: One egg contains the energy template of an entire chicken, so—by weight—eggs are the most yang animal food of all. And back in the day, people weren't slamming back three-egg omelets every morning the way we do now; most families didn't have enough chickens to produce like that. So eggs were spread throughout dishes, like pad Thai, egg drop soup, or fried rice. Eggs have a very strong energy—they are reproductive cells—so it's best to go very easy, if you eat any at all. Unless you have your own chickens, it can be hard to find eggs laid by chickens kept in decent conditions or raised without antibiotics. Even "free-range" means the chicken (and her hundreds of coop-mates) simply have *access* to the outdoors for some unspecified period of time each day. It doesn't mean they go outside.

Fish: First, we are fishing the oceans clean. An international group of scientists who studied our global fishing habits predicted that if we continue to go at our current rate, we will be a world without seafood by 2048.† Second, most of the fish we eat is pretty toxic. Environmental toxins (mercury and other industrial poisons) that are released into the air collect in the clouds and then get rained down onto the ocean, contaminating the algae and other tiny organisms that are eaten by fish. This just goes up and up the underwater food chain, with the biggest and fattest fish—ahi tuna, tilefish, king mackerel, and swordfish—carrying the most deadly gunk. If we weren't so stuck on tuna (canned tuna is the number one seafood eaten in the United States), we'd think long and hard about putting it in our bodies; mercury causes kidney and brain damage. Even the most conservative experts agree it's best to avoid the bigger fish, especially if you're pregnant or nursing. Some MILFs eat fish every once in a while, but it's generally white-meat fish (flounder, cod, sole, tilapia), because it is lower in fat and therefore doesn't have so many toxins socked away. But many MILFs eat no animal protein at all and feel great.

* http://www.drmcdougall.com/free_2d.html.
† http://www.washingtonpost.com/wp-dyn/content/article/2006/11/02/AR2006110200913.html.

Meat attracts sugar and other extreme yin foods. Because meat contains lots of minerals and no carbs, it makes you crave carbohydrates. Next time you eat a chicken salad, or a bacon cheeseburger, notice what you want to consume right after it. Chances are it will be French fries, or alcohol, or some goody chock-full of sugar. *Not* a measly little apple. Meat is extreme yang that attracts extreme yin.

And this loops around to the argument about whether it's meat or sugar that causes heart disease. One of the reasons researchers may be confused is that when meat consumption rises in industrialized countries, the consumption of sugar and refined carbohydrates follows right behind it. Followed quickly by heart disease. So it's become difficult to tease the two factors apart within the data. But to a MILF who's giving both meat and white sugar the heave-ho, it doesn't really matter. The MILF diet is heart healthy.

Kicking Meat 101

Some people give up meat very easily. I've met a bunch of MILFs who became vegetarian (or vegan) after simply practicing yoga for a little while. It's as if their bodies were learning a new flexibility—and freedom—and meat just didn't jibe with their new path.

Because meat is so dense and contracting, women tend to have an easier time letting go of it than men do; meat goes against our very nature, energetically speaking. But that's not always the case. Some MILFs feel stuck in meat.

Unlike with sugar and dairy, which need to be kicked like drugs, you will experience benefits by simply ratcheting down on meat (although I recommend getting off it entirely at some point). If serving tofu at the dinner table tonight will kick off World War III, here are a few tips:

- Start cooking your meat with beans. Meat and beans go very well together (franks and beans, anyone?), and the beans serve as a creamy host to the meaty guest.
- Try any of the whole-grain recipes starting on page 107 with a little meat added, or throw some into soups.
- One of the biggest steps is getting used to grains and vegetables as the big stars on your plate, instead of a hunk of steak. Once you've covered that psychological hurdle, it's really quite easy.
- While you ratchet down, try fish instead of beef, pork, or chicken. White-meat fish is lower in toxins than other fish and much easier to digest than other meat.

Kicking Meat Completely

- Load up on beans and bean products. Have canned beans at the ready if you're not up to speed with cooking them regularly from scratch. Get acquainted with cooking tofu, tempeh, and seitan—all rich, delicious, and very adaptable sources of protein. Try some fake meats if you want to: there are lots of meat substitutes out there, made by many companies. Yves and Gardein both make meat-like foods in many textures and flavors: ground "beef," deli "meats," "chicken" strips, and "bacon." These substitutes should not make up the bulk of your protein, because they are quite processed, but they are great transition foods.
- Learn how to prepare beans well. There are good recipes not only in this book, but also in lots of other great cookbooks out there. Look for vegan or macrobiotic cookbooks for good bean recipes.

What to Look Forward To

Your body will start acquainting itself with plant-based proteins and trying them on for size. Because they are easier on your liver, kidneys, arteries, bones, and joints while delivering the richness, density, and protein you crave, your body will automatically start moving in their direction.

- You will have easier bowel movements. In fact, without meat, your poops should get lighter in color and even float. TMI!
- You will become more physically and mentally flexible.
- If you've had aches in your joints, getting off meat should help significantly. (Losing dairy, sugar, and nightshade veggies helps, too.)
- You will have milder PMS.
- Your skin will look better as you get more circulation to your periphery.
- You will become more sensitive to energy and vibrations.
- You will be happier and feel less internal pressure and intensity. You will become softer and MILFier.

White Sugar and Refined Carbohydrates

What are sugar and refined carbohydrates? Here's the deal: your body is like a car that runs on one fuel: sugar. Yes, you need protein, but protein is a building material, not a fuel. While protein continually does maintenance on your lovely Ferrari, sugar fills it up at the gas station.

Like any fuel, sugar comes in different grades. There's low grade, which is stuff like white sugar and white flour. They are highly refined, which sounds rich and fancy, but they are actually bad news. Drugs are also highly refined; the coca leaf is refined to become cocaine, and the poppy flower is refined to become opium. When substances are refined, certain qualities are lost, while others are wildly concentrated. This makes them less stable than the original plant.

White sugar and white flour are carbohydrates that we call simple, because—having been refined—they have just one or two molecules in their chemical structure. They break down really quickly in the body and keep you on the roller coaster of highs and lows. After you crash on simple carbs, you just want more. Just as with drugs, we can easily become addicted to simple sugars and they begin to run our lives.

Then there's the high-grade fuel: complex carbohydrates. Found in whole grains, vegetables, beans, and some natural sweeteners, these break down much more slowly in the body and deliver a smooth, happy ride. The complex carbohydrates found in the MILF diet are the perfect food for a MILF looking to feel calm and centered, yet full of energy.

All of the following are what I mean when I say "sugar": cane sugar, beet sugar, high fructose corn syrup, evaporated cane juice, brown sugar, turbinado sugar, Florida Crystals, dextrose, sucrose, glucose, and maltose. When you see any of these on a label, run!

"Refined carbohydrates" also include the white flour found in breads, cakes, and pastas. They break down very easily and commit almost every crime that sugar does. You will find a little white flour in a few of the recipes in this book; they are meant for occasional use and celebrations.

How much "sugar" do we eat? A lot. And we keep eating more. Between 1982 and 1999, our sugar consumption increased by 28 percent. According to a study by researchers at Emory University and the Centers for Disease Control and Prevention,[25] the average American eats 21.4 teaspoons of added sugar per day. That's *added* sugar, on top of the naturally occurring carbs found in fruits, vegetables, and grains. That's the equivalent of 7 teaspoons at every single meal, day after day, week after week, year after year. And get this: Teenage males consume 34 teaspoons of the stuff per day.

How do we get it? Well, the biggest source is soft drinks. Thirty-three percent of America's sugar consumption comes from the cans we have glued into our fists. And considering that most soft drinks are now sweetened with high fructose corn syrup, that's a big, fat deal (see below). Candy ranks second at 16.1 percent, followed closely by cake and cookies (12.9 percent), and pulling up the rear are sweetened fruit drinks and punches, dairy desserts (ice cream, anyone?), and other sweetened grain products like cinnamon toast and honey-nut waffles.[26] I get a headache just writing this stuff!

Is sugar more yin or more yang? In general, sweet foods have a yin impact. But white sugar and other refined carbohydrates are *too* yin for the body to process without creating a precarious imbalance.

If we're looking for balance in our lives, sugar is the wrong choice. Because it is stripped of all its minerals, vitamins, and fiber, sugar is not balanced and tends to kick you off the end of the seesaw. Yes, it causes you to feel released, even happy, for a little bit, but then your blood becomes weak and your body goes into overdrive in an attempt to stabilize itself, and you end up tired, depleted, and sad. Like most drugs, it's unnaturally expansive.

---

25. http://thevreelandclinic.wordpress.com/2010/04/21/see-the-amazing-statistics-on-sugar-consumption-in-the-u-s/.
26. http://online.wsj.com/article/SB10001424052970204660604574370851517144132.html.

Fat Rats

These days, there's a new kid on the sugar block: high fructose corn syrup, which is especially dodgy.

Let's start at the beginning: this country makes a lot of corn. In fact, the government subsidizes corn farmers so heavily that their crop—for the most part—has been cheap, cheap, cheap. So cheap that there came a point in the 1960s when we started to apply our scientific skills to figuring out different ways of processing all our extra corn and stuffing it into a million different products. So now we have corn (or some part thereof) in beer, whiskey, cosmetics, candy bars, coffee, tea, paper products, pharmaceuticals, gypsum wallboard, paint, varnish, toothpaste, and even . . . spark plugs. You heard me. Spark plugs. Not to mention just about every processed food on the supermarket shelf. In terms of food, one of the big corn breakthroughs was the invention of high fructose corn syrup (HFCS). This new sweetener was cheaper than cane sugar and started creeping into soda pop, bread, and all sorts of other goodies. But when they created HFCS in the lab, the scientists did something strange. Whereas regular table sugar has a fructose-to-glucose ratio of 50:50, in HFCS the ratio was 55 percent fructose to 42 percent glucose (with the remaining 3 percent being larger sugar molecules called higher saccharides). And that's important. You see, in white sugar, the fructose and the glucose molecules hug each other very happily, and if they are not used as energy, they go into the liver to be stored for later use. If what's stored in the liver *doesn't* get used, it is converted into fat. But in HFCS, the fructose is like a single guy, partying by himself unbound to glucose, and it seems to convert into fat much more quickly.

This is not good. In a study conducted at Princeton University, where rats were fed a HFCS-water solution sweetened to *half* the level of the average soda, *every single rat* became obese over six months.* These rats gained 48 percent more weight than rats on a normal diet and much more weight than rats on a normal diet that were drinking a solution of sucrose (simple table sugar) and water.

Not only did they gain weight, but the weight showed up in the patterns that indicate a condition called metabolic syndrome—including weight concentrated around the belly and high triglycerides in the bloodstream.

It is believed by many experts, including the researchers at Princeton, that the obesity epidemic in this country is strongly connected to the introduction of HFCS into our food supply. In the last forty years, we've gone from eating none of it to consuming an average of sixty pounds a year of the stuff. This is just another example of our arrogance kicking us in our own (big) butts.

* http://www.princeton.edu/main/news/archive/S26/91/22K07/.

What About Artificial Sweeteners?

These guys are just no-nos. They are about as far from Mother Nature's plan as you can get, all having been derived in the laboratory. You know what saccharin actually is? A derivative of coal tar. And aspartame? Invented as an antiulcer drug.

I'm sure when that lucky lab technician dropped some into his coffee by accident, he tasted a sweet, sweet fortune—but not without a ton of problems. Aspartame (in NutraSweet) breaks down to create aspartic acid, phenylalanine, and methanol in the body. These three doozies can lead to headaches, depression, seizure disorders, anxiety attacks, vision problems, and more. Saccharin (Sweet'N Low) was linked to bladder cancer in rats, but its makers managed to get it approved nonetheless. Even sucralose, used in Splenda, is actually chlorinated sugar and hasn't been proven to be safe. But in a world going at mach speed, with every woman believing she needs to be the next Kate Moss, we have been hypnotized by the shiny, speedy, zero-calorie drinks we put these substances in. Go, go, go! Be thin, thin, *thin* . . . and one day you'll be famous, famous, *FAMOUS!!*

Although it's more natural, you'll also find stevia (Truvia) in a discreet white packet these days. This recent addition to the sugar bowl comes from a plant native to Paraguay. Native Paraguayans have been using stevia leaves in their tea since anyone can remember, and the leaves impart a sweet, calorie-free taste. That's stevia in its unrefined form.

But we refine it. The stevia that you or I can buy at a store comes in a powder or a liquid and is 300 times sweeter than sugar. It is not the whole leaf of the plant and sometimes it is just one chemical extracted from the plant. Although it has been shown to have some healthful benefits, like lowering blood pressure and blood sugar, there have also been studies showing it may have an adverse effect on both male and female fertility and may even be related to cancer.*

Things to keep in mind: The FDA, backed by the sugar lobby, tried really, *really* hard to keep stevia off our shelves for about twenty years because it was seen as serious competition to Big Sugar and artificial sweetener companies. In the meantime, Japan has been using it in foods for over thirty years without any scientifically proven adverse effects. So studies linking stevia to this and that disease may be good science, but they may also be funded by those interested in giving it a bad rap. It's hard to tell these days. I definitely think stevia is a better choice than aspartame, saccharin, or sucralose, but I'm not really crazy about any of them.

What I know: Anytime you introduce a refined substance, whether that's sugar, aspartame, or stevia, into your routine—coffee in the morning, dessert at lunch, soda on break, tea after dinner—it becomes a big player in your body, mind, and spirit. Even in tiny amounts, a substance that is introduced with mind-numbing regularity will begin to alter your life. It seeps into every cell. Alters your bloodstream. You may not see it, or feel it, for a very long time, and issues that arise may *never* be consciously connected to that Truvia packet you dumped into your decaf . . . but it's there and, on some level, it's having its way with you. Determining your direction. Pulling you off nature's seesaw. The only things I want to give that type of power to are whole grains, vegetables, and plant-based proteins. Unprocessed or minimally processed, they belong in a human body and I want them to build the foundation of my energy and my life. Not white powders poured out of little packets.

* C. Wasuntarawat et al., "Developmental Toxicity of Steviol, a Metabolite of Stevioside, in the Hamster," *Drug and Chemical Toxicology*, 1998 May; 21(2):207–22.

The Arguments Against Sugar and Refined Carbohydrates

Sugar takes you on a hell ride. White sugar and other highly refined carbohydrates cause a sticky glut of glucose in your bloodstream that gives you a rush like a ten-year-old on an amusement park ride. But then your body freaks out: because the ride is a little too hairy, your pancreas secretes tons of insulin to mop up all the excess glucose. This works for a moment, but because the whole situation is unnaturally extreme, your pancreas puts out *too much* insulin and your blood sugar—once high as a kite—takes a precipitous dive. This leaves you feeling like a five-year-old who's just dropped her scoop of ice cream in the gutter. Constantly seeking balance, your body tries one more trick: the pancreas sends in anti-insulin to balance out all the insulin and to bring you back to center. But because it's all a circus of extremes, you don't end up feeling balanced. You just feel tired. The blood sugar lows can lead to depression, fatigue, nausea, and crankiness. And guess what you crave when you're feeling these things? More sugar. The stuff is addictive.

This roller coaster absolutely wrecks your MILFiness and can make you needy and dependent, on a deep, vibrational level. If sugar really has a hold on you, you may be so weak that you're a sort of black hole walking around in a body.

Much of the mysterious "chaos" that men feel women represent—the flightiness, the indecisiveness, and the overwrought emotions—can be attributed to the white stuff. A more balanced female should actually feel quite grounding to a man, as if she is a warm home he can return to. Balanced mothers should be harbors their children can return to as well.

We are already on our own internal roller coasters, ladies, with our hormones hitting peaks and valleys throughout the month. No need to up the ante.

Sugar contributes to osteoporosis. Sugar creates an acidic condition in your blood and also interferes with your body's ability to absorb calcium and magnesium, your two major bone builders.

So sugar doesn't just cause your teeth to decay, it causes *all* your bones to decay. *Sweeeeet!* There may be another reason behind bone loss as well: the cortisol secreted by your adrenal glands when you chomp on that candy bar also contributes to mineral loss.

Sugar makes you fat. Yes, in the laboratory, every carbohydrate boils down to sugar. But as we've seen, different carbs behave differently in the human body. If you deliver sugar in its natural package—which brings fiber, minerals, and vitamins to the mix—your body handles it normally. And if the food is chewed well, its energy (sugar) actually gets used instead of stored. For example, you use the carbs in your brown rice when you chew it really well. But with refined sugar and flour—stripped of all their attending nutrients—you just get high on the sugar buzz and then the excess energy goes straight to your thighs, making you fat.

And we're not talking about just a pesky ten pounds here; sugar is also implicated in a condition called insulin resistance, which often leads to obesity. It seems that eating refined sugar in the amounts that we do is actually messing with our ability to use our bodies' insulin and is making us fatter than fat. And sick. Insulin resistance can lead to diabetes, high blood pressure, and the new scary condition on the block: metabolic syndrome. Which brings me to my next point . . .

Sugar may be the bad guy behind heart disease. The latest buzz in the world of food is that consumption of refined carbohydrates, principally white sugar, high fructose corn syrup, and white flour, may be the underlying cause of metabolic syndrome. This condition leads to high blood pressure and diabetes, and raises the level of triglycerides in the blood. Nasty little triglycerides cause inflammation of the arteries, which leads to plaque deposits. The connection between elevated blood sugar and heart disease is so strong that diabetics die of heart disease *two to four times* more than nondiabetics do.[27] Although we always looked to meat as raising triglycerides, it may be sugar that really does it.

Sugar weakens your immune system. In a study conducted at Loma Linda University, sugar was

---

27. http://www.diabetes.org/diabetes-basics/diabetes-statistics/.

shown to decrease the ability of white blood cells to surround and attack foreign invaders.[28] If you can't get through a winter without getting colds, kick the white stuff.

Sugar gives you wrinkles. Because sugar weakens your blood, it weakens everything, like the elasticity of your skin. You see, sugar attaches to proteins in your body and creates what are called advanced glycation end products, otherwise known as AGEs. Very funny, scientists! AGEs damage proteins, and they're gunning for the collagen and elastin that keep your skin tight and springy. AGEs also interfere with antioxidants' doing their job in your body, which makes you more vulnerable to sun damage.

Sugar feeds cancer. Mutating cells are hungry little suckers. In fact, reproducing mutant cells eat much more than normal cells do. And what's their favorite snack? Sugar, of course. Sugar is premium gasoline for tumor growth.

Sugar causes inflammation. Sugar expands things, like your waistline. But it also causes tissue to expand and that can lead to painful inflammation. If you have sore joints, or suffer from what you think are normal aches and pains, trade in white sugar for more natural sweeteners and you'll notice a difference.

Sugar will space you out. I can't write when I've eaten sugar. Nor can I retain information very well. All I really want to do is lie on the couch and watch TV. A sugar crash is so yin and expansive that it renders you unable to hold a thought.

Sugar causes decay. Sugar basically wrecks things. It isn't normal. It's like the freaky kid at school that even the teacher doesn't like. Sugar can't be trusted and it just kills things before their time. Not so sweet.

Finally, sugar attracts strong yang foods. After that candy bar demineralizes your blood, the

---

28. http://www.ajcn.org/content/26/11/1180.abstract.

next food you'll want to eat will be something full of minerals—usually meat, or something very salty. Extreme yin attracts extreme yang. You can spend a lifetime on the seesaw of meat and sugar.

Kicking Sugar

Because sugar carries such extreme yin force, sugar addicts are walking around in a very expanded state. So when you choose to let it go, your body and mind will begin to contract very quickly. This can be uncomfortable—and set you up to binge—so the following tips are ways to keep some good-quality yin in your life so the contraction doesn't happen too fast.

- Load up your kitchen, your purse, and your desk at the office with good-quality natural sweets. Make the Chocolate Chip Rice Treats on page 223, the Killer No-Bake Drop Cookies on page 215—you name it. Make sure you have them on hand. There are also some good health-food-store treats that don't contain white sugar. Get some. You can also go crazy with tropical fruits when you're first kicking the sweet stuff. Although they are high in natural sugars themselves, and very yin, they don't have a druglike effect on the body. All this loading up should keep your mind from going into a deprivation spin, which can fuel a sugar binge. Be armed with yummy sweets.
- Use natural sweeteners like rice syrup to your satisfaction. A tablespoon of brown rice syrup, right out of the jar, is legal at any time while you're kicking.
- Trade in white-flour products for whole-grain products.
- Chew your complex carbohydrates well. This will keep you satisfied and less likely to slip.
- Go easy on salt, miso, soy sauce, and pickles. Don't skip them, but season things with a light hand. Too much salt produces cravings for sweets.
- Reduce your meat intake and increase your beans. Meat craves sugar.
- Eat lots of vegetables and less grain to stay loose and yin.
- Drink carbonated fruit juice drinks instead of soda or diet soda.
- Buy some amazake; it's a sweet, relaxing drink made from rice. It's especially satisfying when served warm.

- Eat fruit-sweetened (or naturally sweetened) soy, rice, or coconut "ice cream." Check labels carefully. Agave is okay while you're kicking.
- Use fruit-sweetened jam.
- If you are a chocoholic, get SunSpire (nondairy, grain-sweetened) chocolate chips.
- Check *all* labels carefully, avoiding high fructose corn syrup, evaporated cane juice, and anything ending in "ose."
- Meditate. If you have a meditation practice, now is the time to employ it. Because sugar is addictive, you may have strong cravings for the first three or four days. Meditation can help you sit through cravings and impulses, thereby making it easier when a cupcake floats by at work. For tips on meditation, see page 97.

What You May Experience

Even with all sorts of good substitutes to keep you as relaxed and satisfied as possible, you may experience some withdrawal. You see, sugar causes your brain to release dopamine, which makes you feel good. Without it, you may feel a bit of a crash. Go easy on yourself. Talk to your MILFy friends to get a dopamine hit from another source. Exercise helps, too, although for the first few days, you just might feel draggy and sad.

Other withdrawal symptoms may include fatigue, depression, weakness, nausea, and headaches. Personally, I have really scary dreams and night sweats after about forty-eight hours off the stuff. But I know I'm turning the corner when I experience about four hours of crazy-deep depression followed by a gut-wrenching sob. Seriously. These symptoms of withdrawal come like clockwork. After enduring them, I'm out of the woods. Ahhh, sugar.

What to Look Forward To

After ten days, you will feel free of the sugar monster:
- Your desire for it will lessen *significantly,* because your body doesn't actually want or need refined sugar—it's just been hooked on it.
- You will feel less intense and compulsive about food in general.
- Your emotions will feel less volatile, and yet, at the same time, you will have more clarity about them.

- You will lose weight more easily.
- You will be less susceptible to colds and other illnesses. You will feel stronger.
- After a while, your mind will be sharper and you will get things done more easily.
- Food will taste better.
- You will reduce the symptoms of PMS and any menstrual discomfort you might have.
- If you've felt overheated in the past, your body will feel cooler.
- You will wake up more easily and generally have a calmer disposition.
- But most of all, you will feel free. Your slavery to sugar will be over. *Congratulations!*

By saying good-bye to white sugar and highly refined carbohydrates, you are reducing your risk of diabetes, heart disease, cancer, arthritis, osteoporosis, obesity, and depression. But keep in mind that you may not be out of the woods yet. Sugar is hidden in a lot of foods, and once you're off it, you will taste it more easily (sugar has a sharp, almost superficial taste . . . not mellow or round), and for me, even the sugar in some salad dressings sets me up to want more and even puts me through a mild withdrawal cycle. As far as I'm concerned, I've suffered enough for one lifetime in Sugar Jail and I go to any lengths to avoid it. Being conscientious about sugar is well worth the effort.

Dairy

People often ask me, "If I were to give up just *one* food, which would be the best to give the old heave-ho?"

I look at them closely. They look so innocent, asking me that question. They are all excited to improve their lives, all game to get started. They never expect the punch in the face that's coming.

"Dairy," I say, landing a soft right hook, quickly followed by a left: "Get rid of dairy." I take a deep breath. I know that I have just acted like the therapist who's suggested a divorce from the perfect husband.

Their faces wither, become childlike and confused. "Dairy?" they say, half laughing, half trembling. "Like . . . *cheese?*"

"Yes," I say, handing them a tissue. "Like cheese."

Unlike with meat, I don't worry too much about entering the Dairy Debate. In fact, I drove through Wisconsin one summer proudly displaying a homemade bumper sticker saying, "Dairy is SCARY."

What is dairy? You, as a MILF, should be more acquainted with this than anyone else. Dairy is a natural food, made for baby mammals, that is excreted from the mammary glands, i.e., breasts.

Is dairy more yin or more yang? Dairy, as milk, has both yin and yang elements, but overall, it's pretty yin. It causes relaxation and expansion, is a vehicle for lots of fat, but also contains yang minerals.

However, we wrangle our dairy into lots of different forms, so that can change its yinness or yangness. For instance, add some bacteria and lots of salt and you have hard cheese. This saltiness makes the cheese more yang. Add sugar and fruit or cocoa, freeze it, and you get ice cream . . . much more yin. Softer and less salty cheeses are more in the middle, but that doesn't make them balanced foods for the human body. Dairy, in any form—more yin or more yang—is just strange for humans.

What Are Dairy's Problems?

Dairy is addictive. Let's get back to the fact that dairy food is the mother's milk of a species, secreted from the breast. Perhaps you've done this excreting yourself and seen the lovely stoned glaze of your infant's eyes, felt the lovely vibes between you, and watched that little one grow at quite a rapid pace dining exclusively at the local pub, Ye Olde Boobe.

It feels great. Not just because you are bonding with the fruit of your loins and future leader of the free world, but because Mother Nature has installed certain hormonal payoffs in the act to ensure that the two of you do it: you are feeling the effects of prolactin, which induces lactation and causes you to relax; and oxytocin, which forges that incredible bond between you and your baby.

But there's more: Human breast milk contains two types of protein, casein and whey, in about a 40:60 ratio. Casein contains a special added bonus called casomorphin, a naturally occurring opiate designed to soothe and relax Your Little One. Although it's only one tenth the strength of the morphine you'd find in a hospital, it is an opiate nonetheless and it is absorbed very easily by your baby's immature gut. Casein, a protein found in all dairy products—and the milk of all mammals—always delivers this hit of casomorphin, so dairy is the feel-good food. And cheese is even more potent because its casein is concentrated and the element that refuses to get you high—the boring whey—has been removed. So cheese cranks the casomorphins up, making it the heroin of the food world.[29] No wonder people cry when I take away their Camembert.

Cow's milk (or goat's, or sheep's) is not designed for humans. Of course, at a certain point, Junior stopped nursing. Or you weaned him. It may have been hard—a little emotional for everyone— or maybe it came without much to-do, but no matter how it happened, you are *not* still nursing that kid at sixteen. Or even ten. Or even five. Mother's milk has a very specific role, in a finite window of time, and every human culture seems to follow those parameters.

In fact, all mammals follow these natural rhythms. Oh, wait. Except us. I mean, sure, *you* are not nursing your son at age sixteen, but you *are* encouraging him, your DILF, and especially your daughters to slide themselves under the belly of a cow and suck on one of *her* udders.

Think about it. Mother Nature designed cow's milk for cows, specifically to support the DNA of a bovine. Mother Nature thought up a whole different recipe for us humans, specifically designed to nourish us. That's pretty neat. And we stupidly cross the line and mess with it.

We see animals *eat* other animals. Not many, but we do. And even for humans, there are some climates wherein it's pretty hard to eke out sustenance without leaning on the food chain by eating meat. Creatures are born and creatures die. That is the rhythm. The death of one creature supports the life of another. But stealing the milk from another species' babies? We're the only idiots that do that. Chimps don't. Horses don't. Dogs don't. Just us.

Maybe that's why an estimated *75 percent* of the world's population is lactose intolerant.[30] Most Africans, most Asians, many Latinos, and even a big percentage of the people of milk-

---

29. It's also this opiate effect the makes dairy food constipating.
30. http://www.pcrm.org/health/veginfo/lactose_intolerance.html.

swilling India no longer carry the dairy-digesting enzyme called lactase necessary to break down lactose in the gut. Their bodies stop producing it after infancy. In fact, the term "lactose intolerant" is misleading. People who can't tolerate lactose are actually quite normal.

Only a small percentage of humans still produce lactase into adulthood. The theory is that northern Europeans, at some point in history, had to depend on their herds of cattle for sustenance during times of famine. In order to make this work, they adapted genetically by producing lactase.

But that was an adaptation made in order to live under duress and stressful conditions. For survival. It was not the original plan, nor do most other human bodies around the world do it. In fact, when the "lactose intolerant" ingest dairy, they experience pain, bloating, and even nausea and diarrhea as their bodies struggle to digest it. Although people of northern European descent may not suffer from the digestive stuff, that doesn't mean their bodies handle it well either. You'll see what I mean in a moment.

And please consider that richly layered, powerful, and sophisticated cultures of long standing—like China's and Japan's—were developed without a drop of milk. You won't find a glass of milk in a Chinese, Thai, or Korean restaurant, and people in those societies aren't exactly weak and anemic.

The Arguments Against Dairy

Dairy food contributes to osteoporosis. I know. *What?* That's the exact opposite of what you've been told your whole adult life, right? Well, either I'm lying to you or the National Dairy Council is. You decide, based on the facts.

It is true that cow's milk contains calcium, a mineral you need to keep your bones strong and healthy. Your bones are basically made of calcium. So when the National Dairy Council tells you that milk is a great source of calcium, they are not—technically—lying. That's why they are allowed to say it.

What they *don't* tell you is that the calcium in cow's milk is basically as unavailable to you as George Clooney because it comes with another element called phosphorus that binds with the calcium and makes it less absorbable. Remember, cow's milk is designed for *cows*. Every milk is different, just as the DNA of every species is different, and cow's milk just isn't designed for humans.

Instead, cow's milk contains lots of fat and protein because calves are all about growing; depending on the breed, a baby cow can gain up to 100 pounds *in a month.* So it's a milk that is designed for supercharged growth. But the high protein content of cow's milk isn't right for your human frame and it means that acids build up in your body. Remember, protein is made from chains of amino *acids.* And what does your amazing body do when too much acid is present? It offers up its mineral supply in order to neutralize the acid. And where does your body get these minerals? Well, first from your blood, but then it goes into your mineral warehouse—your bones. We talked about this in the meat section. Oh, yeah. *And* in the sugar section, because both those foods cause an acidic response in the body. But it bears repeating: when you're body gets too acidic, you lose minerals from your bones. Every MILF needs to understand that. As with meat, countries with the highest rates of dairy consumption have the *highest* rates of osteoporosis.[31] And vice versa. The National Dairy Council won't tell you that.

Maybe it's because the National Dairy Council (and all the local dairy councils) want to sound like some intergalactic board of wise old grandfathers devoted to your health and welfare, when they are actually just collectives of dairy farmers figuring out ways to market their product. They are neither doctors nor nutritionists. They sell milk. And they're doing a pretty good job because they've gotten you to believe that you need three glasses of milk a day, and that some cheese on your sandwich is good for your bones, and so is that cottage cheese at breakfast and that skim milk in your coffee . . . KA-CHING!!

But scarier still is that they have convinced you that their product *protects* against bone loss, when it actually contributes to it. That, my MILFy friends, may prove to be the hoax of the century.

Dairy is implicated in all autoimmune disorders. Because cow's milk is designed for another species, the human body actually greets it as an attacker. It's as if an automatic alarm system goes off when the species line is crossed. I mean, hey, Mother Nature won't let us *breed* with another species (there are not "deople" or "pogs," thank goodness), so it makes sense that Mother

---

31. http://www.ajcn.org/content/74/5/571.full.

Nature has some boundaries preventing us from suckling from each other's teats. These alarm bells include allergies, asthma, chronic stuffy and runny noses, and a generally compromised immune system.

A few years ago, I was at my doctor's office and we were looking over my blood work. This guy is a very well-respected physician in Connecticut who also has a background in whole foods and the MILFy way of eating. The only thing that seemed like a red flag on my stats was a low white blood cell count. I asked him if he was concerned about it, and he said, "Naww . . . because you don't eat dairy, your body's not *pissed off* all the time."

And it's not just about white blood cells. Type 1 diabetes is considered an autoimmune disorder because—for some mysterious reason unknown to medicine—the pancreatic cells of the diabetic person are destroyed to the point where the pancreas goes kaput. And because the pancreas is no longer able to produce insulin, the diabetic must inject it.

But studies may be showing us that the problem is dairy: it turns out the casein (protein) molecule in milk is eerily similar to cells that the pancreas makes, and that's a big problem. As I said above, the immune system perceives casein molecules as a foreign invader and attacks them. And some scientists believe that, after fending off all the casein, the immune system goes after the look-alike pancreatic cells. It may then go on to destroy the pancreas's ability to make the cells at all.[32] Ugh. It may be that childhood-onset diabetes is utterly avoidable.

In studies conducted at Toronto's Hospital for Sick Children and the University of Helsinki over the last ten years, babies who were genetically prone to diabetes were split into two groups: one fed a cow's milk–based formula; and the other, a formula designed for lactose-intolerant infants. By the time they had reached age ten, those fed the alternative formula showed markedly lower rates of type 1 diabetes than the kids fed cow's milk formula.[33]

Researchers have also discovered larger trends; in Puerto Rico, where approximately 95 percent of babies are fed cow's milk formula, the rate of type 1 diabetes is a whopping ten times higher than it is in Cuba, where babies are almost universally breast-fed.[34] Wow.

Rheumatoid arthritis and osteoarthritis are also autoimmune disorders, and dairy is also

32. http://www.ncbi.nlm.nih.gov/pubmed/8843812.
33. http://www.thestar.com/news/article/889575—researchers-hail-stunning-breakthrough-in-childhood-diabetes-study.
34. http://www.sciencenews.org/sn_arc99/6_26_99/fob2.htm.

implicated in their development.[35] In fact, the groovier MDs out there will recommend the elimination of dairy (along with some other foods, like nightshade vegetables, meat, citrus, some grains, and sugar) to arthritis patients who ask if diet changes can help. Lots and lots of people find that when they skip the dairy, the pain diminishes significantly. A pissed-off body tends to scream out in pain.

Dairy food exacerbates respiratory issues. Asthma, allergies, chronic colds? Because a dairy-eater's body is always on the defensive, she is prone to a chronic state of mild, or major, allergic response. If you suffer from any of the above, I challenge you to go dairy-free for three months and see how you feel. For most people, their symptoms lessen, or even disappear, very quickly.

Dairy may be a player in heart disease. If we go with the lipid hypothesis, which puts forth the idea that saturated fat contributes to blocked arteries, then dairy is a big no-no for your heart. With lots of saturated fat and absolutely no fiber, that latte may be a cardiac event waiting to happen.

Dairy is linked to cancer. In terms of cancer, many of Dr. T. Colin Campbell's experiments looked at dairy as much as meat. As a food containing animal protein (casein), it too seems to "turn on" cancer genes and enable carcinogens to do their nasty work.

Milk also contains something called insulin-like growth factor 1 (IGF-1), a naturally occurring compound that helps babies (and calves) grow at a rapid rate. Cute. However, IGF-1 may also be a factor in the growth of tumors. Not so cute. And when a cow is pumped full of bovine growth hormone, it gets a big ol' extra dose of IGF-1.

Milk is also connected to hormone-related cancers like breast cancer. Estrogens that are produced in a body—whether it's your body or a cow's—are up to 100,000 times more potent than the estrogen-like compounds found in pesticides, and these body-made estrogens are

---

35. http://eng.anarchopedia.org/vegan_diet_benefits_skeletal_structure.

ridiculously abundant in milk. According to Ganmaa Davaasambuu, a physician who conducted research at Harvard on the topic: "Among the routes of human exposure to estrogens, we are mostly concerned about cow's milk." In fact, she says that we get 60 to 80 percent of the estrogens we consume from dairy.[36]

But it's not like this in every country. The U.S. dairy industry milks cows roughly (in both senses of the word) 300 days a year, and for the majority of that time, the cow is pregnant. The further along she is in her pregnancy, the more estrogen is present in her milk. By the later stages of pregnancy, estrogen levels are *thirty-three times* that of a nonpregnant cow.

In many traditional cultures, milking is not this rigorous. For instance, in Mongolia, cows are milked for only five months of the year, and if that falls within a pregnancy, cows are milked only in the earliest stages. It seems to make a difference: when Mongolian third graders were fed U.S. milk for just one month, their hormone levels jumped.[37]

And how might these hormones affect us in other ways, beyond the issue of breast cancer? Well, there are other hormone-related cancers, such as uterine and ovarian. And prostate cancer, which can fell your DILF, is also hormone-related. Remember, estrogen isn't the only hormone going into cattle; there are also testosterone and progesterone and growth hormones. It's a mess.

Dairy is a source of antibiotics, too. Dairy cows are routinely dosed with antibiotics to treat painful mastitis and these medications are passed on to you. See the meat section to remind yourself of superbugs and other real-life horror-movie facts.

Dairy is bad for animals and the environment. Suffice it to say, it takes a huge amount of food, water, electricity, and fossil fuels to maintain a milking cow. Depending on the size of the cow, how much milk she is producing, and the average temperature of the climate she's in, a milker needs between eighteen and thirty-five gallons of water per day.[38] Every day. A twelve-year study done at Cornell shows that the average cow eats five times as much grain as the average

---

36. http://news.harvard.edu/gazette/2006/12.07/11-dairy.html.
37. Ibid.
38. Michael L. Looper, Extension Dairy Specialist, New Mexico State University, and Dan N. Waldner, Extension Dairy Specialist, *Water for Dairy Cattle, Guide D-107,* Oklahoma State University.

American human,[39] so the vast majority of the grain production in this country is devoted to animals, not humans. Would you like to calculate how much fossil fuel it takes to fertilize, harvest, and transport the grain that feeds the cow that gives us the milk that leads to our splintered bones, hacking coughs, and breast cancer? Me neither.

But the havoc our milker wreaks doesn't stop there; like other cows, good ol' Bessie burps and farts a LOT, creating methane, a greenhouse gas twenty times more potent than carbon dioxide. Not to mention what else comes out her hind end; a single dairy cow produces up to 120 pounds of wet manure a day. That's the equivalent of what twenty to forty people poop in the same time frame.[40] And this manure piles up and runs off into rivers and lakes and leaches into the water table, bringing all its excess hormones and antibiotics with it. All this for a little mozzarella?

So I hope you can see why I'm unafraid to deliver the one-two punch to my friends who ask about dairy. It just doesn't add up; not for our MILFiness, our health, or the future of the planet. I assume the cows agree.

Kicking Dairy

Now that you're eating whole grains, and experiencing your inner balance, dairy may feel like it comes with a heaviness, or fuzziness, that you no longer desire. Guess what, MILF? It's time to give up dairy.

Although dairy contains casomorphin, it's not addictive in the same way sugar is. You won't feel like you're jonesing for a yogurt, jumping out of your skin if you don't get "that slice of CHEDDAR!!!" You may just miss it for a while, like an old friend who's gone away on a long trip. Don't worry. Your longing will soon turn to a mild "good riddance."

Now, in order to give up dairy, you have to really give up dairy. In other words, chucking the cheese and the milk and the ice cream, but still putting cream in your coffee, is not giving up dairy. Making that morning smoothie with low-fat milk is *not* giving up dairy. And I don't say this to be the food police. I say it because your body is extremely sensitive to

---

39. http://www.livablefutureblog.com/2009/08/how-much-does-us-livestock-production-contribute-to-greenhouse-gas-emissions/.
40. http://www.animalsaustralia.org/factsheets/dairy_cows.php.

dairy. Remember how I said that your body experiences cow's (or goat's, or sheep's) dairy as an attacker, a foreign agent? Well, that's true whether you guzzle a half gallon of milk or you just put one shot of cream in your Starbucks. Your body notices and sets off its alarms. Because of this, it's impossible to feel the benefits of a dairy-free existence without going whole hog on the project. So on your dairy-free date, it's no milk, no ice cream, no cheese, no yogurt, *and* no cream in the coffee. In fact, maybe it's time to give up coffee, too! Just kidding. We'll do that in good time.

- Load up on dairy substitutes from the health food store, like various milks: there are now rice, almond, soy, hemp, and oat milks on the market. Try them all; some are richer, some are sweeter. If you're going to use milk substitutes for a while, go easy on the soy milk (see page 326).
- Get fake cheese, but make sure it's casein-free. My favorite is made by a company called Daiya and it comes grated in a bag. This stuff is pretty good, in terms of melting and tasting cheesy. I don't eat it often, but for an occasional comfort-food grilled cheese (see page 230), this is definitely the way to go. It contains no casein, soy, or gluten.
- Follow Your Heart also makes casein-free cheeses, but I prefer slathering their cream cheese alternative on a toasted whole wheat bagel and covering that with St. Dalfour Red Raspberry and Pomegranate 100% Fruit Conserve. Oooh-la-la! This is pure decadence on a Sunday morning.
- Cook with rich ingredients like oil, tahini, nut butters, soft beans, avocados, and soft tofu. Cheese is high in fat and salt, and you can achieve that rich satisfaction by using plant-based foods. You should be set on the rich and creamy front.

As your attachment to dairy lessens, I encourage you to loosen your hold on even the dairy alternatives like "milks" from a box; they're pretty processed and you just don't need them. Our adult love of all things dairy is as much cultural as it is organic. Most of Japan and China doesn't drink milk or eat cheese. Remember, most of Africa is lactose intolerant.

What You May Experience

- If you've struggled with respiratory issues like allergies or sinus problems, they will lessen relatively quickly. Dairy has pressed the "on" button on all your respiratory issues, and now that it's off, your body can go into healing mode.
- Within a few days, you may start coughing up some phlegm. Consider it a good and healthy sign to hack up nasty stuff in the shower. That's your body healing itself.

What to Look Forward To

- Now that you're dairy-free, stubborn pounds should begin to disappear. If you're chewing your food well and eating lots of grains and vegetables, you should actually feel like quite a new person in your body. Enjoy. You've earned it.
- Dairy food has compromised your taste buds. If you've had a white coating on your tongue up until this point, that's dairy. As it lessens (and it might take a few months), you will find that you are tasting food more clearly and enjoying natural food with a new and deeper appreciation.
- In fact, after a while off dairy, the whole world of your senses will sharpen and become more acute. You're coming out of a sort of cocoon designed for a baby, and you're emerging as an adult. Literally. Remember, dairy is baby food and it keeps us soothed and dependent and protected. When you are thrust into the light of a dairy-free day, it may feel as if you're experiencing things at a whole new level of clarity.
- Your mind will be clearer. Don't go looking for this in a nutrition book, but dairy can lead to cloudy, fuzzy thinking. It is not brain food, in terms of cognition. We are not asking babies to do math. So now that you're dairy-free, it might feel as though you have a whole new brain.
- You will feel quicker in your body. Dairy contains a lot of saturated fat, so it has a certain sludginess. Without it, you will feel you can move and respond to your life with more accuracy and speed.
- You will feel sexier. Dairy insulates us from things . . . our own emotions and sensations in our own bodies. By going dairy-free, you are waking up to a new level of sensuality.

- After a while, you should feel a natural revulsion to dairy food. When I see cheese now, my body recoils a little, from both its smell and its oily density. This is natural. Little kids eventually wean themselves off the breast if mom doesn't prompt it. We are *meant* to get over baby food. Rejoice when this happens.
- And finally, remember: By cutting out dairy, you have significantly decreased your likelihood of developing osteoporosis, allergies, asthma, rheumatoid arthritis, heart disease, and many types of cancer, especially breast cancer.

Caffeine

I know, I know. . . . Waking up every morning to the thought of "Here comes my espresso!!" makes life absolutely worth living. I know. I know. Whether it's through coffee, tea, soda, or those newfangled "energy drinks," caffeine has most of the world wrapped around its trembling little finger.

So brace yourself: I think there is nothing that messes with your sexy, smooth MILFiness more than the 'ffeine. Nothing.

Full disclosure: I wrestle with coffee myself. It's not pretty, but it's true. But unlike most people, I am not a chronic caffeine user.[41] Instead, I go on these horrible coffee benders like a mustachioed man in a polyester leisure suit partying at Studio 54. I can go without coffee for months at a time and then, *bang,* I'm ordering a double espresso at Starbucks and topping it up with some rice milk at 6 P.M. Then I'm up all night watching Netflix and cyberstalking old flames.

This lasts for a few days, as Dr. Jekyll slowly morphs into Mrs. Hyde, and, on about day four, I fall to my knees, exhausted and miserable, pleading to the universe to give me my soul back.

What is caffeine? Caffeine is a naturally occurring pesticide. That's right. Mother Nature puts it in plants to paralyze and kill bugs. Which it does quite nicely. I'm not sure if the poor bug

---

41. Although I do eat malt-sweetened dark chocolate every once in a while. In fact, you'll see it in a couple of recipes in this book. I don't feel the effects of the caffeine in chocolate and I don't know why. Some people do. If you're supersensitive, avoid it.

stays up all night and finishes his term paper before keeling over, but I hope so. Killing bugs. That's caffeine's proper use.

Who uses it? Just about everyone. Caffeine is the most widely used psychoactive drug in the world and one of the biggest cash crops on the planet. Next to oil, coffee is the most widely traded commodity in the world. We are all 'ffeine fiends. In the United States, coffee shops are the fastest-growing sector of the restaurant business, with a 7 percent annual growth rate. It is estimated that 90 percent of American adults consume caffeine, in some form, every day.[42] And the kids are buzzing too: in a study published in *The Journal of Pediatrics,* roughly 75 percent of the children surveyed ingested caffeine on a daily basis.[43] All told, Americans consume 146 *billion* cups of coffee per year, making us the most coffee-addled country in the world.[44]

Is caffeine more yin or more yang? Caffeine has both yin and yang characteristics, but the poor-quality versions of both. Caffeine stimulates your sympathetic nervous system, which causes some blood vessels to expand (those going to your arms and legs) and some to contract (those going to your brain). It also causes a big rush of adrenaline; you get tense and your heart beats faster . . . both yang responses. Caffeine also supports lots of thinking—a yang quality—and not so much deep feeling. However, caffeine causes your blood to become acidic, which creates an overall weakness. Like all things, it has both yin and yang qualities, but caffeine has a strong impact in both directions. It's a long, shaky seesaw.

How Does Caffeine Interfere with MILFiness?

Caffeine stresses you out. If MILFiness comes from our ability to relax and to receive and enjoy our female energy, then caffeine is enemy Numero Uno. By stimulating the sympathetic nervous system, caffeine puts us squarely in the fight-or-flight response, causing adrenaline to rush through the body and a state of hyperalertness to develop. This may sound good if you're doing your bills, but basically your body thinks a tiger has entered your

---

42. http://www.dopestats.com/dopestats/template.jsp?drug=13.
43. http://www.jpeds.com/content/JPEDSWarzak.
44. http://coffee-statistics.com/coffee_statistics_ebook.html.

kitchen nook. Using caffeine on a regular basis pushes your precious adrenal glands to the point of exhaustion. That may be fine for a college freshman with energy to burn, but *you* need your adrenaline to handle life's real stresses. Don't waste it.

When there is a *real* threat or stressor in our lives, we are meant to address the threat and then relax completely. Just as a cat reacts quickly to a noise and then melts back into a nap seconds later, we are meant to have that kind of flexibility between stress and relaxation. But with caffeine, we are constantly overstimulated, never allowing our bodies to go back to that deep, lovely MILFy place inside. And because caffeine is addictive and causes withdrawal symptoms, its users rarely kick the stuff long enough to really sink into the restorative, healing parasympathetic nervous system. In other words, it's impossible to connect with your deepest inner yin force while sipping on a Diet Coke.

Caffeine overstimulates the heart and raises blood pressure. Of course, this is a health issue, but it's also a MILF issue. Normally, when you are with another person, there is a certain unconscious alignment that happens between you. You may mirror each other's body language, start to breathe in a closer pattern, and even your heartbeats find a way of relating to one another so that there is a deeper rapport and better communication. This is called entrainment, and it is one of a MILF's deepest strengths. Entrainment with others is a great source of pleasure in life; it builds bonds, families, and communities. It's also part of a good sex life. But with a caffeinated, *bangbangbang* heart whacking away in your chest, you are no longer able to align with certain natural rhythms. Your ability to resonate with others plummets as caffeine controls your vibe. With caffeine in the mix, you are unable to relax to the place where this resonance occurs, and your poor, overworked heart just bangs away in isolation.

Caffeine steals minerals from your bones. Osteoporosis, anyone? One of the major culprits in bone loss—especially in postmenopausal women[45] —is caffeine. Snap!

Caffeine messes with fertility. According to a Danish study,[46] drinking even small amounts of

---

45. http://www.ajcn.org/content/74/5/694.short.
46. http://www.ivf1.com/caffeine-and-fertility/.

coffee affects the ability to conceive. Women in the study who consumed more than the equivalent of one cup of coffee per day were *half* as likely to become pregnant, per cycle, as women who drank less. The more a woman drank, the lower her chances for becoming pregnant. Studies also show that coffee drinking increases the risk of miscarriage.[47]

Let's examine this: Could it be that the relaxed receptivity that is characteristic of our womanhood flies out the window when we're jacked up on the joe? It's well understood that stress affects our ability to climax, can interrupt our menstrual cycles, and can even stop a labor, so why would the chronic state of agitation produced by caffeine *not* mess with our baby making? All of our reproductive functions work better when we're relaxed. I mean, think about it: running from a saber-toothed tiger is not exactly a good time to get knocked up.

Caffeine gives you wrinkles. Caffeine dehydrates. Ever notice that caffeinated beverages make you pee like a racehorse? That's because caffeine is a natural diuretic. I know that sounds like "I'm gonna lose weight!" but what caffeine is actually doing is overworking your kidneys, 24/7. And, honey, you need your kidneys for other things—like cleaning your blood—so don't waste their precious chi on chai. Oh, yeah, and being dehydrated gives you wrinkles. Give up caffeine for a week and you'll see your face relax and plump up, all MILF-like.

Caffeine makes you afraid. We live in a culture that loves us to be afraid—afraid of aging, of global warming, of our kids getting kidnapped. Just watch the news and pay attention to how many times your mind is being bullied into generating fear. By using caffeine, you are much less able to handle this already-stressful environment. Chronic caffeine consumption can lead to chronically fearful, defensive thoughts. Before you get a prescription for Ativan, try kicking the java.

Caffeine makes you bitchy. We all know this on some level, but after years and years of caffeine consumption, you may have begun to actually *identify* with parts of yourself that are simply the by-products of caffeine. You see, after the initial high of the fight-or-flight response comes a

---

47. http://www.nytimes.com/2008/01/21/health/21caffeine.html.

crash. Extreme yang (hyperactivity) becomes extreme yin (exhaustion). Your blood sugar drops, you feel weak, and your mind hits the skids. Suddenly every single person in the office is a total freaking *idiot*! Which is weird, because you loved them all just an hour ago. You are on a roller coaster that is taking not only your moods, but your entire personality, for a scream-inducing ride. Get off caffeine and you will discover whole new dimensions of yourself.

Caffeine makes you self-centered. Think about it: survival is—by definition—self-centered, and by keeping you in the fight-or-flight response all the time, caffeine keeps your brain stuck on the ME-ME-ME channel. Of course, because everyone else is on the *me-me-me* channel, too, and we live in a myopically individualistic culture, this seems normal, but what it's really getting us is isolation, narcissism, a dearth of compassion, and an inability to let down our defenses so we can really receive one another.

One of the characteristics of yin force is that it makes room for other people. It allows others to simply be, and a true MILF is a good listener who enjoys drinking in her friends and family like good Champagne. We are meant to feel a natural connection to and affinity for other human beings. It doesn't have to be cultivated only through religious or spiritual pursuits; it's actually our default mode—*unless* we're jacked up on the 'ffeine, in which case we are acting defensively. Not so MILFy. Ever notice a school of fish or a flock of birds pounding shots of espresso?

Caffeine interferes with deep sleep. You knew this. It's one of the few things we admit to ourselves in our global caffeine trance. If you have any trouble sleeping at all, cut out caffeine and you will see improvement. MILFs need their beauty sleep.

How much is too much? In my classes, when the subject of caffeine comes up and someone says, "But I only have a cup a day," I answer that it's not whether you drink one cup or six (although there is a difference between them). Rather, the crux of the matter is found between one cup and none at all. Any caffeine at all is going to stimulate your sympathetic nervous system and cause you to secrete adrenaline. Only by getting off it *completely* can you see what you're missing.

Kicking Caffeine

First, choose whether you're going to go cold turkey or ratchet down with green tea.[48] If you're ratcheting down, go out and buy some good green tea. Drink it as you would coffee or your regular tea. Then alternate between decaf green tea and the real stuff. Within a couple of weeks, you'll be ready to let go of it altogether.

No matter how you get there, aim for total freedom from caffeine. Yes, drinking green tea (or any mildly caffeinated tea) will make you feel better than you do on coffee, but it's not the same as no caffeine at all. And don't make decaf coffee your final destination, either; it has recently been shown to be bad for the heart.[49] Plus, it'll just bring you closer to the real stuff. I find it easier to just skip the coffee shop experience altogether when I'm off the 'ffeine. Don't make it harder than it needs to be.

Even in the ratcheting-down stage, start to practice the following self-massage technique in bed before you get up:

Rise 'n' Shine Morning Massage
- As you lie in bed, take a nice deep breath, make a loose fist, and tap the top of your skull. Hard. Your head can take it. On your exhalations, tap all over your head. This is a great waker-upper.
- Then massage your ears—pulling on them quite vigorously. Pull your earlobes and generally massage the ear without going into the ear canal. According to Chinese medicine, by stimulating your ears, you are stimulating your kidney energy.
- Tap lightly or massage all areas of your face (except your eyes). Your forehead, brow bones, cheekbones, and jaw can handle vigorous tapping and rubbing.
- Move the tapping down to your shoulders and the muscles between your neck and shoulders. Give them a good going-over. Tap your chest (avoiding boobs, but the rib cage is fine), underarms, down each arm (a few times), and onto the palms of your hands. This really wakes up deep energy in the body and will make you feel very good.

---

48. Personally, I go cold turkey, but I don't have a real job that I have to stay awake for, so you might want to choose the second route.
49. http://www.guardian.co.uk/uk/2005/nov/17/research.health.

- After you've tapped your upper body well, massage each finger individually. Each finger connects to a meridian that an acupuncturist or shiatsu practitioner stimulates, so massaging your fingers is important.
- Continue tapping on your belly, around to your lower back, and down your legs, getting the fronts, sides, insides, and backs of each. Tap the bottoms of your feet. Massage each toe. Meridians end and begin at your toes, too.
- All this tapping should take you no more than five minutes. You will be amazed by how alert and energized you feel. COFFEE NO LONGER NECESSARY!!! This is a great way to wake up for the rest of your life, by the way.

- Another great way of waking yourself up in the morning is the body scrub on page 76. Doing both the self-massage and the body scrub will give you wonderful, clean, and alert energy all through the morning.
- At work, when you're feeling sluggish, tap your skull and anywhere else on your body that needs stimulation. That will perk you up.
- Get exercise. After the first few days of lethargy, make sure you work out. This will replace some of the endorphins and dopamine you're no longer stimulating with the caffeine.
- Meditate. Meditation is 5 million times easier and more fruitful when you're not caffeinated. As is hypnosis, yoga, or any other groovy, MILFy pursuit. Meditation will also slow down your brain (in a good way) and help you not to reach for that Diet Coke.

What You May Experience

The nice thing about caffeine is that it's not as addictive as sugar. You shouldn't crave it like a junkie. However, you will experience withdrawal. This differs slightly for everyone, but make room for a one- or two-day-long headache, fatigue, lethargy, and even some depression for a good week. And remember this: *You are not allowed to judge yourself, or your life, during this week.* You are not the normal "you" and this week is *not* indicative of your caffeine-free future. Your brain has to do some serious rejiggering when you withdraw from the java. But it's all good. After ten days of feeling so-so, you should be back up to speed, but with a mellow, warm, and loving human inside your body. The bitch will be gone.

A decaf life can feel a little dull at first. Caffeine produces tons of drama because it keeps you in your fight-or-flight response all the time. So even if someone at the office isn't being mean to you, you *think* they are because of all the adrenaline pumping through your veins. Don't worry. You will find new dramas, in real life, that need your attention. And on the days that you don't? Enjoy the peace.

What to Look Forward To

- The drama in your head will die down. The angry person will go away.
- You will sleep more easily and more deeply. *Ahhh . . .*
- You will be a softer and kinder human being without really trying.
- You will feel more courage. Caffeine has been taxing your kidneys and adrenal glands and they will start to get stronger, increasing your natural fortitude.
- Your intuition will become stronger.
- You will connect more with your true feelings.
- You will open up to a deep creative energy inside you.
- You will have easier menstrual periods and milder PMS.
- Your fertility will increase and you will reduce your risk of miscarriage.
- You will be in the moment and appreciate little things you don't normally notice.
- You will be more present for sex and have a deeper energy connection with your DILF.
- You will feel that your life works more smoothly, with less effort and drama.
- Others will be more attracted to you as a person because you're not giving off erratic, jagged vibes.

By functioning more from the parasympathetic nervous system, you will develop a whole new type of strength—good-quality, softly enhancing, yin strength. You will tune in to a larger web of information, not through a computer, but through your relaxed nervous system. Finally, if you relate to something you call "God," "Spirit," or "Higher Power" in your life, you will feel closer to it when you lay down that latte. Welcome to the quieter and deeper power of the MILF.

So why do I use caffeine? Sometimes it's because I don't exercise enough and my brain is craving the dopamine that a vigorous workout releases. But more than that, I think it's because I can't handle the profundity of a noncaffeinated existence for too long. I get a little afraid of the magic, afraid of my own power. Afraid of the continual procession of humble successes and victories that a peaceful, connected life brings about. Yes, sometimes I'm perversely afraid of feeling happy, grateful, and confident 24/7. I know that's weird, but maybe you relate. Maybe this is the yin and yang of life itself. I can handle the quiet and stillness at the center of my being for only so long before I have to shake it up like a snow globe. Oh, well.

Weird "Foods"

> What we eat has changed more in the last forty years than in the
> previous forty thousand.
> —Eric Schlosser, *Fast Food Nation*

If being MILFy is all about being beautiful, powerful, and connected to nature, weird and processed foods have got to go. Well, not all processed foods. You see, technically, juicing a carrot is processing it. Ditto pureeing a soup, or pickling an onion. *Cooking* is a form of food processing and when it is done by a MILF with an open heart, it is quite magical.

However, in the last hundred years or so, we've turned food processing over to Big Business. At first it seemed like a smart thing to do; what's so wrong with a little convenience? Processed foods mean easier, more convenient, and often cheaper foods. Processed foods allow a busy twenty-first-century household to keep buzzing at a modern pace. But at what price? Well, unfortunately, that price may never be determined exactly. No laboratory technician is going to peer down the microscope at a slice of a tumor and say, "A Big Mac did this!" because by the time the chemicals in the processed foods have done their bioterrorism, they've morphed into the form of disease and aren't recognizable as the cause.

So let's take a look at America's Great Escape from Nature.

Prior to World War II, this country was fed by smaller, mostly family-owned farms that used trusted, natural compounds as herbicides and pesticides. And many families—just regular folk, not farmers—had gardens from which they plucked parts of their dinners. But after World War II, things got really wonky. Chemicals that were developed for warfare were just sitting around, needing to be used, so they were applied to agriculture. You heard me: toxic chemicals started getting used as herbicides and pesticides in food farming.

You may be thinking, "Okay, they were toxic, but they must have increased efficiency, right?" Well, not exactly. In 1940, U.S. farmers were able to produce 2.3 food calories for every calorie of fossil fuel invested. Postindustrialization, we now produce 1 food calorie for every *10 calories* of fossil fuel used.[50] That means modern farming is a whopping 23 times *less efficient* than the old-school version. But, hey, when we thought this technology up, oil was ridiculously cheap and still spewing out of Texas.

And the chemicals didn't stop there. Postwar chemical inventions also got *into* our food, creating the modern processed foods we've come to know. In 1945, after having entered the workforce while their DILFs were off in combat, postwar MILFs had a taste for freedom, and processed foods were sold as a way of giving women more time for leisure and work outside the home. So women gained a certain type of "freedom" through cake mixes, canned frosting, and Red Dye No. 2. The added chemicals allowed foods to be boxed, bagged, canned, or frozen, or to just sit around on shelves for months. Women could "whip up" meals in a matter of minutes. It was spectacular! Add a dishwasher and a washing machine to the mix and the modern MILF had broken the chains of domestic servitude. Processed foods were as liberating as anything Betty Friedan had to say.[51]

Because we weren't dropping dead after eating these "foods," they were considered safe. So we indulged. Laden with refined sugar, fat, and bad-quality salt, processed foods quickly trained America's palate to their wily, addictive ways. And they grew rapidly in sophistication. Today there is a mind-boggling array of additives being put into your "food," including anticaking, antifoaming, and glazing agents; artificial colors, flavors, and aromas; thickeners, stabilizers, and things called humectants; and "tracer gas," which sounds like something a spy might use. According to the FDA, there are more than 3,000 substances on their Everything Added to

---

50. http://www.panna.org/issues/food-agriculture/industrial-agriculture.
51. If processed foods played a part in women's having the time, energy, and freedom to contemplate gender politics, then I thank Goddess for them. I really mean that. It may be the silver lining in the cloud of processed food.

Food in the United States (EAFUS) list.[52] Although the U.S. government must declare them "generally recognized as safe" (GRAS) before they are used, many seem questionable in terms of safety.[53] And did you know that when the GRAS designation was first introduced in 1958, all 700 additives being used at the time were simply grandfathered in as safe? It's only when problems arise that we seem to get wise: MSG, saccharin, Red Dye No. 2, and sodium nitrite have all been questioned or pulled from the shelves in our lifetimes. And with the average American estimated to ingest more than four pounds of additives each year, those may be just the tip of the iceberg.

In a study conducted by researchers at the University of Southampton in England, children were given what would equal a daily dose of common food additives and then their behavior was monitored for changes; symptoms of ADHD were clearly observed. Professor Jim Stevenson, who headed the Southampton study, said: "We now have clear evidence that mixtures of certain food colors and benzoate preservative can adversely influence the behavior of children."[54]

And we adults are getting our fair share of chemicals, too. According to *The New York Times*, the average U.S. citizen eats 787 pounds of processed foods per year compared with a measly 194 pounds of vegetables. The United States consumes more processed foods than any other country, although Spain, France, and Mexico are not far behind us. Meanwhile, in China, the average person consumes 604 pounds of veggies per year and 116 pounds of processed foods.[55] That's a lot of bok choy.

But we're getting ahead of ourselves. Let's go back to the 1950s and 1960s and more food technology. So we had frozen TV dinners and instant puddings, and, to zap us all into another dimension, the first countertop microwave oven was introduced in 1967. Just eight years later, microwave ovens were outselling gas ranges,[56] and by 1976, microwaves were more commonly owned than dishwashers, with nearly 60 percent of American households nuking their food. Today 90 percent of us own microwaves, and I wish I could tell you that they're safe, but the

52. http://www.fda.gov/food/foodingredientspackaging/ucm115326.htm.
53. http://findarticles.com/p/articles/mi_m0NAH/is_4_33/ai_100732356/.
54. http://www.guardian.co.uk/uk/2007/sep/06/lifeandhealth.health.
55. http://graphics8.nytimes.com/images/2010/04/04/business/04metrics_g/04metrics_g-popup-v2.jpg.
56. http://www.gallawa.com/microtech/history.html.

FDA has studied only the effects of radiation leaking through a faulty microwave oven door. The government has yet to study the effects of microwave cooking on food.[57]

Luckily, others have. A Spanish study done in 2003 showed that broccoli cooked in a microwave lost 97 percent, 74 percent, and 87 percent of three important cancer-protecting antioxidants. However, when it was steamed, the broccoli lost only 11 percent, 0 percent, and 8 percent of the same compounds, respectively.[58] Turns out your healthy food isn't so healthy after being nuked.

As if that's not enough, a Japanese study showed that microwaving meat and dairy reduced their vitamin B_{12} content by 30 to 40 percent.[59] A study conducted at Stanford in 1992 showed that heating breast milk in a microwave destroyed lysozyme, a naturally occurring infection fighter. And it looks as though heating formula in a microwave is even worse, converting a certain amino acid into a substance reputed to be toxic to the kidneys and nervous system.[60]

In 1991, when a Swiss scientist named Dr. Hans Hertel studied the impact of microwave cooking on health, his findings were remarkable: Blood taken from people who had recently eaten microwaved foods showed lower red blood cell counts, with increased white blood cell and cholesterol levels. And what happened to Dr. Hertel? Oh, he was issued a gag order, convicted of "interfering with commerce," and prohibited from publishing more of his results.

I urge you to ditch your microwave. I have never, in my adult life, owned one; I've rented apartments that have had them, but I use their doors as mirrors to check for food between my teeth. Not one MILF I interviewed for this book uses a microwave to cook her food. Not for warming up soup or for defrosting vegetables. Not even to microwave popcorn. They just don't use them.

Microwaves work by agitating water molecules until they heat up. And food—like your body and mine—is made up of lots and lots of water. However, the technology used to do this agitates the molecules at a rate that is much faster and more aggressive than any other form of natural heat. And the water molecules, each of which has both a negative and a positive pole,

---

57. http://www.bls.gov/cpi/cpimwo.htm.
58. "Microwave Cooking Zaps Nutrients," *Journal of the Science of Food and Agriculture,* Vol. 83, p. 1511.
59. F. Watanabe et al., "Study to Evaluate the Impact of Heat Treatment on Water-Soluble Vitamins in Milk," *Journal of Agricultural and Food Chemistry,* 1998;46:206–10.
60. http://pediatrics.aapublications.org/content/89/4/667.

experience a flip in their poles up to *1 billion times per second*. By pounding the water molecules so hard, microwave cooking often destroys the cell membranes of the food. This damage is called structural isomerism. Best-case scenario, the cells are simply rendered without their normal chi (which is bad enough, frankly), but worst-case, they are changed in ways that alter their function, turning good molecules into very bad ones. Yes, normal heating of food changes cells as well, but it doesn't go exploding them quite like this. Remember the poor broccoli you just read about?

Just because Uncle Sam wants to stay in denial about what microwaves might be doing to food doesn't mean you have to. An antioxidant in broccoli reduced by *97 percent*? Antioxidants are why you're eating broccoli in the first place, for goodness' sake!

But our food story isn't just about what we were doing at home. Around the same period as the rise of chemical foods and the mighty microwave, fast-food restaurants were getting their foothold in American culture. Since 1940, when the original McDonald's restaurant opened, the chain has expanded to over 31,000 restaurants worldwide, serving an estimated 64 million customers *per day*.[61] And that's just McDonald's, one of many, many fast-food chains. It appears our Great Escape from Nature has gone global.

Two more leaps in food technology have widened the gap between our bodies and nature: the invention of high fructose corn syrup in 1967 (see page 275 to get a reminder on what that's doing) and, in 1982, the first genetic modification of a plant cell, in a laboratory owned and operated by a company named Monsanto.

First of all, it's important that you know that Monsanto has not always been in the food business. They'd like you to think they have, because they are buying up seed companies all over the world, but Monsanto was originally a chemical company. It has the dubious distinction of having brought the world saccharin, DDT, PCBs, and a cute little defoliant used in the Vietnam War called Agent Orange. Monsanto was in the business of making chemicals until the early 1980s, when it got into genetic engineering.

Monsanto also wants you to believe that we need genetically modified foods because Monsanto wants to feed the hungry of the world. And if you do the math on some of their inventions, it looks like genetic engineering could make feeding the developing world a little

---

61. McDonald's Corporation 2010 Annual Report.

easier. But that doesn't seem to be what they've been concentrating on. . . . Monsanto's biggest contribution to the world has been genetically modified crops that are so resistant to chemical herbicides that farmers can spray up to ten times more on them than they normally would. This means they can be sure to get rid of all the weeds that interfere with your wheat, or corn, or soy.

And who makes all this herbicide farmers are spraying on these crops? Oh, a little company called Monsanto, that's who. Their Roundup Ready seeds are designed to withstand intense spraying of their leading herbicide, Roundup. Roundup is the most-used herbicide in the United States and the biggest-selling herbicide in the world.

And, until recently, no one seemed to be considering that all these extra chemicals were getting into you—the consumer—as well. Or into the flesh of an animal that you might later eat. But in 2011, it was discovered that Roundup's primary chemical, glyphosate, had been found to cause birth defects in laboratory animals at doses much lower than those at which it is currently used on crops.[62] And it turns out Monsanto knew this.

So let's just not use Roundup, right? Well, that's easier said than done. Roundup Ready crops are so resilient—and prevalent—that most farmers *must* buy them in order to remain competitive. And some farmers get into the business through the back door: these genetically modified crops tend to pollinate neighboring fields of non–genetically modified crops, making it hard to avoid contamination.

Genetic engineering has also brought us "suicide seeds" (or "terminator technology"), which constrain farmers as well. You see, Monsanto has designed plants whose seeds are sterile, rendering them useless to plant the next year. This forces the farmer to buy new Monsanto seeds every season. Perhaps this represents the eeriest of our leaps to escape nature: a natural and historic cycle . . . seeds producing plants . . . producing seeds . . . producing plants . . . has been broken.

And even if a farmer refuses to buy Monsanto seeds, it's getting harder and harder for him or her to survive. Monsanto has bought up most of the world's large seed companies, so even non–genetically modified seeds are Monsanto "products." With its deep pockets, the big "M" is pressuring governments to craft legislation to position us all under Monsanto's big green

62. http://www.huffingtonpost.com/2011/06/07/roundup-birth-defects-herbicide-regulators_n_872862.html.

thumb: seed laws, pushed through Congress thanks to Monsanto's lobbyists, are making the cleaning, saving, and storing of seeds both onerous and expensive. And it has started overseas as well. In Europe, farmers using non-Monsanto seeds must register their crops, paying fees and doing paperwork for every type of seed they use. A farm that grows twenty types of olives? Forget it. Too expensive for the farmer to register them all.

And because Monsanto's genetically engineered seeds are patented, they are protected by already existing intellectual property law. You see, seeds are no longer seeds; they are *ideas.* And Monsanto employees go to great lengths as seed detectives by trespassing and stealing samples from crops—even flying over fields to determine if their "customers" are breaking patent law.

Monsanto is very slick about this stuff; its website has devoted extensive space to answering the allegations brought up by the documentary *Food, Inc.,* in which an Indiana man named Moe Parr was sued by Monsanto. Mr. Parr ran a seed-cleaning business, a service farmers have used for decades in order to clean their seeds from one year's crop to plant for the next year's. But that's a problem for Monsanto. The corporation accused Moe of "aiding, abetting, encouraging, and enticing the farmer to break the patent law." Remember, even when not using "suicide seeds," Monsanto "customers" are contractually obligated to buy seed from Monsanto for the next year. So seed cleaning and guys like Moe Parr are a *big* no-no in this Monsanto world.

Vandana Shiva, an Indian MILF, is a powerful and vocal activist against Monsanto. She is following in the footsteps of Gandhi, who flouted the British salt tax by encouraging thousands of Indians to march to the sea and simply take their own salt. Shiva, in the face of newly emerging seed laws, is encouraging people to actively store their own seeds in a nonviolent demonstration against what she calls "a criminalization of the most beautiful activity that humans can engage in—working with the earth and working with the soil."

It used to be that business was business and nature was nature. They were separate. But now a corporation is beginning to own nature, to own the very seeds we grow food from. To get between us and the earth.

One of the most politically radical things you can do is to buy USDA-certified-organic foods, which contain no genetically modified organisms (GMOs). However, that's easier said than done as well. With Congress in bed with Monsanto, there is no labeling of GMOs, so any food—especially soy, wheat, and corn, which show up in almost every processed food—can be genetically modified and the manufacturer has absolutely no responsibility to inform you about it.[63]

And I haven't even touched upon the actual impact that GMOs might have on you, me, or the environment. Forget the herbicides GMOs endure; the genetic modification itself is a creepy, global, heretofore unheard-of experiment in biology. We have *no idea* what the crossing of these genetic lines might be doing to our bodies, or to biodiversity, or to other plants. With no respect for earth's living systems, ecological interdependence, or nature's innate wisdom, we have become drunks in the science lab. All to make a buck.

Monsanto proudly assures us that GMOs have been around for a full *sixteen years,* and that there have been absolutely no problems recorded so far. But how, I ask you, will the problems show up? In the history of the world, we have never been able to zap together a plant gene and an animal gene, until now. We have absolutely no idea what to even look for in terms of problems. We are engaged in a crapshoot with a rich, powerful bully of a teenager. Sixteen years. Wow.

We can argue all we want about why the rates of disease in our country are sky high. Why the richest nation in the world, with the most advanced medical technology, has a population dropping dead from heart disease, cancer, and diabetes at such alarming rates. Why our kids won't live as long as we do. Why, instead of walking down the streets, we are rolling down them. We can debate until we're blue in the face, but the fact remains that these diseases began to spike in absolute lockstep with the mass industrialization of food production and our introduction to processed foods.

And don't forget that we are guinea pigs here. This little experiment has never been perpetrated before in human history and it has taken place over our MILFy lifetimes. No other generation of humans, *ever,* has had the dubious "luxury" of walking into a store and buying a "dinner" complete with irradiated, sprayed, colored, antibiotic- and hormone-injected, genetically modified "foods," and then zapping it in a microwave—rendering it either more toxic or

---

63. They're hopping mad about this in Europe, by the way, with very little genetically engineered farming there and strong pro-labeling laws.

almost useless—only to chase it all down with colored, flavored, fluoridated, and caffeinated water mixed with other synthetic chemicals and sweetened with high fructose corn syrup.

And perhaps your lovely human body, doing its best to harmonize with nature and to resonate with the sun, the earth, and the stars by eating natural foods, could tolerate this assault once, or maybe twice. Cough up the toxins. Poop them out. No problem! But some precious bodies absorb this assault day after day, week after week, year after year . . . and we wonder why we're so sick? Why our culture is going crazy? Why our prescription drug companies are some of the biggest in the world? Don't let convenience kill you.

Kicking Processed Foods

If you are someone who eats fast food all the time, and you've been chewing whole grains and vegetables of late, you've come a *looooong* way, baby. And the goal may not be to get rid of *all* processed foods; we will probably all lean on healthier processed foods from time to time. Fortunately, you can change your health for the better by simply switching from the bad processed foods to the healthier, groovier ones and chewing them well. There are lots of companies out there these days making a healthy life easier, quicker, and more convenient for people like you and me. Yes, it will be more expensive, but the price you're paying right now—if you're eating fast food on any kind of regular basis—is higher. Their price tag includes: headaches, fatigue, body odor, moodiness, skin problems, extra pounds, and a seriously increased risk of heart disease, cancer, and diabetes.

Now let's get started! Go to a health food store and buy (organic whenever possible):

- Nondairy frozen pizzas
- Veggie burgers from various companies
- Tofu hot dogs
- Seasoned canned beans and canned soups
- Dips and spreads like hummus and guacamole
- Fake cheeses like Daiya and Follow Your Heart
- Soy, rice, and coconut "ice creams"
- Corn chips

- Popcorn
- Whole wheat bread, crackers, and bagels
- Soy margarine
- Soy "cream cheese"
- Fruit-juice sodas
- Sugar-free cereals (unsweetened, or sweetened with barley malt, brown rice syrup, agave syrup, or honey)
- Organic frozen meals
- Sugar- and dairy-free cookies

Many health food stores, and Whole Foods Markets, have big precooked deli cases and buffets. Go crazy on them.

Truth is, you can be a very satisfied, nonsugar, nondairy, meat-free MILF eating exclusively processed foods. I'm not encouraging it, but it's true. And I'm glad. There may be some of you who never make it into the kitchen and at least we now live in a world that gives you more choices than the drive-thru.

With the transition, you can expect to:

- Lose weight
- Feel lighter inside your body
- Have more energy
- Feel happier and calmer
- Have better skin
- Experience a cooler temperature in your body

I dived enthusiastically into cooking when I first started the MILF diet, so I don't have firsthand experience with going from crummy processed foods to the groovy ones. In fact, most of them didn't even exist when I started. If you are a MILF who takes this route, write to me and let us all know how it goes!

One Last Thing About Kicking

If you find it really difficult to make some of these changes, in spite of your desire to do so, you may have deeper issues or even an eating disorder. It's important to get help; therapy and support groups like Overeaters Anonymous and Food Addicts Anonymous can be very helpful in unpacking deeper issues and supporting individuals in following healthy food plans. If you've struggled with food issues for as long as you can remember, don't be afraid to reach out. Life's too short to go it alone.

Whole Grains

Whole grains and vegetables are your new yin and yang—the center of your seesaw. You don't need to throw anything out at this point—that will happen quite naturally after you've experienced a saner, softer ride inside your body. For now, we are just going to *add* whole grains and vegetables.

What exactly do I mean by "whole grains"? Well, these days, every cereal company and biscuit broker is touting the "whole-grain goodness" of their products. Recent nutritional research has given props to whole grains, so corporate America—as always—has gone crazy with the dumbed-down version of the real thing. But I am *not* talking about brown bread or Cheerios or wooden spaghetti.

I mean the whole grains *themselves.* The little grains of wheat *before* they are milled into flour . . . the brown rice *before* it's stripped to make white rice . . . the barley *before* it's polished for the soup. These are the earthy, gritty, gutsy forms of carbohydrates and they are the key to an altogether better life.

Are whole grains more yin or more yang? Whole grains are the most centered of all food groups and central to most diets in the history of civilization. Although most grains are very mildly acid-forming, their acidity is nicely buffered by the alkalinity of most vegetables. Their acidity can also be reduced by soaking before cooking and thorough chewing.

Compared with meat, grains are yin because they are parts of plants—containing more oxygen and lighter overall energy. However, compared with most vegetables, grains are more yang, because they are smaller, tighter, and drier than veggies. But hey, you don't need to think too much about the yinness or yangness of grains because they are simply not extreme.

What's So Great About Whole Grains?

Whole grains are balanced foods. In terms of yin and yang, whole grains provide a lovely balanced feeling to the average human being. You see, we—humans in general—are more yang than yin. In other words, we are held together in our bodies; we are walking securely on the earth. . . . The forces of contraction are stronger in us than expansion. Yes, women are more expanded than men, but all together—as a species—we are pretty yang.

But grain plants are just the opposite: practically weightless, aiming toward the sun, seemingly defying gravity with their strong upward push, grains help us to feel poised, light, and balanced. They are more yin than we are and together we make a great couple.

Whole grains are rich in complex carbohydrates. If you've been alive for the last two decades, you've seen carbs get battered in the press. But every time your sister-in-law screeched, "I'm off *CARBS*, Barb!!" she really meant *refined* carbs. And that's cool; it's good to be off refined carbs. But not unrefined carbs. Complex carbohydrates are as vital to you as oxygen, steady friendships, and a decent bra. When chewed thoroughly, complex carbs convert to glucose, which then feeds every cell in your brain and body. By making whole grains and vegetables the center of your diet, you will experience calm, peaceful, and sustained energy. *Très* MILFy.

Whole grains contain tons of fiber. I wrote in the meat section about the benefits of fiber, but they bear repeating: fiber sweeps out your body, taking things like toxic waste and excess hormones with it. It gives you good, easy bowel movements and is believed to help lower cholesterol. Fiber rules.

Whole grains are simply *good* for you. Whole grains are full of vitamins (especially the B's), minerals (including potassium, magnesium, selenium, and iron), antioxidants, and other phytochemicals. In other words, they are specifically designed for your body to use, making them one of humanity's perfect foods. Studies show that consuming whole grains lowers blood pressure and reduces the risk of heart disease, stroke, diabetes, and metabolic syndrome, not to mention a handful of cancers.[64]

---

64. http://www.medicinenet.com/script/main/art.asp?articlekey=55832&page=2.

Whole grains will keep you slim. In a study looking at over 2,000 women,[65] those who ate at least one serving of whole grains per day had consistently lower body mass indexes than those who didn't. Many studies,[66] in fact, point to the truth that people who eat whole grains on a regular basis stay leaner than those who don't.

In 2011, researchers at Harvard who examined the data from The Nurses' Health Study (and its spin-off studies), which looked at the eating habits of over 120,000 health professionals for between twelve and twenty years, concluded that counting calories is not enough; there are good foods and bad foods when it comes to how your body handles those calories. On the bad list? French fries, potato chips, sugar-sweetened drinks, red meats, processed meats, refined grains, other fried foods, 100 percent fruit juice, and good ol' butter. These foods, no matter the amount, tend to slow metabolism and lead to weight gain. And what about the foods that increase metabolism and help you lose weight, regardless of calorie count? Whole grains, vegetables, and fruit.[67] Thank you, Harvard!

Whole grains will calm you down. Loaded with B vitamins, whole grains relax your nervous system. You will feel an inner peace you've never experienced before.

Whole grains are antidepressants. Whole grains increase serotonin levels in your brain.[68] Let's consider this for a minute. Why would an amazingly complex interlocking system like the one we call nature *not* provide perfect foods—foods that make us feel happy—for the creatures created within it? It has developed air, water, and soil that support us physically. Why not emotionally? The system supports itself. That's how it works.

Whole grains will make you one with everything. These little seeds, packed with the life force, will make you feel connected—connected to yourself, to the natural world, and to whatever invisible glue there is between all natural things. Eating whole grains will, over time, help

65. http://www.ncbi.nlm.nih.gov/pubmed/18460485.
66. http://www.nel.gov/evidence.cfm?evidence_summary_id=250304.
67. http://www.nytimes.com/2011/07/19/health/19brody.html?pagewanted=1&_r=1&sq=calorie%20counting&st=cse&scp=10.
68. http://www.livestrong.com/article/360001-foods-that-restore-serotonin/#ixzz1JuZS6QHq.

you to perceive more holistically and function more intuitively within the larger system. If you have a spiritual practice, like meditation, you will find it much easier and more satisfying with whole grains as your fuel. As you continue to eat whole grains—chewing them well—you will see what I mean.

Whole grains have been around the block. Of course, whole grains may sound so good right now that you're thinking, "Why haven't we been eating this superfood before now?" Well, we have. It's only in the last couple of hundred years that we have refined grains to such a great degree—making white rice, white bread, etc. Until relatively recently, humans ate whole, unpolished grains, or at least whole-grain products. White rice wasn't introduced into Japan until the end of the seventeenth century and didn't make its way down to the masses until the beginning of the twentieth. And what followed? A serious vitamin B_1 deficiency called beriberi.

In South America, the Incan civilization was nourished by corn and quinoa; Europe developed on wheat, oats, and barley; Africa fed itself millet, teff, and sorghum. Of course, sometimes these grains were refined—made into whole-grain breads and noodles and chapatis. But they were never refined like the crazy, stripped, lifeless "carbs" we eat now.

Since the dawn of modern agriculture—roughly 10,000 years ago—grains have been cultivated and have brought with them settled communities, the ability to store excess food for times of famine, and eventually the time to sit around to make great art, literature, and even democracy. I'm not saying that whole grains are directly responsible for all that, but they provided the principal fuel.

The Whole Story

Whole grains are unique in that they are both the seeds *and* the fruits of their mother plants. They contain tremendous reproductive potential, like a juicy, fertile MILF. In fact, if you plant a whole grain, an entirely new and beautiful plant emerges, laden with more whole grains. But if you plant a slice of pizza, the only thing that emerges is a hungry college student.

So by eating whole grains, you are eating life itself.

But as soon as whole grains are ground into flour, or stripped of their fiber, or even just sliced in half, this potential for growth is stopped. When a grain is oxidized or pulverized, its magical wholeness dies. Gone. Kaput. That's why you don't see any pizza trees around.

And this wholeness is important; it heals. In fact, the word "heal" comes from the word "whole." To heal is to become whole again.

Think of yourself as a diamond—perfect, intact, and designed to glitter. Chances are, throughout your life, you've experienced trauma and stress that have caused flaws in this inner diamond. Perhaps you split off a little in order to protect a parent or as a result of abuse. Maybe you've heard yourself say, "I feel like there is *a part of me* that wants [or does] X" or "I feel disconnected from myself." You may have broken into "parts," not in a multiple-personality way, but in such a way that you don't feel entirely on your own team. Under certain circumstances, you may even sabotage yourself, not wanting to and not understanding why you do it.

Baffled, you go to therapy. You talk to your MILFy friends. You pray, meditate, maybe take up yoga. Some of these things help—a little—but many of those flaws in the diamond are just too deep, and they persist in making you feel disconnected from your deepest self. Sensing those splits are there and not being able to fix them is awful. But even worse is seeing some of them be passed on to your kids and feeling helpless to stop the transfer.

But fear not, my MILFy friend: . . . (drumroll) . . . Whole grains will fix your diamond.

Now, don't get too excited. This is not a quick fix, and it won't take you off the hook of having to do the emotional work, but eating whole grains on a daily basis has the power to slowly, but surely, heal the inner you.

Because they maintain their powerful spirit—whole and intact—whole grains help you to reclaim your own. As these little seeds become your primary fuel, a natural magic will enter your bloodstream. It will then move to your brain, making your thoughts happier, less fractured, and more focused. These tiny agents of nature—full of reproductive energy—will support and nourish your internal organs, making you stronger and more vital than ever before. Perhaps most amazingly, below the level of your issues and your fancy diplomas, whole grains will begin a subversive, silent campaign to heal you. To heal your spirit. To connect you with your Source. To make you whole. Can I get an "Amen!" for that??!!!

As I said before, this doesn't mean you have no work to do. If you have deep splits inside, eating whole grains may make you notice them even *more*. The unifying force of the grains will bring old wounds up to be healed. But healing the splits will be relatively simple and organic—one or ten gut-wrenching sobs, maybe some vigorous whacking on a pillow, a well-supported confrontation with an abuser, and an old split can be gone. Forever. Whole grains will push you to become whole. They are the perfect fuel for your continual and magical healing of the diamond that is you.*

If this seems too good to be true, consider this: Why would nature have us walking around crippled by old hurts? If nature can heal a physical wound, why would it be unable to heal an emotional one? It is in nature's *interest* to push us forward and to keep us whole and healthy. Look around and you'll notice that the plant and animal worlds have a natural resilience that we seem to have lost: a perennial flower cut the year before does not reappear in the spring cowering and scarred, afraid of blooming. No, no, no. It bursts forth, proud and strong, staring straight into the sun. Life moves forward, with gusto.

And yet, because we humans have developed "foods" that keep us weak, disconnected, and experiencing premature decomposition, we are unable to bounce back from—or work through—pain and difficulty. As a species, we are losing that natural strength and resiliency because we've been building humans out of scary, crappy, unnatural garbage. Especially in the last sixty years or so.

But that's all over now. By eating whole foods, and specifically whole grains, you will recover a vital strength and flexibility you had no idea were there.

* For those of us with more serious issues, a combination of good eating and outside help is key. I have had some form of therapeutic support—on and off—throughout my life, and eating whole foods has been its perfect internal complement. Don't do life alone.

Vegetables

Whole grains and vegetables are a dynamic, powerful duo. They are not everything in a healthy diet, but they are its center. We've discussed whole grains at length, now let's give some time to their partners.

What Are Vegetables?

We are all familiar with vegetables. They are usually the leaf, stem, or root of a plant. However, the term "vegetable" is used liberally; a mushroom, which is actually a fungus, is often referred to as a vegetable, as is a tomato, which is technically a fruit.

Are vegetables more yin or more yang? There is a range of yinness and yangness among vegetables. Roots, because they grow downward and are more contracted, are considered more yang than greens, which grow upward and expand outward. Some are cooling, while others are more warming. However, when all vegetables are compared with all grains, vegetables are considered more yin and grains more yang.

Grains and vegetables make a dynamic combination. Whole grains—tight, compact, and relatively dry—are the perfect energetic complement to the juicy, soft, and expanded nature of the average vegetable. Grains, slightly acidic, are balanced by veggies, which are mostly alkaline. Although they both contain vitamins, minerals, fiber, and complex carbs—making them ridiculously healthy foods—they deliver them in very different packages.

Whole grains tend to support the yang side of your life force (keeping you centered, gathered, and forward moving), while vegetables support the yin side (allowing you to relax and release and be in the moment), although they are both so close to the center that it can take a while to feel this difference between them. Not to worry; by eating both, you will experience easy movement between these two states of being.

Why Are Vegetables So Great?

Have you ever seen a headline in *USA Today* shouting, "The Dangers of Vegetables!" or "Vegetable Consumption Linked to Obesity" or "Do Veggies *Kill?*" Of course you haven't. These are the good guys. No one needs to spend millions of dollars a year and pay off Congress to defend *vegetables.* Our biggest problem when it comes to vegetables is simply eating more of them.

Vegetables contain lots of complex carbohydrates. This makes vegetables the perfect fuel for your MILFiness, not just physically, but mentally, emotionally, and spiritually. Complex carbs will feed your brain the sugar it needs, while making you feel peaceful, calm, and balanced.

Vegetables contain vitamins. "Vitamin." Now there's a great word. Vitamins were originally discovered and named by a biochemist named Casimir Funk while he was studying the disease beriberi. And where did he find his first vitamin (now called B_1, or thiamine), the one that completely prevents beriberi? In a lowly rice husk, that's where.

Upon the discovery of vitamins, the world's eyes opened up to the fact that natural foods contain organic compounds *needed* for normal human growth and activity. Turns out we couldn't just float around on whiskey and smelling salts. Edible plants are *designed* for the optimum functioning of our bodies. No substitutes suffice.

Do I Need Supplements?

Let's "B" frank: just about the only vitamin you cannot get from plant food is B_{12}. And this "B" is a biggie; B_{12} deficiencies take quite a while to develop and can remain undetectable in their early stages but can put you at risk for a heart attack and serious neurological damage. Deficiencies in B_{12} are not MILFy. You see, vitamin B_{12} is synthesized by little critters—bacteria in the soil. Meat contains B_{12} because ruminants, like cows, eat grasses and things that are still dirty and earthy, and their digestive tracts are rich in B_{12}-laden bacteria. Before we scrubbed, pasteurized, and sanitized everything like maniacs, and before we grew things in chemical-laden soil, we would get some B_{12} here and there in our plant food and the bacteria it carried. But today that's not the case.

If you choose to follow the MILF diet without eating any animal protein, then it's important that you take a B_{12} supplement—preferably what's called a "B complex," because it includes all the B vitamins, which work together.

Vegetables contain lots of minerals. I love the idea of minerals. . . . I imagine little metals and crystals in our bodies. . . . It's so science-fiction-y. Minerals like calcium, magnesium, copper, zinc, and phosphorus are all needed in trace amounts to maintain, oh, muscle function, cell repair, and body temperature. Just stuff like that. Vegetables contain lots of different minerals, and sea vegetables contain even more (see page 328).

Vegetables are alkalizing. Your blood is basically salty, like seawater, and it needs to maintain a certain alkalinity measured by what we call pH levels. Foods with lots of minerals help to maintain this alkalinity, but other foods that make the blood acidic (e.g., sugar, meat, dairy, caffeine, alcohol, drugs, certain fruits, and even some veggies mentioned below) stress the body out and make the blood release its minerals. Over time, this weakens you. Most vegetables bring an alkaline pH right to the table. Vegetables keep your blood strong, happy, and stable. *Go vegetables!*

Vegetables have tons of fiber. If you've forgotten how amazing fiber is, go back to page 267.

Vegetables are superheroes. If vegetables had a day job, they would be making your life better—giving you more energy, better looks, optimal performance. Like a good trainer at the gym.

But by night, when they get to don their superhero costume with the "V" across the chest, vegetables become little disease-fighting do-gooders. The science is relatively new on this, but every day it seems we're finding another phytochemical like sulphoraphane in broccoli that, oh, *blocks tumor growth.* Or sinigrin in Brussels sprouts that, get this, persuades precancerous cells to commit suicide! "Yes, Mr. Cell, step *toward* the edge. . . . It's okay, Mr. Cell. . . . *Jump!*" These newly discovered phytochemicals are so truly amazing that they make antioxidants— the cleaner-uppers of DNA-damaging free radicals—seem *soooo* last year. Oh, and by the way, vegetables are chock-full of antioxidants, too! Yes, vegetables are downright cool and getting cooler by the minute.

You can grow your own. There's nothing quite like growing things. The awe, satisfaction, and feeling of security that come from working Mother Earth defy description. And these days, there are other reasons—like the price of organic vegetables, keeping your family's food as clean as possible, and giving the kids a chance to participate—that motivate many a MILF to start either a window box or a full-fledged garden. If you have the time, the space, and the inclination, you have nothing to lose and everything to gain from getting your witchy hands dirty. Remember: you're magic.

Vegetables make for an endless variety. Let vegetables be your new best friends. Okay, vegetables and whole grains. But unlike whole grains, vegetables allow for a million cooking styles, so your relationship to them should only grow and deepen over time. And by experimenting in the kitchen, you will come to respect the magical powers of veggies even more. An onion, when raw in a salad, is spicy. Blanch it, and it's mildly pungent and crunchy. Roast it, and it's *sweeeeet* like candy. A hamburger can't do that.

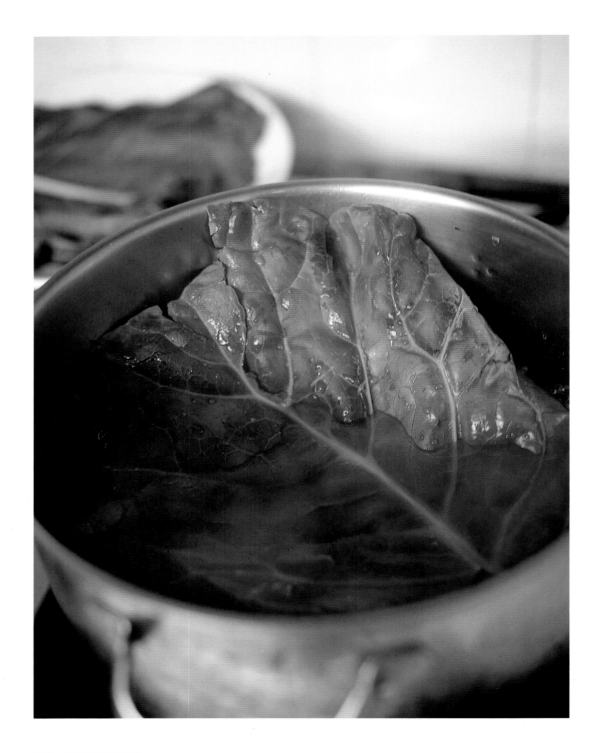

The Yin and Yang of Vegetables

The MILF diet also looks at vegetables a little differently; instead of breaking them down into their nutritional bits and pieces, we look at how they grow and what kind of energy they give to the body.

Upward-growing, green vegetables: Kissed by the sun, green and upward-growing veggies are full of chlorophyll, which helps oxygenate the body and neutralize pollutants. There are lots of upward-growing vegetables, including kale, collards, napa cabbage, leeks, celery, bok choy, mizuna, mustard greens, watercress, and lettuce, although the heartier ones like kale and collards contain the most minerals and chlorophyll. Greens are usually cooked lightly and quickly (or not at all) and make you feel light and flexible, without making you spacey. They are more yin and expansive and are great for the liver and gallbladder.

Round vegetables: These guys generally grow on the earth or just slightly pushed into it. Think cabbage, squash, onions, sweet potatoes, cauliflower, and turnips. These veggies are generally sweet, especially when cooked. They prefer a long, slow cooking that helps to open up their flavors, and the energy they impart to the body is mellow and centering. Great for the stomach, spleen, and pancreas. More balanced.

Root vegetables: Downward-growing and married to the soil, these veggies are rich in minerals and also taste really good when slow-cooked or baked. Think carrots, burdock, parsnips, and daikon. The downward energy of root vegetables actually makes you feel rooted and stable and focused. Their energy is a tonic to the intestines and they are more yang and contracted.

Of course, there is tremendous variety within each category. Bok choy contains lots of water and kale does not. Carrots are great raw, and parsnips . . . not so much. But if you begin to look at the energy character of vegetables—looking through the lens of yin and yang—you will see better how to harmonize with nature.

Again, don't go looking for your nutritionist to confirm this for you. This is not what is taught in Western schools. But ask your inner teacher, your intuition, by playing around with these vegetables. How do you feel after a big plate of greens? How do you feel after a carrot-burdock sauté? A pureed squash soup? Have fun and explore.

Vegetable Dos and Don'ts

Do: Eat veggies fresh and in season. Now, I'm not going to show up at your house with a gun as you pull a bag of frozen corn from the freezer in February. The MILF diet isn't militant. But it just makes sense to eat foods in the season that they ripen. That's like Mother Nature yelling at you, "Hey, MILF, eat this *now*!!!" And the whole point of this book is that when we do what Mother Nature tells us to, we look and feel better on every level.

However, in colder climates, it can be hard to get enough variety during the winter. Don't despair. That's why we have root cellars and cold frames and—if those are simply not on your radar—California and refrigerated trucks. I know the latter's not the most ecologically sound way to go, but if you don't have a cold, dry basement and you're not picking your own kale and parsnips from under a cold frame in your garden, it's hard to get enough variety when the growing season doesn't produce what we need.

And sure, I keep some corn and peas in the freezer. To add to a soup or a fried rice dish when I can't get them fresh. But I don't depend on frozen or canned vegetables. They are used on rare occasions.

Do: Get organic vegetables when you can. I know they're more expensive, but with farmers' markets, CSAs, and supermarkets doing their best to stay competitive with places like Whole Foods, you should be able to get your hands on some. Not only are they more nutritious, they don't carry toxic pesticides, they taste better, and they are not genetically modified. You're worth it.

Do: Explore MILFy variety and balance with vegetables. In order to feel your best, in sync with the natural environment, and to support your health, variety is key. Try and eat vegetables from each category every day, if not at every meal. Also, we're *not* looking for a third-third-third split on these. Because we are women, more governed by upward energy, and because this world is determined to bring us down, we need to get more like half of our total veggies from the leafy green category. You can split the difference between round and root.

Don't go crazy with the following vegetables:

- Potatoes
- Tomatoes
- Eggplant
- Green bell peppers (red bell peppers are better, but not for daily use)

These guys are members of the nightshade family of plants, so they are high in alkaloids, which serve as natural protection for the plant but are mildly poisonous to us. These alkaloids are suspected to leach calcium from the bones and redeposit it in soft tissue. Think kidney stones. They also cause inflammation and are believed to aggravate both rheumatoid arthritis and osteoarthritis. If you have any joint issues, stop eating nightshades and you should see an improvement. Cooking helps reduce the alkaloid content somewhat, but it's just not a good idea to get into a serious nightshade habit. If you are in good health, enjoy them out at restaurants—and maybe here and there in your cooking—but go easy.[69] Arthritic, weak-boned women with kidney stones? Not so MILFy.

Oh yeah, three more. Sorry. Go easy on spinach, chard, and beet greens. They are all high in something called oxalic acid, which is too acidic for everyday use. Use them here and there.

Beans and Bean Protein

I know; I know. Beans seem profoundly unsexy. Even the word "legume" sounds like an old-fashioned hosiery item your grandmother might have worn. "Her varicose veins were supported by a pair of silky *LEGUMES!*"

What are beans? Beans are large plant seeds from a family of plants known as Leguminosae.

Are beans more yin or more yang? Again, compared with meat, beans are yin. They are lighter and plant-based. Compared with grains, most beans are more yin as well, since they are bigger

---

69. There are a few nightshades in the recipes of this book, but they can easily be removed without compromising the taste of the dish.

and softer than grains. Nutritionally, beans are on the yin side, because they are high in protein (yin) and often contain some fat and oils (yin). But like grains and vegetables, beans are such balanced foods that their yinness and yangness is really negligible. Just eat them.

What's So Great About Beans and Bean Protein?

Plant-based proteins are simply better in every single possible way. They just are. Here's the deal:

- Beans are high in protein, making them a great food for building and repairing your body.
- Beans also contain complex carbohydrates, making them an energy food as well.
- Beans contain fiber, which helps to regulate you and your hormones.
- Beans are comparatively low in fat and contain no cholesterol.
- Beans are high in vitamins and minerals.
- Beans are dense and satisfying and delicious.
- Beans are cheap.
- Beans nourish the soil, adding much-needed nitrogen back into the earth.
- Beans, because they come from plants, pull carbon dioxide from the atmosphere and add oxygen to it.
- Beans are sustainable; unlike meat, they don't leave a stinky, toxic, insanely heavy carbon footprint.

And keep in mind what beans *aren't* doing behind your back. Beans

- Do *not* deliver excess hormones to your body.
- Do *not* pass scary bacteria or antibiotics on to you.
- Do *not* contribute to osteoporosis.
- Do *not* contribute to arthritis.
- Are *not* implicated in any cancers; soy even helps prevent cancer (see below)
- Do *not* bring you closer to a heart attack.
- Do *not* trash the planet.

If we look at beans through a holistic lens, they just make sense. It's as if Mother Nature is offering up, once again, the perfect food to help us fit harmoniously within the biggest picture.

Off-Gassing

Let's get clear about passing gas. Farting isn't very MILFy, but it's a fact of life. Everyone cuts the proverbial cheese. Unfortunately, beans get an extra bad rap in this department (along with certain cruciferous vegetables) because they contain special sugars that break down in the gut and gas is created in the process.

Here are some tips for mitigating "legume plume":

- Chew your beans extremely well. You can break down these sugars in your mouth, thereby reducing the need to process them down below.
- Soak beans (except lentils and split peas and other small beans) before cooking.
- Cook beans with a small piece of kombu, which helps to break down their farty sugars.
- When the beans come to a boil, skim off any foam that might rise.

And remember, there's no getting around some ladylike gaseous emissions, created just by life itself. Every person discharges about 1.5 liters of gas a day . . . most of it inhaled while we eat. So don't talk so much while you eat! Another source of gas? Carbonated drinks—their excess gas doesn't only bubble back *up*. So don't go blaming beans for all that.

Beans Are Downright Cool

There is a ridiculous variety of beans in the world, with at least 4,000 types grown in the United States alone. Each bean has a distinct character: Some are dark; some are light. Some are small, some more expanded. Some are speckled, while some are shiny. Nature produces this kind of variety not just to blow our minds, but to provide each food's physical strengths. Some are actually medicinal, like the adzuki bean, which is a tonic to the kidneys. Or the garbanzo bean, which, according to Chinese medicine, is good for the pancreas and heart. Each food applies itself to different organs in the body. If you want to dive deeper into this way of understanding food, there are books aplenty about macrobiotics and Chinese medicine that explore the subject. Food isn't just for your gustatory delight or to fuel your afternoon. Food is medicine.

Is meat medicinal? Sure, every food has its place. In extreme situations of anemia or weakness or demineralization, animal food can give an overall reboot to the system. I mean, heck, you're drinking blood—it's chock-full of the life force. But it's not subtle, as plant foods are. Meat is sort of a punch to the stomach as opposed to a stroke on the cheek. Plants offer a more yin way of exploring nature—an invitation to learn about the exquisite subtlety and refinement of our physical world, both inside and outside your body. They are lighter and clearer and come without toxins. Eating too much meat opens the barn door and lets the animals run roughshod all over your body.

Soy Story

You might have heard a lot about soy lately. We've gone from overvaluing the soybean to devaluing it. Let's get things straight: soy is not bad. In fact, in its whole or slightly processed form, as in tempeh, miso, or soy sauce, soy is very, very, *very* good. Any natural imbalances it might have are mitigated by the fermentation that takes place in processing. It is a complete protein, extremely absorbable, high in calcium, and an elegant food that keeps various dishes tasting fabulous.

Soy has been used for thousands of years in Asian cultures, none of which suffered from the modern diseases we managed to manifest in the last hundred years or so. But keep in mind that the Chinese and Japanese weren't chowing down on soy burgers covered in soy "cheese." Soy consumption averaged about one ounce a day (eight ounces of tofu per week) and soy was processed in a way (usually fermented) that made it digestible and healthy. They didn't *have* soy "cheese," soy "ice cream," soy protein powder—all of which are processed in ways that do *not* deliver soy's goodness and, in fact, deliver lots of bad. Yes, they had soy milk, but it was the by-product of tofu-making, not the processed stuff we buy in a box.

The problem with soy is what *we've* been doing to it. Our overly reductionist scientists have been dicking around, isolating parts of it, hacking it into bits and pieces in a ridiculous attempt to suck the good out of it and to get the most bang for their buck. And that never works. Just as you would never cut out your dog's heart (because "that's Bucky's best asset—his heart, a heart of gold") and expect that organ to represent Bucky, or to even *function* without the rest of him attached, there is no reason on earth to believe that an extracted portion of a whole food would work better than the original entity. Unless, of course, you're creating drugs or poisons, both of which are pretty extreme and have some very serious side effects. These days, soy is subsidized by the U.S. government, so it's a very cheap crop in this country. It is also estimated that *90 percent* of the soybeans grown in the United States are genetically modified. Because soy is so cheap, soy and soy by-products are used as fillers in many, many processed foods. Terms like "soy protein," "soy protein isolate," "hydrolyzed soy protein," "soy lecithin," "soy oil," "soy concentrate," "hydrogenated soy," and "isoflavones" refer to soy by-products that are *not* whole or fermented. And they are used all the time. If the soy alarmists are looking just at this to get their ammo, then I understand their hissy fit. Massive amounts of genetically modified soy by-products in processed foods (including soy "cheese," soy "ice cream," soy milk, and soy powder) are not good. Stay away from most processed food and you'll be fine.

What about phytoestrogens? Okay, this may be the one that worries you the most. Maybe you've heard that soybeans increase the amount of estrogen in your bloodstream, and that breast cancer is related to high estrogen levels. Or maybe it's the idea that soy will make your little Paul into a Paula. Either way, the lowly soybean, kept close to its natural state, is not a problem. Not only do studies show that consumption of tofu, tempeh, and other naturally processed soy products *does not* increase the risk of breast cancer,* there is evidence that eating them may actually protect against it.† You see, the plant-based "estrogens" found in soybeans are naturally occurring and *much* weaker than the hormones that your body makes. Because of this, you might actually want a plant-based estrogen to jam up some of your estrogen receptors in order to prevent your body from absorbing too much of the human kind. This is how the prevention of breast cancer is thought to work.

By the way, flaxseeds outdo soy on the phytoestrogen list. Falling well below soy, but still represented as containing phytoestrogens, are sesame seeds, garlic, mung bean sprouts, dried apricots, and dates. Don't worry. The media will get all alarmist about them at some point, too.

* http://articles.latimes.com/2011/apr/06/news/la-heb-soy-breast-cancer-survivors-20110406.
† http://www.ncbi.nlm.nih.gov/pubmed/11694655.

So what role do beans play in the MILF diet? Well, you'll probably want to have some bean or bean product at least once a day. Unless you're an athlete or pregnant, or both, you'll probably need about one cup of beans per day. But that's just an average; the nice thing about the body is that it lets you know when you need more protein by sending you a little craving for it. Not in a "Pass me that lentil soup now or you'll be SORRY!!!" kind of way, but in just a gentle attraction to the dense and satisfying nature of beans. When it's running on nature's fuel, your body knows *exactly* what it needs.

However, when you first make the shift from meat and dairy to beans, you may find that you simply crave the richness and heaviness of beans (or bean products) as substitutes for your old foods. That's okay. Well-cooked, creamy beans with a delicious seasoning can be very sexy and satisfying . . . and your mouth may want to indulge. But as you continue, allow your body to lighten up—as grains and vegetables will inevitably invite it to do—and really listen to its signals.

Sea Vegetables

The MILFiest thing you can eat is seaweed. I know; I know. That sounds weird, and perhaps a little scary, but it's true. Maybe you've eaten sushi rolls wrapped in nori seaweed at Japanese restaurants. Maybe *you've* been wrapped in seaweed at a fancy spa. Maybe you've not been acquainted with seaweed at all . . . until now.

What are sea vegetables? Sea vegetables are algae that grow mostly in seawater. Some algae are from freshwater lakes, but the ones on the MILF diet are all from the sea.

Are sea vegetables more yin or more yang? Sea vegetables, like all foods, have their yinness and yangness. They are soft (yin) and have a general softening effect on the body (yin). However, because they contain so many minerals, they are also quite yang.

FYI: Keep in mind that sea vegetables are such powerful superfoods that we need only small amounts of them. Don't get all Western on me and decide that "some is good, more is better." Your body doesn't work that way. Recommendations on amounts are coming up.

Why Should We Eat Sea Vegetables?

Plants from the sea are ridiculously high in minerals. I know I've listed some of their functions in other sections, but here are a few more jobs that minerals do: they build and maintain healthy bones and teeth and help your blood to clot. Minerals also maintain the fluid and electrolyte balances in your body, help your cells to function, and support almost every other major biological process. Good-quality minerals are the secret behind strong hair, hard nails, and lovely skin. Minerals are, as the kids say, *rad.*

But minerals keep you strong in other ways, too. They help support your overall life force, or chi. You see, when your mineral stores get depleted, you feel weak. Foods like sugar, white flour, dairy, meat, and coffee deplete mineral stores over time. Add some alcohol and lots of carbonated drinks, and you're even more depleted, retreating from the adventures of life. Take a sleeping pill every night after that pint of ice cream and your treasure chest of minerals gets really empty; your bones get hollow and you sort of start to disappear.

Not only will a person taking in all these demineralizing foods eventually manifest an illness, but her personality will lose its balanced center, her spirit its true strength. And people who are weak on the mineral level tend to suck the spirits of other people. They are like vampires.

You see, in Eastern thought, there is no separation between the physical and the spiritual. Our spiritual strength depends on our physical strength, but I'm not talking about hard abs and ripped quads. It is the strength of our blood, which comes down to the amount and quality of the minerals in our blood, that gives us a strong presence, spirit, and life. Your blood is charged with trace metallic elements like iron and cobalt, and this magnetism gives you a strong force field. You are powerfully attracted to certain people and appropriately repelled by others. Your intuition is razor sharp. Your mind is clear and your memory reliable. So minerals affect not just you and your body, they affect the people around you. If your blood is strong, you are effective and positively charged. You get things done. You are here.

What I notice most about my MILFy friends is that not one of them is a shrinking violet. Nor are they bitchy or manipulative. They are simply here. No question about it. They are moving forward in their lives with confidence in their own intuition and judgment. They are positively charged.

The MILF diet is full of mineral-rich foods like whole grains, leafy green vegetables, nuts, and seeds. But the king of Mineralville? The queen of Mineralia? Sea vegetables. They are ridiculously rich in minerals and are very easily absorbed by your body. *Plus,* they have other magical qualities. . . .

Sea vegetables bind with radioactive isotopes and discharge them from the body. We are bombarded by radiation all the time, and of differing types. If you fly on planes, you're getting exposed to increased cosmic radiation just by being high in the sky. Different parts of the earth emit different levels of radiation because of the naturally radioactive metals in the soil. If you get X-rays, or work with X-rays, you're getting a slightly higher dose, and when nuclear disasters occur, as after the 2011 earthquake and tsunami in Japan, radiation becomes a very real and serious danger.

Fingers crossed, you are dealing only with natural, industrial, and medical radiation, but even with those sources, it's important to be able to release and discharge any of the radioactive material you might be exposed to. Why? Because radiation alters our DNA and causes genetic mutations and—in high doses—can cause serious, even fatal illness. Although we use radiation for medical treatment, it is a very strong measure used in extreme circumstances where the pros and cons of radiotherapy have been carefully weighed.

Even when radiation becomes a serious threat, sea vegetables have helped to minimize it. After Nagasaki and Hiroshima were bombed in 1945, Dr. Tatsuichiro Akuziki at St. Francis's Hospital in Nagasaki fed his patients a strict diet of brown rice; miso soup; wakame, kombu, and other sea vegetables; winter squash; and salt. He also denied them any sugar or sweets because he knew these suppressed the immune system. No one at his hospital died of radiation poisoning, while those at hospitals much farther from the blast site did.[70]

MILF's Favorite Sea Vegetables

The first two sea vegetables listed pack the biggest mineral punch and a small portion (⅛ to ¼ cup, cooked) should be eaten of one or the other twice a week. Feel free to cook an arame or hijiki dish once (your first serving) and eat from it as a leftover the next day (your second serving). Also, it's best to alternate them week to week, as they have slightly different qualities.

Arame: This is a mild sea vegetable that comes in little shreds. It is best cooked with sweet vegetables, usually as a long sauté (see page 171). Arame is elegant and delicate, and you'll develop a taste for it quickly.

Hijiki: This is the granddaddy of sea vegetables. With a whopping 34 grams of minerals per 100 grams of hijiki, rumor has it that hijiki is responsible for the long, thick, and lustrous hair of Japanese women. It beats the crap out of a glass of milk, and all its minerals are digestible.

There has been some controversy surrounding hijiki of late, as it seems to contain inorganic arsenic. The Canadian government has issued warnings on the packaging. I have looked into this topic and there seem to be some mitigating factors. First of all, although hijiki does contain

---

70. Tatsuichiro Akuziki, MD, *Nagasaki, 1945* (London: Quarter Books, 1981).

inorganic arsenic when tested, it also contains *organic* arsenic, which binds with the inorganic and renders it harmless. It seems that what is happening in the lab is not necessarily what is happening in the body. There have been no known cases of hijiki causing arsenic-related illnesses in humans, and it's eaten in Japan all the time in moderate amounts.[71]

Wakame: This is mainly used in miso soup, although it's also great served chilled with cucumbers or other vegetables. If you've ever ordered miso soup in a restaurant, it has had wakame floating in it.

Kombu (kelp): This is used mostly in the cooking of beans. It helps to soften the beans and add minerals to the dish. It generally dissolves in the cooking, but you can also pull it out at the end if you don't like it, because it's done its job by the end of cooking. Kombu can also be baked and crushed into a salty condiment.

Nori: This is what sushi rolls are wrapped in. You can buy it in sheets at the health food store. Look for "sushi nori" or "toasted nori." These days, you can find seaweed "snacks" in health food stores that are made of nori with added oil, salt, and spices. I would not get into the habit of eating these, as the salt and oil may not be of the greatest quality and the salt is raw. Just buy toasted nori and eat half a sheet a day, whether it's rolled around rice or a leftover, or just dry like a potato chip. Nori is tasty!

Agar-agar: This is used to gel things like puddings and aspic. In fact, you've probably eaten a lot of another sea vegetable called carrageenan, which shows up in many processed foods as a thickening agent. Agar-agar is mostly used in desserts and other gels.

Dulse: This iron-rich red sea vegetable is a favorite in Ireland and the maritime provinces of Canada. It's great shredded in salads, or in soups, or baked and crushed into a condiment.

---

71. http://www.edenfoods.com/articles/view.php?articles_id=79. Use the edenfoods.com website for more information on the hijiki debate.

One last thing: Because sea vegetables are still widely consumed in Japan, MILFs have tended to depend on Japanese companies to supply them. Plus, sea vegetables like nori and hijiki are cultivated or harvested only in Asian waters.

At this writing, it remains to be seen if, or how, the Fukushima nuclear power plant disaster in Japan has affected the quality of sea vegetables harvested in the area. I realize that I've just explained how sea vegetables help to discharge radioactive isotopes, but that doesn't mean they should come with their own!

Many of the sea vegetables from Asia are cultivated off the coast of China, which isn't vulnerable to the currents carrying radioactive water from the nuclear plants in Fukushima. Personally, I trust that respected distributors of healthy food in this country, like Gold Mine Natural Foods, will carry only products that are tested as safe. I know the woman who runs Gold Mine. She's a MILF.

And keep in mind that there are some top-notch harvesters of sea vegetables in North America. They can supply you with most of your sea veggie needs:

- Maine Coast Sea Vegetables
- Mendocino Sea Vegetable Company
- BC Kelp

Fermented Foods

I hate to break it to you, but you and everyone you love are basically walking, talking compost heaps. And that's really cool. You see, *trillions* of bacteria in your intestines chomp on and digest the food you eat. And they are not the only microscopic friends you have: colonies of bacteria throughout your entire body—and even on your skin—help your immune system stay strong and vital. But we're living in a world slathered in sanitizing hand gel, and we seem to have forgotten that we desperately *need* the microscopic bacteria we carry in and on our bodies. They are critical in our personal defense against disease and they also help us to harmonize with nature.

What are fermented foods? Letting a food interact with airborne bacteria causes it to ferment, and fermentation helps it to break down. This is a form of predigestion, which makes the food easier to assimilate and introduces good-quality bacteria into the gut. Full-throttle fermenters like Sandor Katz, author of *Wild Fermentation: The Flavor, Nutrition, and Craft of Live-Culture*

Foods, argue that without this bacterial culture, our lives lose a depth and a richness no pill can reproduce.

How did fermentation get started? Well, it was probably hard to avoid fermented foods for most of human history. With no refrigeration, foods were exposed to the air and stuff just got funky. Also, it has long been known that salting a food both ferments and preserves it. So fermentation served as a way of prolonging a food's life while also enhancing some of its qualities.

Every traditional culture developed fermented foods. Whether it is pickled herring in Scandinavia, sauerkraut in Europe, olives around the Mediterranean, or a slightly alcoholic corn-drink called *chicha* in Peru, we consume fermented foods in the West. Asia's been in on this, too: think kimchi in Korea, pickles in Japan, and a wide variety of fermented items in China. Yogurt, kefir, injera—even wine and cheese—you name it, the world's cultures, without even having the Internet to tell one another about it, all developed some form of fermented food. The older the culture, the more it seems to honor its fermented foods.

Bottoms Up! Alcohol

Alcoholic beverages have a strongly expanding impact on the body. One drink and you feel mellow and relaxed; two drinks and you're talking to a perfect stranger about your new iPad; three drinks make you slur your words and six drinks make you numb enough to have surgery on the floor of the restaurant. That's expansion! Many cultures use alcohol in moderation on a regular basis as part of their cuisine. The French couldn't imagine a meal without wine, just as my ancestors—Canadians—take real pride in their beer. The problem with alcohol comes with issues of quality and volume. Booze that has been adulterated with sugar or has had chemical preservatives added to it . . . not so good. So check the label and remember that it's best to go organic. Too much alcohol of any kind will tip you in the yin direction, making you prone to depression, weakness, and yin physical problems. Drinking is great for a party or a wedding, but getting into a daily habit may start to affect your overall balance.

This may be why youthful America doesn't really have many fermented foods—at least not the medicinal ones. We pasteurize our pickles and our cheese (and even though I have completely slammed dairy, unpasteurized cheese and yogurt are probably the most digestible form of it). I guess if you count coffee and chocolate as mildly fermented (they are), we do ingest a lot of the stuff, but not as digestives or medicinal foods. Even wine and beer, probably our most popular and recognized forms of fermentation, are often adulterated with chemicals.

Are fermented foods more yin or more yang? Both. Fermentation itself is upward, bubbly: yin. But if the fermentation is caused by salt, the food becomes more yang as well. Most pickles have a salty agent, but some are also sweetened, giving the pickle a strong yin and yang kick. Pickles made with vinegar (not umeboshi vinegar, which is salty) are more yin than salty pickles. All told, pickles should be eaten in moderation because they are strong foods, in both yin and yang directions.

How much should I eat? Eat just a tablespoon of pickled food per day. If the pickle is salty, rinse or even soak it to reduce the salt content a bit. Pickles go particularly well with grains, as they help to alkalize the grain and help you to produce more saliva for chewing.

In terms of miso, shoyu, umeboshi, and natto, here are the rules of thumb:

- To season a soup, use no more than 1 teaspoon of shoyu or miso per cup of broth for optimum health benefits. Miso should never be boiled and needs to simmer for 2 to 3 minutes. Shoyu should be simmered for 4 to 5 minutes. For parties or to convert salt lovers, you may want to use more, but you should dial the daily seasoning down over time for maximum MILFiness.
- Go easy on the shoyu when seasoning vegetable and grain dishes. It should enhance the flavors rather than dominate them.
- It's fine to have 2 or 3 umeboshi plums per week, either as your daily pickle or in medicinal drinks. But be sure to break them up into smaller pieces and divvy them up throughout different meals; a whole umeboshi plum at once is probably too much.
- If you can find natto—and like it—it's fine to have half a cup per week. It's great mixed with mustard, scallions, shredded nori, and a splash of shoyu.

Here are some MILFy fermented foods to bring this ancient, powerful "cooking" style back to your body and your kitchen:

Shoyu (soy sauce): When soybeans are fermented, some of their strong properties are lessened, so good-quality shoyu is a healthy friend in the kitchen. Like all fermented foods, it helps with digestion, but it is also mineral-rich and high in antioxidants. The best shoyu is raw and unpasteurized (often labeled *nama,* which means "raw" in Japanese). If you are gluten intolerant, use tamari, which is made without wheat.

Tip: Season soups using 1 teaspoon of shoyu per cup of broth and simmer for 5 minutes. Season vegetable dishes with a light hand; shoyu should enhance flavors rather than dominate them.

Miso (unpasteurized, aged at least two years): Miso is a miracle food. A salty paste made from fermented beans, and sometimes a grain, salt, and a bacterial starter called koji, miso packs a huge medicinal punch. Full of natural probiotics, it's great for digestion. But it also contains something called genistein, which inhibits tumor growth. Like sea vegetables, miso also binds with radioactive isotopes and flushes them from the body, not to mention that it's full of vitamins, minerals, and protein. Miso, in moderate amounts and used correctly, is very MILFy.

Tip: Season soups using 1 level teaspoon miso per cup of broth and simmer over low heat for 3 minutes. Do not boil.

Unpasteurized pickles: You can make these at home; they are easy, fast, and delicious. By pickling your own vegetables, you ensure they remain unpasteurized, which is key to their power remaining intact. You see, fermented foods are live foods and once you've pasteurized a fermented food, it's basically dead; most of the goodies you were hoping to get from it are no longer there. You can find unpasteurized pickles in better health food stores (or a pickle store if you live near one), but they're not always available. At the risk of your teenage children rolling their eyes and your DILF thinking he's married a witch, I'd like you to start a pickling crock. It doesn't have to be fancy—a mason jar will do—but it will bring a whole new dimension of wellness to your family.

Tip: Eat the equivalent of 1 teaspoon pickle per day. Rinse or soak first if the pickle is salty.

Umeboshi plums: These little pickles are amazing. Reddish-pink in color with an extremely salty and sour taste, umeboshi plums are strongly alkalizing. If you've overdone it on white sugar, alcohol, or any other food that makes for an acidic condition, umeboshi can zap you back to alkalinity quickly. The umeboshi tonic on page 246 is a great cure for diarrhea, nausea, and other ills, but umeboshi isn't just for emergencies: eating a little piece of a plum a few times a week as a pickle with your grain makes for stronger digestion, which supports your overall health.

Tip: Limit umeboshi to 2 or 3 plums per week. They are very strong.

Natto: If you're a very brave MILF, you might want to find something called natto soybeans. They are available at Japanese markets and restaurants, so if you live in a big city, you should be able to find them. Sticky, slimy natto is a good source of all the essential amino acids, is great for digestion, contains calcium and iron, and is even purported to dissolve blood clots. *And* it smells like dirty socks. Or moldy cheese. The world divides itself between those who love and those who absolutely *hate* natto. I happen to love it, but it tends to have such a divisive reputation that whenever I order it at a Japanese restaurant, the server always looks me straight in the eye and checks, to make sure I know what I'm in for: "You *know* natto?"

Tip: Half a cup of natto per week is perfect (if you like it).

Natural Sweets

I promise that your sweet tooth will be satisfied on the MILF diet. In fact, you'll find that natural sweets deliver a fuller, more satisfying sweetness than highly refined carbohydrates and artificial sweeteners. Because they contain complex carbohydrates and minerals, natural sweets are actual *foods*—instead of drugs—and they will offer you real and satisfying nourishment. Plus, eating them in moderation will keep you deeply satisfied, helping you to avoid overeating or going back to the old extremes.

What are natural sweets? When I say "natural" sweets, I mean sweet foods and sweeteners that are closer to the middle of the seesaw. They generally contain more complex carbohydrates and fewer simple sugars. They do not put you on the roller coaster.

Are natural sweets more yin or more yang? All sweets cause a yin response in the body because sugar makes us relax. But with good-quality natural sweets, it is a mild expansion that doesn't make us crazy. However, sweets that are baked flour products (cookies, cakes) can also have a strong yang effect on the body, as baked flour is drying and causes contraction.

Your New Best Friends

Brown rice syrup: This is made from brown rice that has been fermented with a special bacterial starter called koji. This process makes a thick, golden syrup that delivers a very satisfying sweetness. You can use it in dessert recipes and teas and even treat yourself to a tablespoon of it now and again straight from the jar. Rice syrup contains almost 60 percent complex carbohydrates, so it will give you nice energy without taking you for a ride.

Barley malt: This dark and malty syrup has a stronger flavor and is great in baked beans or for a stronger-tasting dessert. Made from fermented barley, it contains lots of minerals and delivers a bit of a sour flavor along with its sweetness. It is sometimes less available than rice syrup, but you should be able to find it at better health food stores, or order it online.

Maple syrup: This old standby has a sweeter taste and delivers a stronger hit to your blood sugar. It's great for a MILF and her family making the transition from white sugar.

Amazake: This is a creamy drink made from a variety of brown rice called sweet rice. You can find amazake at Whole Foods or better health food stores in the refrigerated or frozen section. It comes in a bunch of different flavors and is like a mildly sweet milkshake. *Mmmm* . . . a couple of cups of amazake a week keeps a MILF very sweet and happy. It's even better served warm.

Fresh fruit: On the MILF diet, fruit is more like a treat than a three-pieces-a-day staple. Don't get me wrong: fruit is great, but it's high in simple sugar, is generally cooling to the body, and should be treated with respect. Too much of it can make you feel weak and spacey, so ratchet up the vegetables and go easy on the fruit. To stay balanced, choose organic fruit that grows within your climate. One piece a day should be plenty.

Dried fruit: When a fruit is dried, its sweetness gets concentrated, so it packs a very nice punch for cooked desserts or as a quick snack or a handy treat when you travel.

Sweet vegetables: I know vegetables don't sound very exciting, but after you kick white sugar, you will begin to taste the lovely sweetness of winter squash, cauliflower, and even long-cooked onions and carrots. Sweetness is more than a taste; it's deeply relaxing and delivers a very soothing energy to the digestive organs. Eating sweet vegetables on a regular basis will keep you feeling centered and happy.

Now and Again

Agave nectar (aka syrup): There is a real debate around agave nectar. This very sweet and high fructose sweetener comes from the agave plant and is used often in health food store desserts and treats. Some say it's hard on the body, while others swear by it. I eat agave occasionally; if it shows up in a dessert, I'll eat it, but I don't use it much in my daily cooking. It doesn't seem to put me on the roller coaster that white sugar does.

Honey: A strong sweet that delivers fast energy, honey comes with tiny amounts of vitamins and minerals, antimicrobial properties, and even some antioxidants. Honey has been used for thousands of years. However, vegans don't use honey because it is technically an animal product. I don't use honey because it's too sweet. As with agave, if it shows up in a dessert when I'm out to dinner, I won't take a pass, but I prefer the slower, mellower hit of brown rice syrup for daily cooking.

Chocolate: Of course, because MILFs avoid dairy and white sugar, the chocolate we choose is dark and malt-sweetened. SunSpire makes great chocolate chips that are MILF-friendly, and they're used in a couple of recipes in this book. Chocolate has a very strong yin force, so it's great for a MILFy treat here and there, but go easy on the stuff. A couple of servings a month is plenty.

In Conclusion

Well, well, well. We've really had a MILFy mental workout. First the right hemisphere of your brain got connected with your intuitive sense of balance, your place in the larger scheme of things, and your special MILFy powers. I hope you feel good about that.

And you learned how to chew . . . and chew . . . and chew . . .

Perhaps you've even started cooking like a MILF, exploring the new MILFy foods and your relationship to the kitchen. Or maybe you've just thumbed through the recipes, getting all excited.

And now you've just finished all the left-brain info. The facts. The lowdown. Turns out this stuff isn't so woo-woo after all.

Thank you so much for the time and attention you've taken to read this book; it has been a great pleasure and honor to write it, and I hope it becomes a well-used, stained, and dog-eared friend in the kitchen.

I encourage you to come back to its ideas as much as to its recipes, because as you eat MILFy foods, your relationship to this information will get deeper and deeper. You will start to really "get it" on an intuitive level. And that's good. Because, Ms. MILF, we need you on our great MILFy mission.

9

. . . .

MILFs
Save
the World

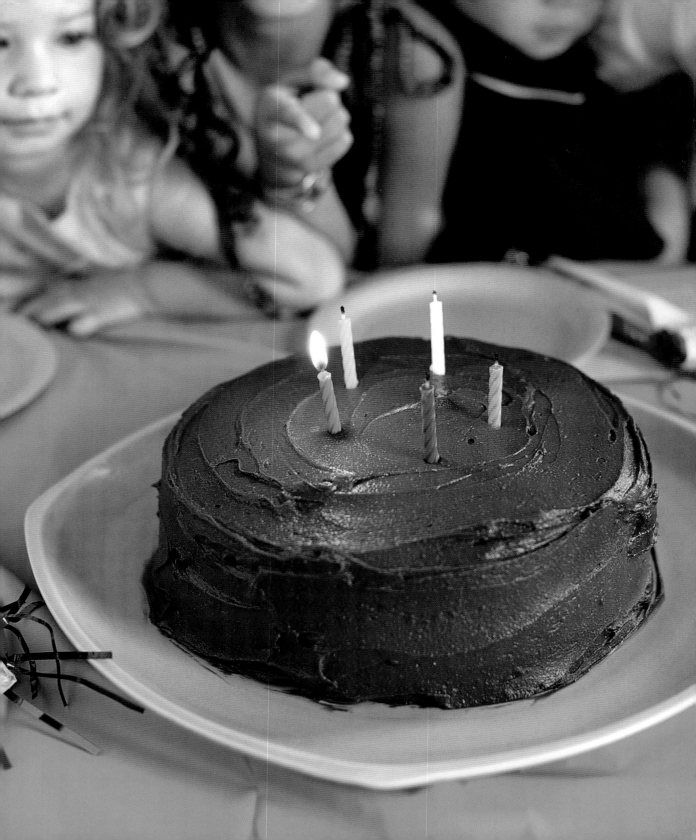

We have power, my friends. Lots of power.

On a material level, by following the MILF diet, you are reducing your carbon footprint. You are saving oil, water, the rain forest, and the atmosphere with every meal that doesn't include meat and dairy. You are building instead of destroying. You are acting with faith that we are here not to kill this planet but to support it.

But you are exerting power in more subtle ways as well: by feeding yourself whole foods, you are becoming more whole. And that's no joke. You are feeling more peaceful and sane. You are beginning to resonate with your truest self, the natural world, and the universe itself. Over time, whole foods will push you to discover your personal genius and bring it to the fore—maybe you'll start a business, lead a charity, or paint a masterpiece. In a world that is spinning out of control, hopelessly out of touch with itself, you will be tuned in.

Experiencing this connectedness is a big deal. Quantum physicists have studied people and how "coherent" their vibrations are. It turns out that some of us resonate nicely with ourselves, while others feel chaotic inside. People with more "coherence" give out stronger signals and have a bigger positive impact on the world around them. They can even influence loved ones at a distance, or over time. This is real-world witchcraft that the scientists are just discovering.

By eating foods that come straight from the buzzing, pulsating earth, you are improving your personal coherence and becoming a stronger radio transmitter in the world. You are putting out a steady, clean, and magical thrum, which brings everyone around you closer to coherence. You are literally harmonizing the vibrations of those around you. How cool is that?

Of course, by feeding your family whole grains and vegetables—cooked with love—you are influencing your entire brood. Raising children means not only feeding them but "raising" their minds, their spirits, and their hearts with good-quality energy. Your yin power is bringing an invisible dimension to their lives, allowing them to relax, look inside themselves, and trust the unseen. You are making them saner, more peaceful, and happier people. You are strengthening the human fabric of the world.

As you feed your DILF more whole foods, he will change as well. Like you, he will feel calm and centered, but his good-quality, natural yang force will become more potent on all levels: he will experience precision, effectiveness, and constructive forward momentum. With natural food fueling him, he will also open up to more sensations, emotions, and even "vibes." You are helping your DILF to find balance.

And finally, we have natural yin force on our side: by eating this way, and spreading the word, MILF to MILF, we are creating a collective vibration. Imagine every household in the world, with a juicy MILF at its center, channeling the fierce and fecund power of nature. Every home buzzing with the electricity of life. And each MILF vibrating with all the others, connecting through this natural witchcraft throughout the neighborhood, the community . . . the country. Raising the world.

This is neither a quick fix nor a flashy one. It requires patience, humility, and surrender. Remember: we are tapping the quiet, holy, and unstoppable power of nature.

We've got that power. Let's use it.

Acknowledgments

This book is the product of the time, attention, and encouragement of many people. I hereby gratefully thank

My late mother, Susan, for teaching me that being a girl is special.

My father, Julian, for handling four daughters like a champ.

My sisters, Sue, Catherine, and Julia, for being unique and brilliant beings.

My stepmother, Anna, a MILF and a loving mentor.

My stepfather, Bob, for changing all our lives in such a beautiful way.

Michio Kushi and his late wife, Aveline, for showing the way of freedom and peace through natural food and lifestyle habits. Your teaching has transformed the lives of countless people.

The MILFs introduced in this book: Maggie, Meredith, Lisa, Simone, Gabriele, Chauvon, Krista, Laura, Karen, Jane, Ally, Aine, Amy, Melanie, Suzanne, Mayumi, Sanae, Eliza, Anna, Toni, and Sarah. Thank you for sharing yourselves so honestly and inspiring me and many others.

Emily Bestler, my MILFy editor and publisher, and her team at Simon & Schuster, for believing in this book and giving it a chance.

My agent, Michael Carlisle, for being a kind, wise, and savvy gentleman.

Lauren Smythe, for being smarter than any of us were at her tender age.

Joshua Shaub, for being the calm, confident, and daring photographer extraordinaire . . . I'm so grateful to have found you.

Aaron Steinbach, for being a great friend, a great chef, and my Garage Band coproducer.

Bini Sharman, Anna Walters, Amy Glen, and Kate Thompson, for shopping and schlepping and cooking.

Leigh Builter, for her love, encouragement, and laughter, even in the hardest times.

Bill Spear, for being a true friend in every situation.

Christina Pirello, for her loving friendship and indomitable spirit.

All my macrobiotics teachers, who've devoted their lives to giving back.

Thursday Silver Lake Last Dancers . . . this is what happens when we stay awake!

Phil Klein, the best lawyer a lady could have.

Elinor Whitmore, Tara Ellis, and Janet Ozzard, my MILFy friends who've held my hand for so long.

Jane Heath, for her kind, intelligent feedback and support.

Gerald L'Ecuyer, for seeing the path ahead of me.

Ari and Whitney, for making me feel extra MILFy.

Howard Wallen, for all his good work and twisted humor.

Amy Jenkins, who pushed me to start a new book.

Christy Morgan, for all her help and support and for getting me through the bluemails.

Others who are simply kick-ass: Tamara Silvera, Meredith Jordan, the Goddard family, Emily McDowell, Lou Frederick, John Buchan, Trey Teufel, Jeffrey Marcus, Stephen Muzzonigro, Carlo Petrini, Bonnie Nelson, Evelyn Vannozzi, Julie and Rob Maigret, Dick Money, Zarra Hermann, Neil Sattin, Lynne Rowe, Jon Radtke, Jenny and Matt Lunt, Roberto Donati, Erin Jones, the Tuesday Ladies, Ellin Sanger, Sheila Jackson, Julia Kirby, and The Writers Junction.

Finally, thank you to Marie Mongan, my mentor and inspiration in shamelessly supporting women in a world that's starting to forget how.

Appendix

Attribute	Yin	Yang
Tendency	Expansion	Contraction
Function	Diffusion	Fusion
	Dispersion	Assimilation
	Separation	Gathering
	Decomposition	Organization
Movement	More inactive, slower	More active, faster
Vibration	Shorter wave, higher frequency	Longer wave, lower frequency
Direction	Ascent and vertical	Descent and horizontal
Position	More outward and peripheral	More inward and central
Weight	Lighter	Heavier
Temperature	Colder	Hotter
Light	Darker	Brighter
Humidity	Wetter	Drier
Density	Thinner	Thicker
Size	Larger	Smaller
Shape	More expansive and fragile	More contracted and harder
Form	Longer	Shorter
Texture	Softer	Harder
Atomic particle	Electron	Proton
Climatic effects	Tropical	Colder climate
Biological	More vegetable quality	More animal quality
Sex	Female	Male
Organ structure	More hollow and expansive	More compacted and condensed
Nerves	More peripheral	More central
Attitude, emotion	More gentle, negative, defensive	More active, positive, aggressive
Work	More psychological and mental	More physical and social
Consciousness	More universal	More specific
Mental function	Dealing more with the future	Dealing more with the past
Culture	More spiritually oriented	More materially oriented
Dimension	Space	Time

Bibliography

Brizendine, Louann, M.D. *The Female Brain*. New York: Broadway Books, 2006.

————. *The Male Brain*. New York: Three Rivers Press, 2011.

Campbell, T. Colin, Ph.D., and Thomas M. Campbell II. *The China Study: Startling Implications for Diet, Weight Loss and Long-term Health*. Dallas: BenBella Books, 2006.

Katz, Sandor Ellix. *Wild Fermentation: The Flavor, Nutrition, and Craft of Live-Culture Foods*. White River Junction, Vt.: Chelsea Green Publishing Company, 2003.

Kushi, Gabriele. *Embracing Menopause Naturally: Stories, Portraits, and Recipes*. Garden City Park, N.Y.: Square One Publishers, 2006.

Kushi, Michio. *The Book of Macrobiotics: The Universal Way of Health, Happiness and Peace*. Tokyo and New York: Japan Publications, Inc., 1987.

————. *The Gentle Art of Making Love: Macrobiotics in Love and Sexuality*. Garden City Park, N.Y.: Avery Publishing Group, Inc., 1990.

McTaggart, Lynne. *The Field: The Quest for the Secret Force of the Universe* (Updated Edition). New York: Harper Paperbacks, 2008.

Pollan, Michael. *In Defense of Food: An Eater's Manifesto*. New York: Penguin Group, 2008.

Sax, Leonard, M.D., Ph.D. *Why Gender Matters: What Parents and Teachers Need to Know About the Emerging Science of Sex Differences*. New York: Doubleday, 2005.

Taubes, Gary. *Good Calories, Bad Calories: Fats, Carbs, and the Controversial Science of Diet and Health*. New York: Anchor Books, 2007.

Other Resources

For more information on great cookbooks, food sources, websites, and more, visit my website at milfdietbook.com.

The MILFs

The women who helped me with this book are powerful ladies, many of whom have done great things or written their own cookbooks. Here's the skinny on the MILFs who helped me on this journey.

Ally Becherer is thirty, the mother of one, and was born and bred in Alaska on the MILF diet. She lives in Austin, Texas.

Krista Berman lives in Winter Park, Florida, where she teaches healthy cooking classes.

Chauvon Collins is a yoga teacher in Los Angeles and recently gave birth to her first child. She has been eating the MILFy way for five years and she is simply gorgeous.

Martha Cottrell is eighty-three years old, is a medical doctor, and has more energy on a dance floor than anyone else I know. She is the mother of three and has been eating like a MILF for more than thirty-three years. She contributed to *The Cancer Prevention Diet* by Michio Kushi.

Eliza Eller is the woman I mention in the beginning who has been eating this way since she was six and is now, at forty-six, the mother of thirteen children, all born of her MILFy body. She lives in a macrobiotic community in Alaska called Ionia and is one of the strongest, most vibrant, and most positive people I know.

Gabriele Kushi is the mother of one and wrote *Embracing Menopause Naturally,* which is a great book about a healthy approach to menopause, physically, mentally, and spiritually. Gabriele has eaten like a MILF for forty years and gives online cooking classes at Kushiskitchen.com. She lives in Minneapolis.

Suzanne Landry has three boys—now men—and has written her own cookbook, *The Passionate Vegetable.* She lives in Ventura, California.

Sarah Loring is the mother of four and has been eating the MILFy way for thirty-three years. She teaches whole foods cooking to both adults and kids, emphasizing a healthy relationship with food and one's body. She is also the nutritional advisor to Dr. H. Robert Silverstein's Preventive Medicine Center in Hartford, Connecticut.

Aine McAteer has been a chef to Hollywood celebrities for many years. She hails from Ireland but is currently living in Indonesia. Her book, *Recipes to Nurture*, is a brilliant and beautiful cookbook, but sadly, it's out of print. Maybe if we make some noise, the publisher will bring it back.

Meredith McCarty teaches whole foods and MILFy cooking in the San Francisco area and has been eating this way for thirty-seven years. I have loved Meredith's cookbooks for a very long time. They include *Sweet and Natural, Fresh from a Vegetarian Kitchen,* and *American Macrobiotic Cuisine.* She's an insanely talented cook. You can see her in a photograph on page 351 with her legs slung over her head in plow pose. She's sixty-five.

Mayumi Nishimura is the mother of two and has been Madonna's private chef for the last ten years. She has been eating healthy food for over thirty years. Her beautiful cookbook is called *Mayumi's Kitchen: Macrobiotic Cooking for Body and Soul.* Her food is classic, elegant, and truly amazing. Just like her.

Simone Parris is an American who lives in India and plans to adopt children there. Her website, Simoneskitchen.com, shows off some of her amazing recipes. Simone has been eating the MILFy way for over twenty years and is a fabulous cook and the picture of health.

Jane Quincannon Stanchich is a southern belle who lives in Asheville, North Carolina, with her DILF, Lino. Together they laugh, chew, and spread the wisdom of macrobiotics.

Amy Rolnick lives in Portland, Maine, where she teaches healthy-cooking classes as the "Natural Food Enthusiast" and has also performed magic in the dirt. Her garden is shown off in this book, as well as her clear eyes and beautiful skin. She's forty-six and is the mother of three.

Anna Romer is the MILF whose life was turned around through chewing. She lives, and chews, in Los Angeles.

Tonya Sattin lives in Yarmouth, Maine, where she is the mother of two and grows a spectacular garden with the grace of a modern Audrey Hepburn.

Lisa Silverman is the mother of my goddaughter Ella and runs the 5 Seasons Whole Foods Cooking School in Portland, Maine. She is the heart of the MILFy community there. I keep telling her to write a book, but she hates writing.

Sanae Suzuki and her chef husband, **Eric LeChasseur,** own a very popular vegan/macrobiotic restaurant in Los Angeles called Seed Kitchen. They have also produced three amazing books: two are mouthwatering cookbooks—*Love, Eric* and *Love, Eric and Sanae*—and the third is Sanae's own book about her recovery from ovarian cancer using a healing version of the MILF diet and lifestyle, *Love, Sanae.* Sanae has been eating like a MILF for eighteen years.

Laura Taylor and **Karen Bryson** teach macrobiotic cooking classes together in Los Angeles. They have both been MILFy for a very long time.

Melanie Brown Waxman is the mother of seven and has written a number of cookbooks. They include gems like *Eat Me Now!: Healthy Macrobiotic Cooking for Students and Busy People; Bless the Baby; Yummy Yummy in My Tummy;* and *The Little Carrot,* a book for kids. She got into MILFy cooking when she was twenty-two and is now fifty-three. You can see her bending forward like a pretzel in this book on page 49.

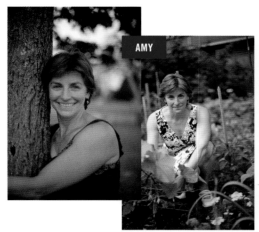

AMY

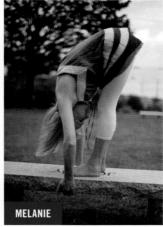

MELANIE

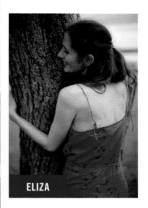

ELIZA

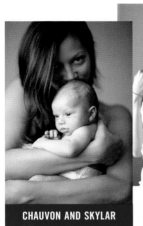

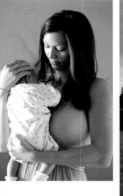

CHAUVON AND SKYLAR

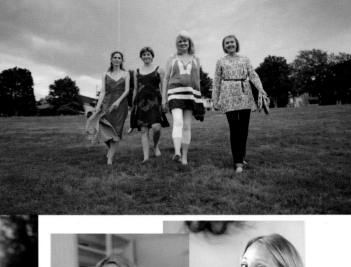

MEREDITH

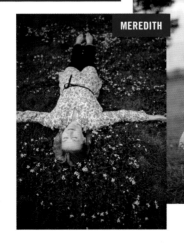

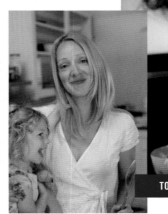

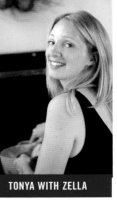

TONYA WITH ZELLA

General Index

Agent Orange, 305
aging, 78–79
Akuziki, Tatsuichiro, 330
alcohol, 333
alkalinity, 318
amenorrhea, 90
amino acids, 259, 263
antibiotics, fed to livestock, 264–65, 289
antidepressants, whole grains as, 313
antioxidants, 319
Arom, Ari, 249
artificial sweeteners, 275, 276–77
aspartame, 276
autoimmune system, 286–88
autumn:
    balanced meal in, 54
    changing diet with season, 58

B

balance, 25–26
    in every meal, 59–60
    yin and yang, 26, 33, 60
beans, 323–27
    in balanced meal, 50
    in DILF diet, 68
    and gas, 325
    once a day, 327
    and soy, 326–27
    substituting for meat in diet, 271, 272, 327
    varieties of, 325
    what's so great about, 324–26
    what they are, 323
    yin and yang of, 323–24
beauty, 75–79
Becherer, Ally, 346
bedtime, eating before, 66–67
behavior:
    yang, 30
    yin, 31–32
beriberi, 314, 317
Berman, Krista, 221, 346
Be the Fountain (exercise), 85

bitchiness, and caffeine, 296–97
blood pressure, and caffeine, 295
body scrub, 67, 76–77
bones, osteoporosis, 263–64
bovine growth hormone, 266
brown rice, chewing, 22–25, 278
Bryson, Karen, 196, 348
Buddha, yin force of, 46
B vitamins, 318

C

caffeine, 293–301
    arguments against, 294–97
    and bitchiness, 296–97
    and blood pressure, 295
    consumption of, 294
    and fertility, 295–96
    kicking, 298–301
    and osteoporosis, 295
    and self-centeredness, 297
    and sleep, 297
    and stress, 294–95, 296
    too much, 297
    what it is, 293–94
    and wrinkles, 296
    yin and yang of, 294
calcium, 263–64, 277
calmness, 313
Campbell, T. Colin, *The China Study,* 262–63, 288
cancer:
    and artificial sweeteners, 276
    and dairy foods, 288–89
    and estrogen, 266, 289
    and meat, 262–63
    and sugar, 279
carbohydrates:
    arguments against, 277–80
    complex, 273, 312, 317
    and heart disease, 261
    and meat, 267, 270–71
    refined, 273–74, 277, 312
    simple, 273
    and sugar, 278
    in vegetables, 317

what they are, 273–74
    and whole grains, 312
casein, 284
celiac disease, 103
chakras, 27
changes, 92–99
chewing:
    beans, 325
    benefits of, 24–25, 278
    brown rice, 22–25, 278
    instructions, 23–24
    phase two, 41
    tips, 24–25
    and weight loss, 66
chi, 28, 328
chickens, free-range, 270
cholesterol, 261
clarity, 95–96
Collins, Chauvon, 119, 346
Community Supported Agriculture (CSA), 58
connectedness, 342
corn syrup, high fructose, 275, 305
Cottrell, Martha, 346
creativity, 96

D

dairy foods, 282–93
    addictive nature of, 283–84
    and antibiotics, 289
    arguments against, 283–90
    and autoimmune system, 286–88
    and cancer, 288–89
    and the environment, 289–90
    and heart disease, 288
    kicking, 290–93
    milk from animals, 284–85, 286
    and osteoporosis, 285–86
    and respiratory issues, 288
    substitute products for, 291
    what they are, 283
    yin and yang of, 283

Recipe Index

(Page references in *italics* refer to illustrations.)

F

fennel: Arugula Salad with Fennel, Bosc Pear, and White Balsamic Vinaigrette, 135
fruit:
  Ari's "Tender Mix" Juice, 249
  dried, 338
  Enlightenment Smoothie, 250
  fresh, 337
  Fruit Topping, 196–97, *197*

G

garlic:
  Cashew-Garlic Aioli, 230, 232
  Garlic-Rosemary Millet with Mushroom Gravy, 116–17, *117*
  Oven-Roasted Root Vegetables with Garlic, Cumin, and Herbs, *132,* 133
  Roasted Garlic, 140
ginger:
  Carrot-Ginger Dressing, 240
  Shoyu-Ginger Dipping Sauce, 146, *147*
  Sweet Ginger-Shoyu Dipping Sauce, 146, *147*
gluten, 103
grains, 102–19
  cooking chart, 105
  dry-roasting, 106
  and gluten, 103
  salting, 105–6
  soaking, 106
Granola, Power Crunch, 209
Green-Life Veggie Dip, 241
greens:
  Leafy Green Vegetable Roll, 128
  Tempeh-Collard Wraps with Peanut Sauce, 154, *155*

H

herbs and spices, 252
hibiscus: Sweet-and-Sour Hibiscus Dipping Sauce, *162,* 163

hijiki, 330–31
  Hijiki, Fresh Corn, and Tofu Salad on Arugula with Toasted Sesame Dressing, 172
honey, 338
Hopi Blue and Yellow Indian Corn Muffins, 210, *211*
Hurry-Curry Vegetables, 142

K

kale:
  Crispy Kale, 220
  Palak Seitan Murg, 238
kelp (kombu), 150, 331
Ketchup, Sun-Dried Tomato, 110
kids, 214–26
  Banana Wontons, 221
  Chocolate Chip Rice Treats, *222,* 223
  Crispy Kale, 220
  Divine Corn-Crust Pizza, 224–26, *225*
  Killer No-Bake Drop Cookies, 215
  "Mac 'n' Cheese," 218
  "Mac 'n' Cheese" #2, 219
  Seaweed-Nut Crunch, *216,* 217
  Simply Delicious Alphabet Soup, 214
kitchen setup, 51–52
kombu (kelp), 150, 331
Kukicha Tea, 244

L

Lace Cookies, *194,* 195
Leeks au Gratin, 141
leftovers, 55
lemons, lemon juice:
  Creamy Lemon Pudding, 193
  Lemon-Poppy Seed Dressing, 240
  Lemony Quinoa Salad, 119
  Lemony Vegetable Salad, 130
lentils: Fake Chicken Soup for the Soul, 178

M

"Mac 'n' Cheese," 218
"Mac 'n' Cheese" #2, 219

maple syrup, 337
millet, 103
  Garlic-Rosemary Millet with Mushroom Gravy, 116–17, *117*
  Millet Croquettes, *108,* 109
  Super-Delicious Mystery "Cheese" Cake, 196–97, *197*
Minestrone, Really Good, 180–81
mirin, 252
miso, 251–52, 334, 335
Miso Pickles, 149
Miso Soup, 176, *177*
Miso-Tahini Sauce, 239
mochi:
  Mochi Flips, 205
  Squochi, 143
muffins: Hopi Blue and Yellow Indian Corn Muffins, 210, *211*
mushrooms:
  Buckwheat Pilaf, 115
  Fried Noodles, 120
  Fried Rice, 111
  Garlic-Rosemary Millet with Mushroom Gravy, 116–17, *117*
  Grilled "Cheese" Sandwiches with Portobello Mushrooms and Cashew-Garlic Aioli, 230–32, *231*
  Really Relaxing Tea, 247
  Seitan Stroganoff, *234,* 235
  Soft Polenta with Braised Wild Mushrooms, 121
  Tom Kha Ghai, *182,* 183

N

natto, 334, 336
noodles:
  Fried Noodles, 120
  "Mac 'n' Cheese," 218
  "Mac 'n' Cheese" #2, 219
  Really Good Minestrone, 180–81
  Simply Delicious Alphabet Soup, 214

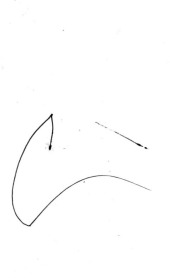